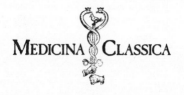

MEDICINA CLASSICA

SIR D'ARCY POWER
SELECTED WRITINGS

SIR D'ARCY POWER

SELECTED WRITINGS

1877–1930

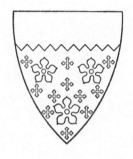

AUGUSTUS M. KELLEY · PUBLISHERS

NEW YORK 1970

First Published 1931
(London: At The Claredon Press)

Reprinted 1970 By
AUGUSTUS M. KELLEY, PUBLISHERS
NEW YORK, NEW YORK 10001

By Arrangement with
OXFORD UNIVERSITY PRESS

SBN 678 03750 7

Library of Congress Catalogue Card Number

78-95632

Printed in the United States of America

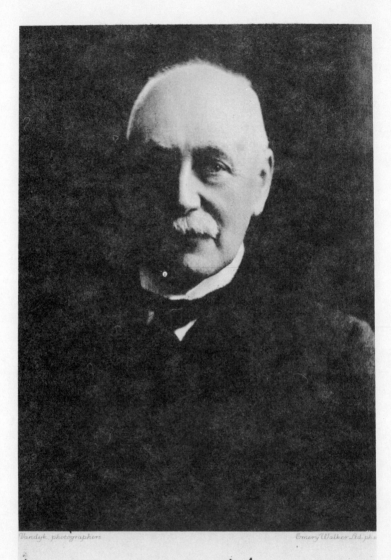

D'Arcy Power

THIS VOLUME

OF THE SELECTED WRITINGS OF

Sir D'ARCY POWER, K.B.E., F.R.C.S.

WAS GIVEN TO HIM BY HIS FRIENDS

ON THE OCCASION OF HIS

SEVENTY-FIFTH BIRTHDAY

11 NOVEMBER 1930

CONTENTS

LIST OF PLATES

LIST OF TEXT-FIGURES

I

JOHN HUNTER: A MARTYR TO SCIENCE [1]

Mihi quidem miserandi magis quam beati videntur ut qui sese perpetuo torqueant. Addunt, mutant, adimunt, reponunt, repetunt, recudunt, ostendunt, nonum in annum premunt, nec unquam sibi satisfaciunt: ac futile praemium, nempe laudem, eamque perpaucorum, tanti emunt, tot vigiliis, somnique rerum omnium dulcissimi tanta jactura, tot sudoribus, tot crucibus. Adde nunc valetudinis dispendium, formae perniciem, lippitudinem, aut etiam caecitatem, paupertatem, invidiam, voluptatum abstinentiam, senectutem praeproperam, mortem praematuram, et si qua sunt alia ejusmodi. Tantis malis sapiens ille redimendum existimat, ut ab uno aut altero lippo probetur.

ERASMUS, *Encomium Moriae*, cap. 1.

MR. PRESIDENT AND GENTLEMEN,

Brought up, as I have been, at St. Bartholomew's Hospital, in the straitest sect of the Hunterian School, I might fairly claim some knowledge of the pioneer in surgery, the anniversary of whose birthday we are assembled to celebrate to-day.

Sir William Savory, my revered master, learnt from Sir William Lawrence, and he from John Abernethy, who himself sat at the feet of John Hunter and was ever afterwards his eulogist. But much as I had heard of John Hunter, a reperusal of his works has shown me how little I really knew about the originality of the man, of his limitations, or of the handicaps under which he laboured. It is on these subjects that I shall speak to you to-day, and my wish to do so is the greater because the principles of surgery which he laid down have fallen somewhat into the background, being overshadowed by advances in chemistry, physics, and physiology, by the advent of bacteriology, and by the work of Lister.

Hunter as a Pioneer

I want you to think first of John Hunter as a pioneer in the philosophy of surgery, not as a skilled operator.

[1] The Hunterian Oration delivered at the Royal College of Surgeons of England, on Saturday, 14 February 1925.

Like all pioneers he lived and worked alone, for none of his contemporaries could think as he thought or see what he saw. Like Vesalius and Harvey he had to educate a new generation to foster his ideas and expound his thoughts.

The limitations of John Hunter are obvious. He was hampered by a defective education. He had an almost medieval respect for words as words. He could not express himself clearly, either in writing or by word of mouth, when he dealt with the more difficult problems of surgery, which he knew existed but was unable to solve for want of the ancillary sciences. He was a gross teleologist. His metaphors were often strained and sometimes wholly false. He was confessedly ignorant of the work of his surgical colleagues and foreign contemporaries, and—as I shall show presently—he suffered from frequent and severe attacks of illness which would have incapacitated any one possessed of a less dauntless spirit. But when we have said this we have said all there is to say against him as a man.

Now consider his handicaps. In his day there was no chemistry; no physics; no acquaintance with minute anatomy, for the microscope was not yet in common use; no knowledge of animal cells; hardly even a theory of fermentation to account for disease, because humoral pathology and the doctrine of climatic conditions still held sway. Joseph Black discovered 'fixed air' or carbon dioxide in 1754; Priestley prepared 'dephlogisticated air' in 1774. Three years later Lavoisier called it 'respirable air or oxygine', and taught the true nature of the interchange of gases in the lungs. Hunter by this time had done much of his work on respiration. The want of a well-calibrated thermometer vitiated many of his experiments on animal heat. He was obliged, therefore, to stumble along and explore the fields of surgical knowledge as best he could, for he was half a century before his time. He would have gotten the true explanation of many of his facts had he been born in 1778 instead of in 1728. With all these

limitations and handicaps he often arrived very nearly at
the truth, and his writings are full of the most astounding
presages of knowledge to come, presages which have been
fulfilled for the most part by the advance of science,
although some still await their accomplishment.

Hunter's methods and the advances he made are nowhere seen to better advantage than in his experiments
and observations on animals in regard to their production
of heat. Just a century earlier his great predecessor,
William Harvey, who equalled him in originality of
thought and excelled him in logical exposition, had dealt
with the subject of animal heat in the seventy-first essay of
his treatise *De Generatione Animalium*. John Mayow had
solved the problem at Oxford in 1674, but he died young,
and the *Tractatûs Quinque* fell stillborn from the press. He
left no successor; his discoveries had to be made afresh
and applied by others more than a hundred years later.
Albert Haller, who did so much to advance physiology in
general, was not particularly interested in the subject of
animal heat, so there had been no material change of
thought about it in the century which separated Harvey
from Hunter. It is fair, therefore, to compare the two
monographs, bearing in mind that Harvey was already well
stricken in years when he wrote on 'calidum innatum',
whilst Hunter—aged 38—was in the prime of life when
he performed his experiments, although they were not
elaborated and published until twenty years afterwards.

Harvey is trammelled throughout by his knowledge of
history, and his treatise is filled with quotations from
Aristotle, although he arrives at the very practical conclusion that the heat of the blood in animals during life is
neither fire nor derived from fire as the ancients thought.
It is a principle inherent in the blood; but he then loses
himself in speculating whether or not the blood is the Soul
or Life itself.

Hunter starts in a very different manner. The lapse of
a hundred years had given him an instrument of precision
—the mercury thermometer—invented by Fahrenheit in

1720 [1]—whilst the work of Black had afforded some insight into the composition of the atmosphere and the interchange of gases. But the science of physics had not advanced sufficiently to enable Hunter to appreciate the relationship of heat to cold. He speaks of animals which 'seem to possess a power of generating cold', whilst heat, as in the time of Harvey, was still a principle. How new an instrument the thermometer was is shown by a letter to Jenner on 6 July 1777, in which Hunter says: 'The thermometer is very useful when understood. You will observe the scratch upon the glass stalk, perhaps about two inches from the globe, which is the freezing-point. Put o or nought which is upon the ivory scale two degrees below the scratch, then o becomes the thirtieth degree, and the scratch, being two degrees above it, stands at the freezing-point; then from that count upwards; or, if the cold is below 30, then put 1 or 2 at the scratch and count down; every number is ten degrees. What the devil becomes of your eels in the winter? But try them in the summer and see what you can make of them.' [2] Jenner does not seem to have been very fortunate in his management of the thermometer, for a few years later Hunter writes chaffingly: 'You are very sly, although you think I cannot see it. You very modestly ask for a thermometer. I will send you one, but take care that those damned clumsy fingers do not break it also.' [3] Nevertheless, even with such inadequate instruments Hunter set out to determine experimentally the cause of animal heat not only in different vertebrata and invertebrata, but also in the vegetable kingdom. He came to the conclusion that 'animal heat is owing to some decomposition going on in the body in pretty regular progression, though it is not the process of fermentation'.[4] He thus, for the first time, gave the correct answer to a problem which had baffled philosophers from

[1] 'Barometri Novi Descriptio', *Phil. Trans.*, 1724–5, xxxiii. 179.
[2] Ottley's *Life* in *The Works of John Hunter, F.R.S.*, ed. J. F. Palmer, i. 63.   [3] Baron's *Life of Jenner*, i. 69.
[4] *The Works of John Hunter, F.R.S.*, in 4 vols. ed. J. F. Palmer, i. 284.

the earliest days. He then adds the very important statement: 'I expect the blood has an ultimate standard heat in itself when in health, and that nothing can increase that heat but some universal constitutional affection.'[1] Ignorance of the functions of the nervous system prevented him from studying the mechanism of heat regulation in animals, though he distinguished clearly between the homoiothermic and the poikilothermic—the warm- and the cold-blooded—for he says, 'the expression should rather be animals of a permanent heat in all atmospheres and animals of a heat variable with every atmosphere'.[2] A strange perversity led him to spoil his result, for he limits the place of heat production to 'some part of the body, perhaps the stomach',[3] and by ill fortune it did not occur to him to measure the fever in disease.

The shifts to which John Hunter was put to explain the general principles of disease in his ignorance of micro-organisms are both interesting and ingenious. He was in the position which we occupied until lately in regard to tubercle and syphilis, and where we still stand about cancer. He knew the clinical facts, but could not interpret them, for he had no knowledge of the part played by micro-organisms.

How near he got to the truth is shown by his definition of disease when he says: 'The most simple idea I can form of an animal being capable of disease is that every animal is endued with *a power of action* and *a susceptibility of impression*, which *impression* forms a *disposition*, which disposition may produce *action*, which action becomes the immediate *sign* of the disease; all of which will be according to the nature of the impression and of the part impressed.'[4] This seems at first sight to be a mere cloud of words hiding nothing, but interpret it by latter-day knowledge, and it shows how far Hunter had advanced in surgical pathology. What he calls the *power of action* we now speak of as the *predisposition* to disease or the *diathesis*;

[1] Op. cit., i. 385.   [2] Op. cit., iii. 16 note.
[3] Op. cit., i. 384.   [4] Op. cit., i. 301.

the *susceptibility of impression* is the *infective organism*; the *disposition* is the *exciting cause*, and the *action* is the *manifestation of the disease by signs and symptoms*. Take tuberculous arthritis as an example: the tuberculous diathesis (*power of action*) allowed the tubercle bacillus (*the susceptibility of impression*) to settle in the joint in consequence of a sprain (*the disposition*), and the joint then became hot and swollen (*the action*).

He says, indeed: 'A true specific disease is one that probably cannot arise but from one cause and which probably belongs only to morbid poisons.' [1] He gives as an example: 'Scrofula, which is one of those diseases which is supposed to be hereditary, but it is only the readiness to fall into this peculiar action, when properly irritated that is hereditary; and when such a cause does not exist we find no scrofula.' [2] Surely, 'nil nisi clavis deest', the key alone is wanting, and the key was not forged until Pasteur and Lister, the master locksmiths, came to maturity more than seventy years after the death of John Hunter. He was even a little in advance of the earliest Listerian teaching, for he showed by experiment that 'air, simply, has no power to excite inflammation'.[3]

He returns over and over again to the problem of the cause of disease when he is considering the causes of inflammation. Thus he says: 'It is the cause producing inflammation which is the disease and not the inflammation itself, for all inflammations that can be called diseases have specific causes.' [4] And he is driven at last to confess that 'inflammation may arise from a vast variety of causes with which we are at present totally unacquainted; nay, which we do not perhaps even suspect: and this last opinion would seem to be the most probable because we can frequently put back these spontaneous inflammations, which would not be the case if they came from the destruction of a part, or anything else, whose stimulus was similar to it, for no such thing can be done with wounds, if they

[1] Op. cit., i. 342.   [2] Op. cit., i. 358.
[3] Op. cit., iii. 352–3.   [4] Op. cit., i. 371–2.

are not soon united by the first intention they must suppurate'.[1] He has to confess his ignorance at last, for he
says: 'I cannot perceive why bleeding should have such
an effect on inflammation as it often has. We cannot
account for it simply on the mechanical principle of lessening the quantity of blood, because this can never remove
the *cause* of the inflammation.'[2]

He is in similar difficulties when he tries to explain the
action of mercury in the treatment of syphilis, and again
he gets very near the truth. 'Mercury by its irritation', he
says, 'will produce diseased action in a healthy part; the
venereal poison, by its irritation, will also produce diseased
action in a healthy part; but from the application of mercury to a part already affected with diseased action from
venereal irritation, an action results different from that
which would be produced by the application of it to a
healthy part; for, from the conjoined action of the two,
results the action of health; but, if carried beyond that it
may do harm, producing its own specific action.'[3] This is
a striking example of the Master's clarity of thought and
poverty of language. What he wanted to say was that
when mercury had done its remedial work in the body it
again became a poison if its use was continued.

The Hunterian School

If Hunter was born half a century too soon to allow
of his genius giving the best results, the span of his life
coincided with the time needed to establish a school of
scientific surgery in this country. No great surgeons
existed in England from the death of Richard Wiseman in
1676 until William Cheselden began to make his reputation by teaching anatomy privately in 1711. The industry
of Mr. G. C. Peachey[4] has shown that Hunter was not the
first to hold private classes, as a demand had already grown
up for more advanced teaching than was provided by the
formal lectures at the United Company of Barbers and

---

[1] Op. cit., iii. 407.   [2] Op. cit., i. 405.   [3] Op. cit., i. 478.
[4] *A Memoir of William and John Hunter*, Plymouth, 1924, p. 8.

Surgeons—lectures which had once been of the greatest service to surgery, but which in process of time had become obsolete. Cheselden, Nourse, Chovet, Sharp, and Pott (Plate I *a*) had lectured to large classes before Hunter, but they dealt only with their own experience and with surgery in its clinical aspects. It was left to John Hunter to invent surgical pathology. His teaching only appealed to a few, and his lectures were sometimes attended so scantily as to give point to the story of his ordering the skeleton to be brought into his lecture theatre that he might address the audience with the usual prelude, 'Gentlemen'.

How, then, did the school spread from such small beginnings? His few pupils became the leaders of the next generation of surgeons. Sir William Blizard of the London Hospital, Henry Cline of St. Thomas's, Astley Cooper at Guy's, John Abernethy at St. Bartholomew's, Anthony Carlisle at the Westminster, Philip Syng Physick and his nephew John Syng Dorsey in Pennsylvania, received the Hunterian teaching with enthusiasm. These great surgeons transmitted their knowledge to Sir Benjamin Brodie, Sir William Lawrence, Joseph Henry Green, John Collins Warren, and Valentine Mott, who in their generation became teachers at great schools of medicine in England and in America. The teaching of John Hunter was thus disseminated amongst the rank and file of the profession, whilst the doctrines he enunciated were so novel, so ingenious, and seemingly so heterodox as to become the subject of acrimonious discussion (Plate I *b*). Attention was thus drawn to them, and they quickly found their way into a text-book so widely read as Benjamin Bell's *System of Surgery*. They thus became public knowledge both at home and abroad even during the lifetime of their author.

But something more is needed to account for the rapid diffusion of Hunter's teaching. It is to be found in the spirit of devoted affection which he inspired in his pupils and in all with whom he was brought into personal contact. Those who, like myself, have been pupils of Huxley,

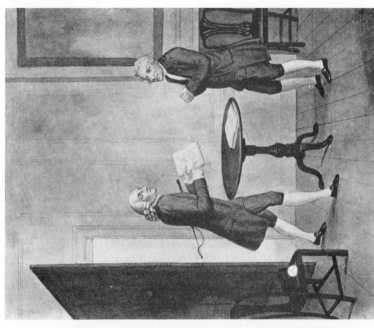

I b. 'Petrus Camper Hunterum corrigit'

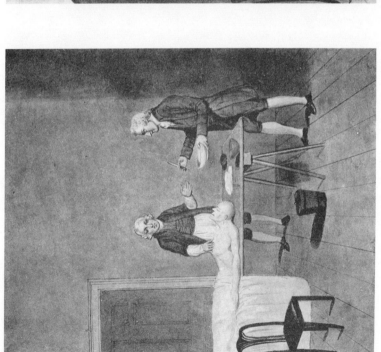

I a. 'Poor Hunter gone to Pott at last'

By permission of the Wellcome Historical Medical Museum

of Rolleston, and of Ray Lankester, can easily enter into their feelings of hero-worship. Adams says of him, 'He was almost adored by the rising generation of medical men, who seemed to quote him as the Schools, at one time, did Aristotle'.[1]

Rough, coarse, and prone to anger as he was in later life, he had the personal magnetism inherent in every great teacher, whether of religion, philosophy, science, or even quackery—a magnetism which attracts kindred spirits, rarely amongst contemporaries, generally in a younger generation. Thus it was with John Hunter. To his pupils he was 'The Dear Man' with whom they were in constant communication either by letter or by word of mouth, and to whom they looked for guidance and instruction in the experimental methods he had taught them to use in scientific surgery.

The Hunterian tradition passed down the next century in two great streams, theory and practice, uniting some-times, but for the most part flowing separately, because it was only occasionally that a single mind could embrace the whole. Both streams took their source from a sound knowledge of human anatomy gained by daily dissection. The streams parted early. Blizard, Astley Cooper, Hey, Physick, Gibson, and Dorsey became great operating sur-geons and advanced the teaching of Hunter along the lines of arterial surgery, the anatomy and treatment of hernia, the pathology of fractures and dislocations. John Aber-nethy, on the other hand, developed the physiological side of surgery and investigated the causes of disease and its non-operative treatment, for he took but little pleasure in the manipulative part of his profession.

Sir Benjamin Brodie was great enough in the second generation to combine the science with the art of surgery —the theory with the practice. He was equally good as a morbid anatomist and as a clinical surgeon, whilst his general knowledge of science enabled him to fill with dis-

[1] Joseph Adams, M.D., *Memoirs of the Life and Doctrines of the late John Hunter, Esq.*, London, 1817, p. 172.

tinction the important position of President of the Royal
Society. Joseph Henry Green, the Hunterian Orator in
1840, alone followed Hunter on the metaphysical side,
and delved so deeply into philosophy that he soon lost
himself in speculation and did but little to advance the
practice of surgery.

Sir James Paget, in the third generation, developed
surgical pathology on truly Hunterian lines; whilst Sir
William Savory was more interested in the teaching and
dissemination of the surgical principles laid down by John
Hunter, though he was a skilful surgeon and dearly loved
to tie an artery or extirpate a tumour so placed as to
demand all his knowledge of anatomy.

You, Sir, like myself and many others in the fourth
generation, hold firmly to the teaching of John Hunter.
We recognize with thankfulness the great work which he
accomplished; but we realize that it was the work of a
pioneer, and that the fields he pointed to are being ex-
plored by methods and by instruments of which he had no
conception. The Museum, Sir, has always been your
especial care, but you have not neglected the equally important subject of teaching both by example and precept.
You have shown, too, so enlightened an interest in the
habits and the customs of the beasts of the field and the
fowls of the air as would have drawn you very near to the
heart of John Hunter had you been privileged to sit at his
feet. To you also he would most certainly have been 'The
Dear Man'.

A Martyr to Science

The attitude of Hunter to Nature and the human body
always had something of the poetic in it, and was akin to
the feeling expressed by Longfellow when he wrote of
Agassiz:

> And Nature, the old Nurse, took
> The child upon her knee,
> Saying, 'Here is a story book
> Thy Father has written for thee.

Hunter looked upon Nature as a conscious personality. He says: 'Everything in Nature involves two consequences, the one beneficial, the other hurtful. But if we understood thoroughly all the remote causes we should probably see its utility in every case.'[1] He speaks of muscles as 'being conscious of their actions and almost endowed with reason'.[2] 'Nature', he says, 'acts purposively in the repair of dead bone',[3] and the 'clot adheres to the side of an aneurysm from a consciousness on the part of the artery of the weakness of its wall'.[4] In like manner he states that 'Nature lays claim to and removes what she pleases',[5] and he speaks of two surfaces lying in contact with each other and 'agreeing mutually not to inflame; or, perhaps more properly expressed, by being in contact there is a mutual harmony which prevents their being excited to inflammation'.[6] He also maintains that the first and immediate cause of the absorption of tissues is 'a consciousness in the parts to be absorbed of the unfitness or impossibility of remaining under such circumstances, the action excited by the irritation being incompatible with the natural actions and existence of the parts, whatever these are; wherefore they become ready for removal or accept of it with ease'.

The blood, too, is for him so living a tissue that the clot 'has the power of becoming vascularized in itself',[7] and when blisters and setons have been used as derivatives to draw off the humours he 'is unable to ascertain fully how they act, that is, how far the real disease is invited and accepts the invitation'.[8]

I wish now to draw your attention to a new aspect of John Hunter's life. It has always been assumed that the statement was the truth, the whole truth, and nothing but the truth, which was made by Sir Everard Home in 1794, the year after his brother-in-law's death, that 'the symptoms of Mr. Hunter's complaint for the last twenty years

[1] Op. cit., iii. 481.   [2] Op. cit., i. 524.   [3] Op. cit., i. 526.
[4] Op. cit., i. 546.   [5] Op. cit., i. 576.   [6] Op. cit., iii. 293.
[7] Op. cit., iii. 351.   [8] Op. cit., iii. 395.

of his life may be considered as those of angina pectoris and form one of the most complete histories of that disease upon record'.[1] Reading the account of his illness in the light of modern knowledge it seems to me that John Hunter died of syphilitic disease of his arterial system, and that, in addition to the angina pectoris due to this cause, he suffered for many years from cerebral syphilis. Both conditions were due to the action of the spirochaetes with which he deliberately inoculated himself in May 1767. He may be looked upon, therefore, as one of the great martyrs to science. Personally I do not think that he was justified in this martyrdom, for the consequences of his action were visited upon his children as well as upon himself, whilst the whole of surgery suffered by a shortening of the life which was advancing its bounds in every direction.

On a Friday in May 1767[2] Hunter inoculated himself with pus from a patient with gonorrhoea to determine whether the poison of gonorrhoea was identical with that producing syphilis. Surely that Friday must have been 22 May, a well-recognized 'Egyptian Day' or Dies Maledicti,[3] when it was most unfortunate to embark upon any new undertaking. The prepuce and glans were scarified, and it was noticed that the incisions itched on the second day, 24 May. The prepuce was inflamed on 26 May, and on 2 June a small ulcer appeared and was cauterized. A slough separated on 6 June, and the sore was cauterized a second time. The glans itched on 7 June, and on the following day a second slough detached itself from the prepuce whilst the sore on the glans ulcerated and was cauterized. Sloughs separated from the glans and pre-

---

[1] Life of the author prefixed to the quarto edition of Hunter's *A Treatise on the Blood, Inflammation, and Gunshot Wounds,* 1794, p. xlv.

[2] *A Treatise on Venereal Disease,* London, 1786, p. 324.

[3] The Fridays in May 1767, as my friend Mr. R. T. Gunther tells me, fell on the 1st, 8th, 15th, 22nd, and 29th of the month. Hunter states that he made the experiment on a Friday in May 1767, but does not specify the exact date. I have assumed for the sake of convenience that it was the only Egyptian day in a notoriously ill-starred month.

puce on 12 June, and the ulcers healed, leaving a scar. The lymphatic glands in the right groin enlarged during the week ending 13 June, but they did not suppurate.

The rapidity with which the two sites of inoculation ulcerated, and the appearance of a bubo, suggest that the pus may have contained Ducrey's bacillus, causing two soft sores. Spirochaetes were also present, because the gland in the groin began to enlarge again after a time, and in July the right tonsil ulcerated. Copper-coloured spots appeared upon the skin in September, and the tonsil ulcerated a second time. The administration of mercury soon healed the ulcer, but it returned a third and fourth time. The rash on the skin appeared on three separate occasions, and mercury was then 'taken in a sufficient quantity and for a proper time', Hunter says, 'to complete the cure. The time the experiments took up, from the first insertion to the complete cure, was about three years'. How complete the cure was will be shown! It is certain, therefore, that Hunter also inoculated himself with the *Spirochaeta pallida* and that his mercurial course was insufficient. The gonococcus, having been inoculated on a skin surface, did not multiply.

He married Miss Anne Home on 22 July 1771. There is nothing to show that she became infected as it was then understood; but John Banks Hunter was born in June 1772 and lived until 1838; Mary Anne, born in December 1773, lived only two months; James, born in November 1774, died in February 1775; Agnes, the youngest child, born in 1776, lived until 1838. It may be remarked that neither of the two surviving children left offspring, and neither was above the average in mental attainments.

Except for an attack of pneumonia in 1759, and occasional poisoned wounds from which every anatomist suffers from time to time, Hunter was a healthy man until he inoculated himself in 1767. In the spring of 1769 he had some toxic disturbance which, in accordance with the fashion of the time, was diagnosed as 'a fit of the gout'. It returned in the three following springs, but not the fourth. Its place was taken in the spring of this year (1773) by his first attack of serious illness. The account reads:

'In the spring of 1773, having met with something which very forcibly affected his mind, he was attacked at ten o'clock in the forenoon with a pain in the stomach about the pylorus. It was the sensation peculiar to those parts and became so violent that he tried change of position to procure ease. He sat down, then walked, laid himself down on the carpet, then upon chairs, but could find no relief. He took a spoonful of tincture of rhubarb with thirty drops of laudanum without the smallest benefit. While he was walking about the room he cast his eyes on the looking-glass and observed his countenance to be pale, his lips white, giving the appearance of a dead man. This alarmed him and led him to feel for his pulse, but he found none in either arm. The pain still continued and he found himself at times not breathing. Being afraid of death soon taking place if he did not breathe, he produced the voluntary act of breathing by working his lungs by the power of the will; the sensitive principle, with all its effects on the machine not being in the least affected by the complaint. In this state he continued for three-quarters of an hour, in which time frequent attempts were made to feel the pulse, but in vain; however, at last the pain lessened and the pulse returned, although at first but faintly, and involuntary breathing began to take place. In two hours he was perfectly recovered. 'In this attack there was a suspension of the most material involuntary actions, even involuntary breathing was stopped, while sensation with its consequences, as thinking and acting with the will, were perfect and all voluntary actions were as strong as before.' [1]

This attack of epigastric angina occurred six years after the inoculation with syphilis. It may have been caused by toxic changes in the smaller blood-vessels supplying the vagal nuclei, or it may have been the first indication of syphilitic inflammation at the root of the aorta. I am inclined to think that it was due to cerebral changes rather than to inflammation in the large arteries, for it would hardly have passed off so rapidly without leaving any marked ill-effects. It is noteworthy, too, that from this

[1] *A Treatise on the Blood, Inflammation, and Gunshot Wounds*, pp. xlv–xlvii.

time until his death twenty years later he drank little if any wine, not, we may be sure, because he liked abstinence, but because, as he says, it went to his head.

Four years later—in 1777—and again in the spring, he was seized with a very severe and dangerous illness in consequence of anxiety of mind from being obliged to pay a large sum of money for a friend for whom he had gone security, when circumstances made it extremely inconvenient.

'At two o'clock in the forenoon he ate some cold chicken and ham and drank a little weak punch; immediately after this he went eight miles in a post-chaise. While he was on the journey he had the feeling of having drunk too much, but passed the remainder of the day tolerably well; at twelve o'clock at night his stomach was a little disordered, for which he took some caraways and went to bed. He had no sooner lain down than he felt as if suspended in the air, and soon after the room appeared to go round; the quickness of this motion seemed to increase and at last was very rapid. It continued for some time, then became slower and slower till the whole was at rest. This was succeeded by vomiting, which was encouraged, and gave him a good night's rest. Next day he was tolerably well but fatigued. The morning after, thinking himself quite recovered, he went out before breakfast, drank some tea and ate some bread and butter which he was not accustomed to do. At eleven o'clock he felt his stomach in much the same state as before; in about half an hour the sensation of the room appearing to turn recommenced and continued for some time, but not with such violence as in the last attack. He became sick and vomited. The sensation of himself and everything else going round went off, but that of being suspended in the air continued with a giddiness. He could now hardly move his head from the horizontal position, and about two o'clock was brought home in his carriage, the motion of which was very disagreeable, giving the sensation of going down or sinking.

'After he went to bed the giddiness and the idea of being suspended in the air increased, and the least motion of the head upon the pillow appeared to be so great that he hardly durst attempt it; if he but moved his head half round, it appeared to be moving to some distance with great velocity; the idea he had of his own size was that of being only two feet long, and when he drew up his foot or pushed it down it appeared to him to be moving a vast way. His sensations became extremely acute or heightened; he could not bear the least light, so that although the window-blinds were shut, a curtain and a blanket were obliged to be hung up against it, the fire to have a screen before it, and the bed curtains to be drawn. He kept his eyelids closed; yet if a lighted candle came across the room he could not bear it. His hearing was also painfully acute, but not so much increased as his sight. The smell and taste were also acute, everything he put into his mouth being much higher flavoured than common, by which means he relished what he ate. His appetite, at first, was very indifferent, but soon became good. His pulse was generally about sixty and weak, and a small degree of heat on the skin, especially on the hands and feet.

'He remained in this state for about ten days and was obliged to be fed as he lay. By this time he was rather better, that is, he could move his head more freely. At the end of ten days all his ideas of his present state became natural, the strange deception concerning his own size was in part corrected, and the idea of suspension in the air became less. But for some time after the fire appeared of a deep purple red. When he got so well as to be able to stand without being giddy, he was unable to walk without support, for his own feelings did not give him information respecting his centre of gravity, so that he was unable to balance his body and prevent himself from falling. He gradually recovered from this state, and as soon as he was able went to Bath at the end of August, stayed there until the middle of November and drank the waters, which were thought to be of service to him, but did not stay long enough to give them a fair trial. He returned to Town much better and in a few weeks got quite well.' [1]

Soon after his arrival at Bath he received a visit from Jenner, who was so much shocked at the alteration which he noticed in him that he wrote to Heberden in 1778 saying, 'When I had the pleasure of seeing him at Bath last autumn I thought he was affected with many symptoms of angina pectoris. . . . As I have frequently to write to Mr. H., I have been some time in hesitation respecting the propriety of communicating the matter to him (i.e., changes in the coronary arteries). . . . Should it be admitted that this is the cause of the disease I fear the

---

[1] *A Treatise on the Blood*, &c., pp. xlvii–l.

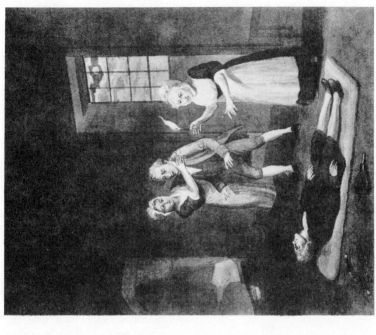

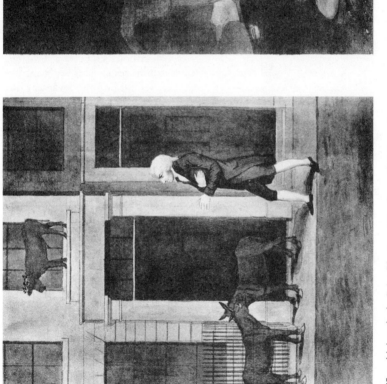

II a. 'Adoration'. John Hunter at the door of his house in
Golden Square in 1763

II b. 'John Hunter in his own Trance'

By permission of the *Wellcome Historical Medical Museum*

medical world may seek in vain for a remedy and I am fearful (if Mr. H. should admit this to be the cause of the disease) that it may deprive him of the hopes of a recovery'.[1]

Here again the symptoms point rather to cerebral than cardiac disturbance, to syphilitic inflammation of the smaller cerebral arteries, perhaps in the nature of a syphilitic peri-arteritis. There was vertigo, but neither tinnitus nor deafness, so that the auditory symptoms were due to inflammation of the vestibular nerve rather than to changes in the labyrinth. The photophobia was of retinal origin, and was due to hyperaesthesia such as led to exaltation of the senses of smell and taste. The lesions were multiple, and although their results lasted for some time, as in the case of the purple-red fire, yet they became compensated in the end. The unsteadiness of his gait does not appear from the description to have been of an ataxic character.

Hunter's brain adapted itself fairly well to the altered conditions for the next eight years, although his arterial system was undergoing progressive degeneration. His friends noticed with concern that he was ageing rapidly.

'At the beginning of April, 1785, he was attacked with a spasmodic complaint which, at first slight, became afterwards very violent and terminated in a fit of the gout in the ball of the great toe. Like the previous attack it was brought on by anxiety of mind. The first symptom was a sensation of the muscles of the nose being in action, but whether they really were or not he was never able to determine. This sensation returned at intervals for about a fortnight, attended with an unpleasant sensation in the left side of the face, lower jaw, and throat which seemed to extend into the head on that side and down the left arm, as low as the ball of the thumb, where it terminated all at once. These sensations were not constant, but returned at irregular times. They soon became more violent, attacking the head, face, and both sides of the lower jaw, giving the idea that the face was swelled, particularly the cheeks, and sometimes they slightly affected the right arm. After they had continued for a fortnight they extended to the sternum, producing the same disagreeable sensations there and giving the feel of the sternum being

[1] Baron's *Life of Jenner*, i. 39 and 40.

drawn backwards towards the spine, as well as that of oppression of breathing, although the action of breathing was attended with no real difficulty. At these times the heart seemed to miss a stroke, and upon feeling the pulse the artery was very much contracted, often hardly to be felt, and every now and then the pulse was entirely stopped. He was afterwards attacked with pain in the back about that part where the oesophagus passes through the diaphragm, the sensation being that of something scalding hot passing down the oesophagus. He was next seized with a pain in the region of the heart itself, and last of all with a sensation in the left side, nearly in the seat of the great end of the stomach, attended with considerable eructations of wind from that viscus. These seemed to be rather spasmodic than a simple discharge of wind—a kind of mixture of hiccough and eructation, which last symptoms did not accompany the former, but came on by themselves. In every attack there was a raw sore feeling as if the fauces were excoriated. All these symptoms (those in the stomach and nose only excepted) were in addition to the first, for every attack began with the first symptoms. The complaint appeared to be in the vascular system, for the larger arteries were sensibly contracted and sore to the touch, as far as they could be touched, principally in the left arm. The urine at these times was in general very pale.

'These symptoms increased in violence at every return, and the attack which was most violent came on one morning about the end of April and lasted above two hours. It began as the others had done, but having continued about an hour the pain became excruciating at the apex of the heart. The throat was so sore as not to allow the attempt to swallow anything, and the left arm could not bear to be touched, the least pressure upon it giving pain. The sensation at the apex of the heart was that of burning or scorching, which by its violence quite exhausted him, and he sunk into a swoon or doze [Plate II b] which lasted about ten minutes, after which he started up without the least recollection of what had passed or of his preceding illness. He then fell asleep for half an hour and awoke with a confusion in his head and a faint recollection of something like a delirium. This went off in a few days.'[1]

These attacks appear to have been of a more complicated nature than the previous ones. They were due in the main to syphilitic changes taking place in the aorta and

[1] *A Treatise on the Blood*, &c., pp. 1–lii.

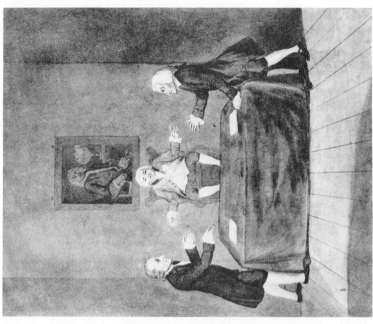

III b. 'The Grand Appeal'. William and John Hunter arguing before Sir Joseph Banks, President of the Royal Society in 1780

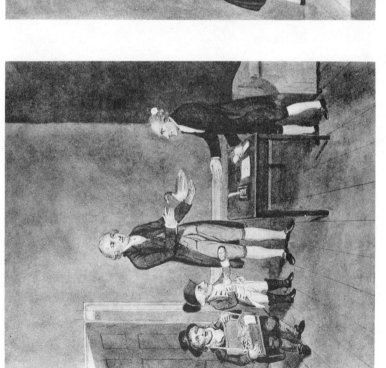

III a. 'Aura Popularis'. John Hunter with three of his freaks

By permission of the Wellcome Historical Medical Museum

heart, and were thus anginal, but in part to alterations in the cerebral circulation.

He went to Tunbridge in the August of this year, 1785, but finding no improvement there he travelled to Bath in September, and in December he was back in London, where he performed his first operation for the cure of aneurysm by ligaturing the artery in its continuity. The attacks of angina continued, though they did not increase in severity throughout the year 1786, until he became so accustomed to them that they formed a part of his life. He was unable, in consequence, to take much exercise, and passed his time in superintending the printing and publication of the *Observations on Certain Parts of the Animal Oeconomy* and the *Treatise on Venereal Disease*, which were issued from his own press in Castle Street, Leicester Square, and in the following year Sir Joshua Reynolds painted the striking portrait which has made his appearance so familiar to all of us.

He wrote to Jenner in May 1788,[1] saying that a severe indisposition for three weeks had prevented him from writing, although 'when two guineas rouse me I cannot resist'.

It is noteworthy that the first appearance of these symptoms was produced by an affection of the mind, and every subsequent attack of any consequence arose from the same cause. Although bodily exercise or distension of the stomach brought on slighter attacks, it still required the mind to be affected to render them severe, and as his mind was irritated by trifles these produced the most violent effects on the disease. His coachman being late, or a servant not attending to his directions, brought on the spasms, while a real misfortune produced no effect.[2]

'About the beginning of December, 1789, he was attacked with a total loss of memory when he was spending the evening with a friend. He did not know in what part of the town he was, nor even the name of the street when told it, nor where his own house was. He had not a conception of any place existing beyond the room he

[1] Ottley's *Life*, i. 110.   [2] *A Treatise on the Blood*, &c., pp. lviii–lxi.

was in, and yet was perfectly conscious of the loss of memory. He was sensible of impressions of all kinds from the senses, and therefore looked out of the window, although rather dark, to see if he could be made sensible of the situation of the house.

'This loss of memory gradually went off, and in less than half an hour he was perfectly recovered. About a fortnight afterwards as he was visiting his patients in the forenoon, he observed occasionally a little giddiness in his head, and by three o'clock it was attended with an inclination to vomit. He came home and drank some warm water, which made him vomit severely, but nothing came off his stomach except the water. The giddiness became severe, but went off again about seven or eight o'clock. About nine or ten it returned with more severity, and when going to bed about eleven o'clock he had entirely lost the centre of gravity, although he could move his limbs as the will directed. Light became offensive and everything had a kind of yellow cast; sounds were more acute than natural; objects had lost their true direction. A perpendicular, for instance, seemed to him to lean to the left, making, as nearly as he could conjecture, an angle with the horizon of fifty or sixty degrees. Objects were also smaller than the natural recollection of them; his idea of his own size was that of being only four feet high; objects also appeared to be at an unusual distance as if seen through a concave glass. He had a slight sound in the right ear at every stroke of the pulse. Motion of his head was extremely disagreeable. He therefore moved it with great caution, although coughing and sneezing did not affect it. It is difficult to describe sensations, especially when they are not common. The sensation which he had in his head was not pain, but was rather so unnatural as to give him the idea of having no head; but with all this neither the mind nor the reasoning faculty were affected, which is not the case when such effects are produced from liquor. Objects in the mind were very lively and often disagreeably so. Dreams had the strength of reality so much so, as to awaken him—and the remembrance of them was very perfect. The disposition to sleep was a good deal gone, an hour or two in the twenty-four being as much as could be obtained. These symptoms were much the same for about a week and began gradually to diminish, so that in a fortnight he was able to sit up, and in three weeks went for an airing in his carriage. He felt a pain in the joint of his great toe, which inflamed gently, but soon left it. During the attack he was unable to make water from ten o'clock in the evening till the same time next evening, the quantity being very considerable, although not so much as would have been made in the same time had he been in health.'[1]

His recovery from this indisposition was less perfect than from any of the others. He never lost entirely the oblique vision. His memory was in some respects evidently impaired, and the spasms became more constant.

These attacks were probably due to cerebral changes similar to those which caused the first symptoms in 1777, more than twelve years before, and perhaps not far from the areas originally involved, although there is no doubt that the disease in the large arteries had made considerable progress. I am not a neurologist, but, so far as a surgeon can guess, the lesions may have been situated in the immediate neighbourhood of the basal ganglia or even still nearer the cerebral cortex. They were certainly not in the cortex itself, nor in the spinal cord, nor in the peripheral nerves. The subjective sensation in the nose, and the pain in the great toe, might help to localize them more accurately. Sir William Macewen, in his address on Brain Surgery, delivered as President of the British Medical Association in 1922,[2] quoted some cases which bear upon this point. He says that in a 'girl under his care a protospasm of the hallux was preceded by sensory impressions and pain in the great toe. The lesion was found mainly in the upper portion of the ascending parietal convolution. In another case a sensory impression in the right foot heralded the invasion of the upper parietal convolution of the opposite side. The pain and discomfort in the foot entirely disappeared after the removal of a wedge-shaped portion of the brain tissue, and was replaced by numbness'.

The illusions as to size and shape may perhaps be accounted for by changes occurring in those 'silent areas' of the brain which it is so difficult to explore experimentally. It is certain that a generation which knew nothing of the individual functions of the brain and which attributed every form of toxic absorption to 'gout' explained the pain

[1] *A Treatise on the Blood*, &c., p. lxi.
[2] *Brit. M. J.*, 1922, ii. 158.

in John Hunter's toe by that disease, just as in later years we have been contented to say that he suffered from angina pectoris, without looking farther for a cause. The permanency of the defect in vision, and the impairment of memory, also point to widely spread changes in the brain which were almost certainly vascular, for no gross lesion was found after death. The sleeplessness and the increasing irritability must be attributed rather to changes taking place in his larger arteries than to alterations in the brain.

He never went to bed at this time without having an attack which was brought on by the act of undressing himself. They came on in the middle of the night, and the least exertion in conversation after dinner was attended by them. He felt, therefore, obliged to confine himself within a certain sphere of action and to avoid dining in large companies. Even operations in surgery, if attended with any nicety, now produced the same effects.

In the autumn of 1790 and in the spring and autumn of 1791 he had more severe attacks than during the earlier periods of the year, but of not more than a few hours' duration. In the beginning of October 1792 one was so violent that Everard Home who was present thought that he would have died.

'On October 16th, 1793, when in his usual state of health, he went to St. George's Hospital [Plate IV *b*], and, meeting with some things which irritated his mind and not being perfectly master of the circumstances, he withheld his sentiments, in which state of restraint he went into the next room, and turning round to Dr. Robinson, one of the physicians of the hospital, he gave a deep groan and dropt down dead.[1]

'The post-mortem examination showed that the pericardium was thickened, the heart very small, and there were two patches of a whitish colour and opaque appearance upon the under surface of the left auricle and ventricle. These two patches were covered by an exudation of coagulated lymph which at some former period had been the result of inflammation there. The muscular structure of the heart was paler and looser in its texture than the other muscles of the body. The coronary arteries had their branches in the state

[1] *A Treatise on the Blood*, &c., p. lxi.

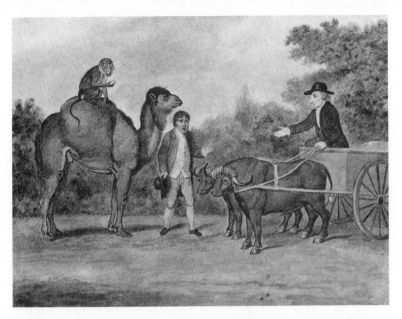

IV *a*. John Hunter in his Buffalo Cart

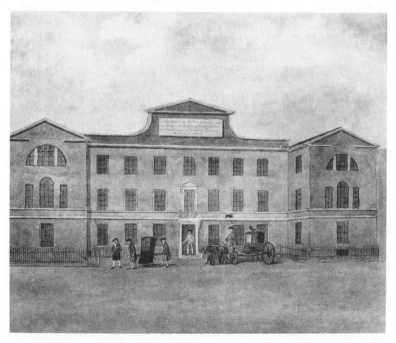

IV *b*. 'John Hunter's Exit'. The body of John Hunter is being conveyed home from Lanesborough House in Mrs. Hunter's sedan chair, immediately after his sudden death on 16 October 1793. His carriage and pair follow behind and Jesse Foot has malignantly represented his own feelings by introducing two magpies into the drawing

By permission of the Wellcome Historical Medical Museum

of bony tubes which were with difficulty divided by the knife, and their transverse sections did not collapse but remained open. The valvulae mitrales where they came off from the lower edge of the auricle were in many places ossified, forming an imperfectly bony margin of different thicknesses, and in one spot so thick as to form a knob, but these ossifications were not continued down upon the valves toward the chordae tendineae. The semilunar valves of the aorta had lost their natural pliancy, the previous stage to becoming bone, and in several spots there were evident ossifications.

'The aorta, immediately beyond the semilunar valves, had its cavity larger than usual, putting on the appearance of an incipient aneurysm; this unusual dilatation extended for some way along the ascending aorta, but did not reach so far as the common trunk of the axillary and carotid artery. The increase of capacity of the artery might be about one-third of its natural area; and the internal membrane of this part had lost entirely the natural polish and was studded over with opaque white spots, raised higher than the general surface.

'On inspecting the head, the cranium and dura mater were found in a natural state. The pia mater had the vessels upon the surface of the two hemispheres of the brain turgid with blood, which is commonly found to be the case after sudden death.

'The internal structure of the brain was carefully examined, and the different parts both of the cerebrum and the cerebellum were found in the most natural and healthy state; but the internal carotid arteries, as they pass by the sides of the sella turcica, were ossified, and several of the ramifications which go off from them had become opaque and unhealthy in their appearance. The vertebral arteries lying upon the medulla oblongata had also become bony, and the basilar artery which is formed by them had opaque white spots very generally along its coats.'[1]

A review of these facts about the illness and death of John Hunter shows, I think, that he died with widespread disease of his arterial system—the largest as well as the smallest arteries being involved. He may have inherited some family weakness of the vascular system, for his brother William had died ten years before of a cerebral haemorrhage, after suffering the vague symptoms associated with arterial degeneration, at exactly the

[1] Ibid., pp. lxii–lxiv.

same age of 65. The post-mortem examination of John Hunter's brain showed no gross lesions—such as a gumma —which were not likely to be overlooked by the trained anatomists who carried it out. The cerebral symptoms from which he began to suffer two years after he had inoculated himself with syphilis until the time of his death twenty-six years afterwards were, therefore, of a microscopic character. They were caused by cerebral syphilis of the interstitial variety, that is to say, they were due to the action of toxins produced by the *Spirochaeta pallida* in the lymphatic sheaths of the smaller cerebral blood-vessels. These changes in the outer coat of the arterioles interfered with their vasa vasorum, and so with the nutrition of the middle coat, thus leading to thrombosis or even complete obliteration of the little vessels as a consequence of the 'endarteritis'. Such a sequence of events recurred several times, and became more frequent and severe as he grew older and the arteriosclerosis became more pronounced. We can only be thankful that the stress of the disease fell upon the deeper parts of the brain, and that his intellectual faculties were so little impaired that he could give sound judgement in consultation, invent new methods of operating, and retain those powers of collecting which enabled him to form his magnificent museum.

Many of the experiences which I have quoted are undoubtedly recorded in John Hunter's own words. Sir Everard Home says: 'Each symptom was described at the time it occurred and was noted either by myself (himself?) or was dictated to me when Mr. Hunter was too ill to write. They will, therefore, be found more accurately detailed than in ordinary cases.'

It never seems to have occurred to Hunter to associate any part of his ill health with the inoculation experiment of 1767; indeed, he says expressly: 'It would appear that some parts of the body are much less susceptible of the lues venerea than others; and, not only so, but many parts, so far as we know, are not susceptible of it at all. For we have not yet had every part of the body affected; we have

not seen the brain affected, the heart, stomach, liver, kidneys, nor other viscera, although some cases are described
in authors.' [1]

How great, therefore, would have been his joy if his
cerebral cortex could have looked down upon the great
basal ganglia of his brain and recognized that some parts
of them were suffering from the effects of the venom which
he had himself introduced into his system so many years
before. We look upon him as a martyr to science; he
would rather have considered that the fresh knowledge
was worth the penalty he paid to gain it. To us it is marvellous that he could accomplish so much, crippled as he
was mentally and physically.

Hunter being Dead yet Speaketh

Whilst praising John Hunter and his pupils for what
has been done in the past, it is the duty of the Orator to
point to the influence of his teaching upon the present
generation of surgeons and to call attention to any outstanding work which may have been done since the last
Oration was delivered in his honour. His spirit still lives
and exerts its influence upon those of the younger generation of surgeons who are endowed with a portion of his
originality of thought and action, stimulating them to
attack and make advances along old lines which many had
long since abandoned as useless.

John Hunter, like his brother William (Plate III *b*), was
always interested in the surgery of the blood-vessels. To
many surgeons of to-day the name of John Hunter as an
operating surgeon is associated solely with ligature of the
femoral artery by a method which is no longer in use for
the cure of aneurysm. They look upon it as a mere stroke
of genius, being ignorant of the time, thought, and experience which had been given by many surgeons in
England, France, Germany, and Italy to the cure of
aneurysm for more than twenty years before Hunter tied

---

[1] *A Treatise on the Venereal Disease*, London, 1786, p. 305.

the femoral in its continuity. As early as 1750 Francis Thierry, of Toul, was inquiring in an inaugural thesis, 'An tutior faciliorque vulgari detur aneurysmatis Chirurgica curatio?'[1]

Pupils in the Hunterian school naturally shared in the enthusiasm of their teachers, and the surgery of the blood-vessels became a favourite subject of research and of practice during the opening years of the last century. Abernethy, Astley Cooper, Blizard, Wardrop, and Anthony White in England; Liston and Syme in Scotland; Colles and Crampton in Ireland, tied many of the large arteries, although the opportunities for doing so were not very numerous. It was far otherwise in America, where wounds of arteries were not rare and the surgical practice was concentrated in a few hands. The teaching of John Hunter was carried across the Atlantic by Wright Post to New York, by Physick to Philadelphia, by Gibson to Baltimore, and by Warren to Boston. In the New World so many opportunities occurred, and they were seized upon with such avidity, that one surgeon alone—Valentine Mott—ligatured the common carotid no fewer than forty-three times, the external carotid once, the first part of the subclavian once, and the third part of the subclavian four times—operations carried out before the introduction of anaesthesia, and for the most part successfully.[2] It is no matter of surprise, therefore, that the tradition of the surgery of the blood-vessels is stronger in the United States than it is in this country, although the excellent work of Sir George Makins and Sir Charles Ballance has done much to keep it alive amongst ourselves. Professor Rudolph Matas has nobly maintained the tradition at New Orleans by his reparative treatment of aneurysm, which is based upon experimental surgery in the true Hunterian spirit.

Sir Lauder Brunton in a short communication to the

[1] Haller, *Disputationes Chirurgicae Selectae*, tom. v, cxxxix. 211.

[2] John A. Wyeth, M.D., *Essays in Surgical Anatomy and Surgery*, New York, 1879.

Lancet in 1902 [1] suggested the possibility of treating mitral stenosis by surgical methods. He had already performed some preliminary experiments in the deadhouse and upon animals, but ill health, and the generally expressed feeling which is always against any new operation involving great risk to life, prevented him from carrying his design into execution on the human subject. Nothing further was done in this country, although it had long been known to physiologists that the healthy heart, even of mammals, could be handled with impunity, [2] whilst surgeons have had many opportunities of suturing wounds of the heart. At any rate nothing more was done in this country, and it was left to Professor Elliott C. Cutler, of the Western Reserve University, Cleveland, Ohio, with the help of Dr. S. A. Levine and Dr. Claude S. Beck, to subdue the diseased human heart to the hand of the surgeon. [3]

Lately, whilst visiting the United States, I had the good fortune to make the acquaintance of Professor Cutler and to see him operate upon a dog. As the original idea was put forward by Sir Lauder Brunton (although it had already entered the minds of Dr. Lauriston Shaw and Sir Arbuthnot Lane), who held in linear succession the office occupied by William Harvey, we must regret that it did not bear fruit at St. Bartholomew's Hospital. But no one who knows Professor Cutler, young, generous, enthusiastic, painstaking, and scientific, will grudge him the laurels he has earned by his brilliant and successful operation, and all will wish him 'God-speed' in what we hope will be a long and prosperous career.

---

[1] 'Preliminary Note on the Possibility of treating Mitral Stenosis by Surgical Methods', *Lancet*, 1902, i. 352.

[2] Robert Grove (1634–96), afterwards Bishop of Chichester, in his *Carmen de Sanguinis Circuitu*, gives a detailed description of Harvey's demonstration of the action of the heart in a living dog. Grove is probably the only bishop of the English Church who actually took part in a vivisection to show the tolerance of the heart to mechanical stimulation.

[3] 'Cardiotomy and Valvulotomy for Mitral Stenosis', *Boston Med. and Surg. Jour.*, 1923, clxxxviii. 1023–7, and 'The Surgical Treatment of Mitral Stenosis', *Arch. of Surg.*, ix. 689–821.

My task, Sir, is ended, and in bringing it to a conclusion I would ask you to remember that if Hunter with the knowledge and means at his command seems to us to-day to walk haltingly, or even often to have gone astray, shall we not seem to have done the same to those who read our story a hundred years hence? It is one of the lessons of history that each age steps on the shoulders of the ages which have gone before, and that the value of each age is in great part a debt to its forerunners.[1]

[1] Sir Michael Foster's *Lectures on the History of Physiology*, p. 299.

The illustrations are taken from water-colour sketches in an extra-illustrated copy of Jesse Foot's 'Life of John Hunter' in the possession of the Wellcome Historical Medical Museum. The drawings are scurrilous, but are not caricatures, and they are interesting because they represent Hunter as he appeared to his contemporaries, and not as he was idealized by Sir Joshua Reynolds. Their accuracy in detail is well shown in Plate III b. Newton's portrait by Vander Banck still hangs behind the President's chair at the Royal Society, but the globe, here plainly seen, is now only faintly visible owing to successive restorations of the picture.

We are indebted to Dr. Henry Wellcome for photographs of these sketches and for permission to reproduce them.

II

ENGLISH MEDICINE AND SURGERY IN THE FOURTEENTH CENTURY [1]

THE Harveian lecture was established in 1875 to pro-
mote the diffusion of exact scientific knowledge, and
the office has always been held by one who has done
pioneer work in the subject upon which he has lectured.
I felt it an especial honour, therefore, when your council
not only asked me to lecture, but invited me to choose
some topic connected with the·history of medicine, a
branch of knowledge which had not previously been
selected by any lecturer. I accepted the invitation with
pleasure, and the more so as it obliged me to carry out
a piece of work which I had long been wanting to do and
might not otherwise have undertaken.

England in the Fourteenth Century

I chose 'English Medicine and Surgery in the Reign
of Edward III'. This king was born, as you know, in
1312, came to the throne in 1327, and died in 1377. He
lived, therefore, practically through the fourteenth century
—a century which closed medieval history in Europe. It
was heir to the wonderful advances in scientific knowledge
which marked the twelfth and thirteenth centuries; it immediately preceded the equally wonderful revival in art
and literature known to us as the Renaissance, a revival
which took place at the expense of what is now called
'research' and 'original work' in favour of art and literature. The men of the fourteenth century were in touch
with the older beliefs and traditions, whilst they were endowed with the knowledge of science which had been
gained by Roger Bacon and Robert Grosseteste. The King
of England still flew the Wessex dragon, the old Saxon

[1] The Harveian lecture, delivered before the Harveian Society of
London on Thursday, 12 March 1914.

flag of England when he went to battle, and his wounded men were treated as often by spells and wort-cunning as by clean dressings and primary suture of the bowel.

The fourteenth century is thus worthy of careful study, and nothing in it is more worthy than the practice and the practitioners of medicine. The country was at war with France for a hundred years, and the upper and lower classes were as familiar with the Netherlands, France, and Spain as our own men are with South Africa. Trade was active and large sums of money were constantly changing hands. The Black Death, too, in the middle of the century was followed by a long train of epidemic illnesses. All classes of the medical profession profited, and all had abundant opportunity of practising their calling, whilst foreign victories by raising the national blood-pressure made them sanguine enough to experiment and advance upon the older methods. The younger generation, too, proved receptive. It watched the results of its teachers and was ready to adopt all means which had proved successful. Surgery, perhaps more than medicine, was in a fair way of becoming a science; then suddenly came the Wars of the Roses, chaos, and all was lost for very many years.

John Arderne

The fourteenth century was an era of really great surgeons throughout Europe. Lanfranc, the most distinguished pupil of William de Salicet, died in 1306; Henri de Mondeville lived from 1260 until 1320; Gui de Chauliac, prince of the medieval writers on surgery, died in 1368; Jan Yperman, the Flemish surgeon, died in 1350. These great surgeons were foreigners. We had in England at least one original surgeon—John Arderne— worthy to be classed with them. Born in 1307 he practised for many years at Newark, then a centre for England and a meeting-place for Parliament. He came to London in his old age and died at the end of the century. Typical of the fourteenth century he was skilful in leechcraft, a believer in spells, as befitted one brought up in the older school of thought, and yet a skilful and original surgeon, owing no allegiance to authority, profiting by his experience, able to invent wholly new operations. I desire to speak of him for a short time because the kindness of Dr. Henry S. Wellcome enables me to show you a manuscript of his works which has not hitherto been thoroughly examined (Plate V).

The original manuscript is in the Royal Library at Stockholm. It is said to have been bought in London in 1759 for the sum of £15 by the Swedish Minister at St. James's, and it was presented by him to the king on his return home.

This manuscript is a roll of eight skins of vellum sewn together. It measures 17 ft. 8 in. in length by 15 in. The writing is arranged in two and sometimes in three columns which are separated by coloured figures illustrating the text. It is written in an early fifteenth-century hand, and there is no reason to doubt the information added later that it was made in the year 1412. The roll has been exposed to considerable vicissitudes during the 502 years it has been in existence, and parts of it are quite illegible. I am, however, very greatly indebted to Mr. Eric Millar, of the Manuscript Department at the British Museum, for the great pains he has taken in transcribing all that can still be deciphered. It is clear from this transcript that the roll is a Latin version of a part of the works of John Arderne made a few years after his death by a copyist who had some knowledge of the *Lilium Medicinae* written by Bernard Gordon in 1305. It is, in fact, what the publishers would now call a revised edition of the works of the late Master John Arderne with additions. Like so many revised editions it is completely spoilt. It has lost its savour. Many additions have been made which Master Arderne would have resented, whilst much is omitted upon which he justly prided himself. Fortunately so many manuscripts of Arderne's works still remain—I have myself seen about sixty—that we need not be troubled because this one has been edited.

I do not propose to weary you with a detailed account of the roll, and I will only give a few short extracts that you may be able to gain some idea of its nature and contents. The work is an abstract of Arderne's *Liber Receptarum* arranged in the same order as the corresponding chapters in Bernard Gordon's *Lilium Medicinae*, which at the time was the ordinary manual of surgery throughout Europe; it cannot be called the text-book of surgery because it circulated in manuscript, as printing was not yet known. Arderne's roll deals with diseases of the head, throat, eye, ear, chest, lungs, digestive organs, liver, spleen, kidneys, and male organs of genera-tion. There is a section on gout, details of cases treated by the author, and some midwifery. Like all Arderne's works it is remarkable in containing no account of fractures and dislocations, and its early character is shown by the very slight reference made to astrology. The religious character of the age is well shown in the short prayer to be said before giving any medicine. It runs—I give you merely the translation—'O Lord, who marvellously madest man and more marvellously reformed him, who hast given physic to regulate the health of men's bodies, pour down from heaven thy blessing upon this remedy or electuary or draught, &c., that into whosoever's body it shall enter they may be worthy to receive strength of mind and of body through Christ our Lord. Amen.'

A single example will show the use made of charms or spells. It is recommended in epilepsy that the words Jasper, Melchior, and Balthazar be written with blood drawn from the auricular or little finger of the patient. The paper bearing the words should be worn by the patient, who was to say daily for a month three Pater Nosters and three Ave Marias for the souls of the fathers and mothers of these three kings. He was also to drink the juice of peony in beer or wine for a month. There is no doubt that Arderne had to treat the equivalent of panel patients, for he says, in speaking of constipation, 'Let the man drink "de brodio",' which was the equivalent of beef-

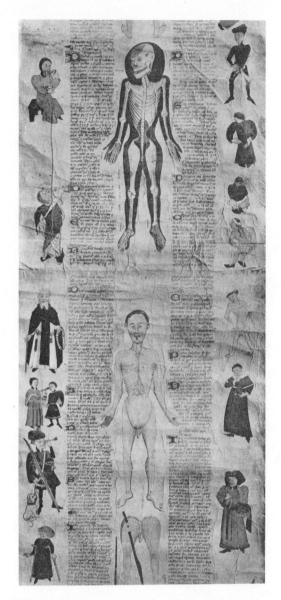

V. MS. of De Arte Phisicali et de Cirurgia of Master John Arderne (1412)

By permission of the Wellcome Historical Medical Museum

tea, 'if he be rich, but if he is a pauper he may just drink his own urine.'

These, however, are mere sidelights, for the manuscript contains a record of valuable experience. Arderne says that the following are fatal signs in quinsy: 'If the patient foams at the mouth, if the corners of the eyes become black or green, if the pulse cannot be felt, if the extremities become cold, and if a cold stinking sweat exudes from the armpits; because in these cases the patient will die on the same day.' He adds in another manuscript that he had treated very many cases of sore throat where the patient died suffocated in three or four days, so that he had probably seen some unrecorded epidemic of diphtheria.

The following case shows his surgical ability in a case of stone impacted in the urethra. He says:

'I saw a young man with a stone as big as a bean so lodged in his penis that it could not escape through its eye, neither could it be pushed back, but it remained in the middle of the organ as it is here shown. I cured him easily with an incision, for I put him on his back and tied his member with linen threads on each side of the stone to prevent it shifting, and after making a small cut with a lancet over the stone I squeezed it out. I then sutured the skin with a needle and thread over the hole, and dressed it with white of egg and finely ground flour, and having wrapped up the penis in a piece of old and thin linen I let him go in peace for three days. I cut and removed the thread at the next dressing, and in less than a fortnight I had cured him completely. There is no need for alarm in these cases, even though the urine escapes from the wound for three or four days after such an operation, for the patient will certainly be cured.'

In like manner his treatment of a case of serious primary haemorrhage was equally surgical, and was far in advance of his time, for he used cleanliness and sponge-pressure when most of his contemporaries would have employed astringent ointments; for ligatures and forceps to stop bleeding had not been thought of. Speaking of fistula in ano, Arderne says:

'I cured a man from Northampton who had three holes in the left buttock and three in his scrotum, as is here shown. The blood escaped very freely after the rectum was divided, because the fistula had tracked deeply. I put a sponge into cold water and stopped the bleeding with it. I then stuffed a good-sized sponge into the bowel and made him sit on a chair. The bleeding stopped directly, and as soon as the patient had eaten a meal and had been put to bed he slept well all night without any farther haemorrhage.'

Another manuscript gives the name of this patient as John Colyer, mayor of Northampton, and the records of the city show that he was mayor in 1327, and again in 1339–40.

The roll also contains a very interesting section on midwifery which is well worthy of more careful study. It gives a series of 'birth figures' like those found in Rösslin's *Byrth of Mankynde*. Each figure is accompanied by a short description which in many instances takes the form of question and answer, as if it had been designed for the oral instruction of midwives. The usual formula runs:

'Quartus partus est si ambas manus foras ei invenerit. Quid facere debet obstetrix? duobus humeris ejus manus suas ex utraque infigens retrorsum eum revocet, sicut superius dixi, manibus compositum et apprehenso capite paulatim et leviter eum adducat. Si infans caput habet et si duas manus ejicit, oportet obstetricem prius missa manu sua caput ad orificium corrigere et comprehensis manibus infantis conari debet ne caput orificium vulve non obstipet, sed facillime omne corpus infantis exire possit quo priores manus exierant.

'(The fourth birth or position is when both hands present. What should the midwife do? Grasping the hands with the arms on either side let her push back the child arranged with its hands as I have said above, and having seized the head, let her draw it down slowly and gently, &c.)'

And so I could go on with extracts for a long time, but as it would be at the risk of wearying you I shall pass on to more general matters.

Medical Practitioners in the Fourteenth Century

The treatment of the sick in England during the fourteenth century was in the hands of the same classes of practitioner as it is at the present time. It was shared by the physician, the surgeon, the family medical attendant, and the quack. The apothecary, then as now, was a tradesman. In country places the ladies did what they could to relieve the illnesses of their poorer neighbours.

The English Medieval Physician

The physician was usually, but not necessarily, a churchman. He learnt abstract science in the monastery schools and the scientific side of medicine in a university. He then returned to his monastery, where he either remained as physician or received preferment, becoming attached to the household of some great man. Dr. Norman Moore [1] gives the names of eight physicians practising in or near London during the reign of Henry III (1216–72). Two were physicians to the Queen—it is not stated whether or not they were in orders; two were canons of St. Paul's. Two were priests resident at St. Albans, and it is to be noted that one of these priests was the son of 'Adam the Physician', who was not therefore a priest. The last of the eight was a doctor of medicine, a doctor of laws, and a doctor of theology, a professor at Paris and Oxford, physician to the King of France and to the Bishop of Lincoln.

We know that no great change had taken place in the status of the English physician in the next hundred years, because John of Gaunt had two physicians in his retinue, John Bray and William Appulton. John Bray was John the Minorite, 'Johannes de ordine Minorum, in armis bellicis strenuus, in physicâ peritissimus, domino Johanni duci Lancastriae familiarissimus' ('John of the order of the Minorites, courageous in war, most skilful in physic, most acceptable to My Lord, John Duke of Lancaster'). It was precisely because he was such a friend of the duke that the London mob beheaded him on Tower Hill after the Savoy was burnt in 1381. His colleague was Frère William de Appulton, 'physician and surgeon', who received xl marks in time of peace from the honour of Pomfret; in war time other xl marks and ranked as a gentleman, clerk, esquire,

[1] *The History of the Study of Medicine in the British Isles*, 1908, p. 16.

or a chamberlain, having four horses and two grooms allotted to him. Bray had received £10 a year, with 3s. a day travelling allowance. He ranked as a chamberlain with an allowance of two horses and the wage of one groom.

The physicians attached to John of Gaunt, therefore, held a good position in his household. They were men of affairs and took an active part in counsels of war. It is clear from the description of Frère William that he was prepared to act as a physician or as a surgeon,[1] so that the line of division between the two branches of the profession was not so absolute as is usually described. The popular idea of a physician as he is represented in Plate VI *a* was generally accurate. He was a learned man who taught pupils, gave advice, prescribed drugs, and ordered active treatment when he considered it necessary. In this particular case[2] the physician is represented in an ecclesiastical dress with a biretta (Plate VI *a*). He is watching a patient who has been ordered to take a dose of medicine. The stool with the basin beneath it shows the primitive sanitary arrangements of the time. It was not even a close stool, the first mention of which is in 1410, or more than fifty years after the time we are considering.

My friend Dr. H. P. Cholmeley has recently (1912) issued an admirable account of the English medieval physician in his book on John of Gaddesden, who lived from 1280 to 1361, and as the book is easily accessible I need say no more about him except that on the two occasions when Arderne, his contemporary, refers to him it is in connexion with the diseases of women, so that he was evidently held in estimation as a gynaecologist.

The Operating Surgeon

The operating surgeon—as a class—was in a lower position than the physician, and during the fourteenth century he was in a transition state. He was still itinerant because he went from house to house to do his cure—that

---

[1] Vide *John of Gaunt's Register*, Camd. Soc. ed., 1911, Part i, No. 836.
[2] *Le Régime du Corps*, by Aldobrandino of Siena, Sloane MS. 2435.

is to say, he undertook for a certain fee to operate and attend the patient until he was well. This involved personal service, occasionally for long periods of time, and the fees charged were relatively large because it was impossible to have more than one case in hand at a time. The fee was paid partly in cash, partly in kind, and partly in the form of an annuity which the surgeon received so long as the patient lived. The operating surgeon travelled extensively, lived with the moneyed classes, and if he was a good fellow was received by his patients on a friendly footing. He also gained a large income.

Most of the operating surgeons in this century had seen war service, I imagine, and although there were a few in the provincial towns, the majority congregated in London where they became members of the Gild or Fraternity of Surgeons. Membership of this Gild gave them the right to call themselves 'Master' or 'Magister' with a special cap and robe, and for a few years they arrogated to themselves the prefix 'de', so that John Arderne when he was elected into the Gild became Magister Johannes de Arderne. Many operating surgeons had taken orders and were consequently unmarried, but they do not seem to have held Church preferment, as was the case with physicians. The attitude of mind of the lay surgeons was, however, sincerely religious when they belonged to the better class, and their religion was certainly not a pose. Arderne, writing in 1376, used to say, 'I did my cure to him and the Lord being mene (*Deo favente*) he was helid perfectly', in exactly the same humble-minded spirit as Ambroise Paré—two hundred years later—said, 'I dressed him, God cured him.'

The Master Surgeons as a gild exercised control over the practice of surgery in London. Isolated notices of them occur as early as 1312, and the record of 1354 shows definitely the use to which the authorities put their knowledge. It says:

'Be it remembered that on Monday next after the feast of St. Matthias the Apostle (24th Feb. N.S.) in the 28th year of the reign of King Edward iiird, the Prior of Hogges, Master Paschal, Master Adam de la Poleterie, and Master David de Westmerland, surgeons, were sworn before the Mayor, Aldermen and Sheriffs, to certify them as to a certain enormous and horrible hurt on the right side of the jaw of Thomas de Shene; whether or not such injury was curable at the time when John le Spicer of Cornhulle took the same Thomas under his care to heal the wound aforesaid. Who say upon their oath, that if the aforesaid John le Spicer at the time when he took the said Thomas under his care had been expert in his craft or art or had called in counsel and assistance to his aid, he might have cured the injury aforesaid; and they farther say that, through want of skill on the part of the aforesaid John le Spicer the said injury under his care has become apparently incurable.'

I am inclined to think that John le Spicer was an apothecary seeking to practise surgery and that he was a member of the Fraternity of Spicerers.

The duties of the officers of the Gild had become stereotyped into an oath as early as 1369, but I quote the oath of 1390 because it states that women as well as men practised surgery in the City of London. It runs:

'On Monday, 10th April in the thirteenth year of King Richard the Second, Master John Hynstock, Master Geoffrey Grace, Master John Bradmore and Master Henry Suttone, surgeons, were admitted in the Court of Guildhall in London before William Venour, Mayor, and the Aldermen. They were sworn as Masters Surgical of the aforesaid city well and truly to serve the people in working their cures, taking of them reasonable recompence, &c. To practise truly their trade and to make faithful oversight of all others both men and women, occupied in cures or using the art of surgery, presenting their lack both in practice and medicine so often as needs be to the aforesaid Mayor and Aldermen. They shall be ready when warned thereto to take charge of the hurt or wounded and to give faithful information to the servants of the City of such hurt or wounded as are in danger of death or not.'

The Master Surgeons themselves were held in some estimation and consorted on fairly equal terms with the physicians, but the reputation of operating surgeons as a whole was not good. Their wandering life very often made them literally vagrants, and if a case was not doing well

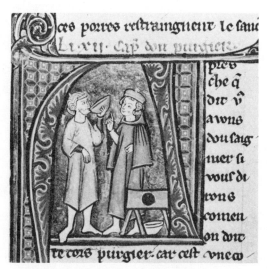

VI *a*. The Physician

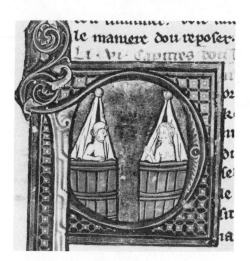

VI *b*. Bathing

they had an unpleasant habit of slipping away and leaving the patient to Providence. In the popular estimation they were drunken, lascivious, boastful, and quarrelsome thieves.

The best of the operating surgeons, however, did good work in the fourteenth century, and they almost succeeded in making surgery a profession. Their skill and boldness may be judged from this extract from the manuscript of an unknown surgeon whose work still lies unprinted at the British Museum.[1] The section treats 'of wounds of the gut and liver'. It says:

'Yf a gutte passe out of the wounde and it be not wounded reduce him in again, and yf you may not reduce him procede in this manner. ffirst chaufe ye guttes that ben oute and mollifie hem with a gret sponge [wetted] in water of ye decoccion of camomülle & anys & enoynte hem with hoote oile of camomulle & when they be chaufed with the aforeseid sponge putte hem in agen as well as you may & yff you may not reduce hem by this weye open ze wound a litell more liztly & widely & then reduce hem & sewe ye wounde & yf the gutte that passe out be wounded then that wounde ben dedlye but yet leve not the resonable cure of the wound.

'An ye guttes be kutte all otmest so that ther leve nothyng hoole thane natheless the wound is mortal and may not receive no curacion; but yf ze guttes be kutte on lengthe other in partie on breadth but not fully cut in sonder hardily conduce ye parties of ye gutte that is kutte, whether that it be kutte ye lengthe other brede, & sewe hem in ye manner as skynners sewen ther furroures [furs], for in this case it is ye best maner; & anone as it is sewed lay on a poudir that mo cleve together to the guttes & the sewing the weche is made in this manner: Take Mastic, draganth & gum arabick, &c.'

In the same manner it is recommended that a ruptured liver should be treated by suture.

The Barbers

The term 'leech' was used familiarly as the term 'doctor' is at present, and was applied to all members of the medical profession. The general or family practitioner, at any rate

[1] *Galien's Book of Operacions*, Sloane MS. 2463, Fol. 116.

in London, was obliged to be a member of the gild or fraternity of Barbers. He was a Barber and was called a Barber or, at the best, a Barber practising surgery, for there were no Barber Surgeons, since the Barbers and Surgeons did not unite until 1540. Some jealousy existed between the operating surgeon and the barber who practised surgery, for Arderne says, in speaking of the treatment of thrombosed piles by incision: 'And be the lech ware that non of tham that standeth ny about perceive when he openeth the lancet for if barbours know this doing they would usurp this cure, appropriating it to themselves unto unworschip and no little harm of the Master (surgeons).' It is clear, too, that the barbers held a somewhat lower position, for it is told of a fishmonger, who spiked his arm on the swingdoor of the Carmelite Church in Whitefriars, that 'he was almost dead what with the aching, swelling, burning and improper treatment of a barber that put into the wound irritating tents of linen and had covered them with diachylon. All these dressings I took away and about evensong replaced them with a simple dressing of oil. And before cockcrow the patient was relieved and in the morning he slept well and I cured him finally and thereby I got much honour.'

Here is a case showing the ordinary course of surgical routine and the relationship between women, barbers, and surgeons in the fourteenth century. The priest had a cancer of his breast. John Arderne tells the story in one of his minor works. He says:

'To a preest of Colstone faste by Bynghuame [Colston Bassett in Notts] ther felle a sore in the ryghte pappe withinne the skyne uppone the heed of the pappe as it were a litill knotte & in manner of a pese with ycchynge & so the forseyd knotte bi contynywaunse grew foorth tyll it was of the gretnesse of ane henne egge & that it came to the foorme & lyknesse of a topp. The colour of this sore was lyvyd medlyd with rednesse & waterynesse & hard in felynge & whane ii yere were passyd he was tawghte of a lady to leye ane emplastre therto & to drynke of the drynke of Antioche and whane he perceyved that the forseyde medicines prevayled hyme nowgth he went uneto the towne of Notynghuame to be leten blood & whane the barbour perceyved the forseyd knotte he asked of hyme whether that he wolde be holpen therof & tolde hyme that he hadde a cure therfore & coowde hele hyme therof. The preest seyd he wolde fayne be holpen but nevertheless he seyde to him he wolde aske counsell yf it myghte be done as he seyd unto him. And in the same towne ther was a wyse sirurgyane of the weche the seyd preest hadde wetynge & wente to hyme to aske counsell yf that he were curable or if that he myghte suffre ony kuttynge or corrosyne or ony suche other medicines. And the seyde leche warned him that he schulde in no manere wyse putte no corrosyve ne non other violent medicines ne lete no kuttynges come ther-ny for yf he dyde he promysed that yt wolde brynge hyme to the deeth withouten ony rekevere.'

The barbers acted in their public capacity as health officers of the City of London. They had charge of the gates of the City and were formally appointed gatekeepers. They knew who came in and who went out, and their medical knowledge enabled them to segregate the lepers who were so fruitful a source of anxiety to every community throughout the Middle Ages. The barbers also had the superintendence of the Bagnios, which were little else than licensed brothels, and it is for this reason that in 1308 Richard the Barber, on his presentation to the Court of Aldermen as Supervisor of the Barbers, made 'oath that every month he would make scrutiny throughout the whole of his trade and if he should find any among them keeping brothels or acting unseemly in any way and to the scandal of the trade he was to distrain upon them'.

These duties interfered to a certain extent with the duties required of every citizen—the serving on juries and keeping of watch and ward. Both were irksome, and the early records of the Barbers are full of attempts to gain exemption. The City watch was especially onerous, for in times of unrest, and they were frequent throughout the thirteenth and fourteenth centuries, the streets of London were patrolled at night by a guard which the chroniclers tell us was as many as 10,000 men armed and grouped into bands under the different aldermen. In ordinary times a dozen men from each ward sufficed, but they had to be properly armed and accoutred so that they were a source of continual expense. The barbers obtained exemption both from serving on juries and from watch and ward, and the exemption, as you know, still holds good for us so long as we are in the actual practice of our profession.

The barbers took no responsibility with their patients. Every person under their care who was 'in peril of death or maim'—that is to say, who was seriously ill or likely to suffer from permanent disablement—had to be seen by the Master or Wardens of the Barbers' Gild within three days of the first attendance. Any barber who neglected this rule of 'the presentation' of patients was fined and might be imprisoned, whereas if he obeyed it he was held blameless—except in very gross cases of malpractice— whatever happened. The rule worked well, and for 300 or 400 years there is no record of the attending barber being supplanted by the Master and Wardens whom he had called in to assist him. The women members of the Barbers' Gild and Company did not exercise their art and mystery, but were the wives, widows, and daughters of members who kept on the apprentices or received what would now be called a pension.

Subordinate Grades

In the subordinate ranks of the profession were many different grades. They chiefly flourished in country places and travelled from town to town. The dentist, as is seen in Plate VII *a*, was known by the belt which he carried to display the number of successful extractions he had performed, but it is evident that his tools were of the rudest, even if allowance be made for inaccurate drawing. The coucher for cataract, the cutter for stone, and the curer of ruptures were well-recognized itinerant occupations, whilst cupping, or 'garsing' as it was called, was left to a special class, of whom the last survivor disappeared from the Blackfriars Road well within our own recollection. It seems, however, that only the operative part was left to

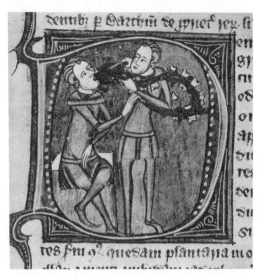

VII *a*. The Dentist

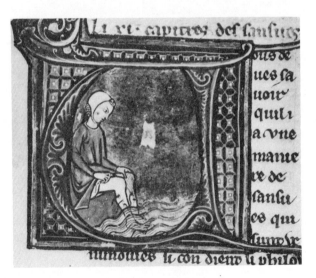

VII *b*. Leeching

these practitioners, for the surgical manuals of the time deal with the treatment of diseases of the eye, with the signs and symptoms of stone in the bladder and kidneys, as well as with hernia. The method of leeching seems to have been simple, if Plate VII *b* may be trusted, for the patient is sitting with her feet in the pond until the leeches fasten upon her legs.

Bathing in like manner was reduced to its simplest form, as is here shown (Plate VI *b*).

The Apothecary

Very little is known of the apothecary in the fourteenth century. He practised a separate trade in London as a member of the Spicers' Gild—for the Gild of Grocers was not yet formed—and in all probability he was an offshoot of the confectioners. The Ward Robe Rolls show him as a court official who in the reign of Edward II, in 1313, received 7½*d*. a day. His name was Odin the Spicer, and when Madame the Queen was ill at Westminster in the November of that year, he bought things for her. He is called definitely 'Odinus Apothecarius Reginae'. In 1345 Coursus de Gangeland, an apothecary of London, was granted 6*d*. a day by Edward III for taking care of and attending his majesty during his illness in Scotland, so that by this time he was definitely engaged in medical practice. In 1360 Peter of Montpellier was apothecary to Edward III, and Freind says, in his *History of Physick* (vol. ii, p. 292), that J. Falcand de Luca in 1357 was the first apothecary to sell medicines in England.

The apothecary held a well-recognized position as the 'physician's cook', and Chaucer says in his prologue, when speaking of a Doctour of Phisike:

> Ful redy hadde he his apothecaries,
> To send him drugges, and his letuaries,
> For ech of hem made other for to winne;
> Her frendship was not newe to begynne.

John Arderne makes several references to 'the potecary'. Writing in 1372–6 he says: 'Euforbium is a gumme that

potecaryes sellen', and in another place: 'Agryppa is ane
oyntment that potecaryes sellen, and it is whyte of coloure';
and yet again: 'Thou mayest put to a wounde common
unguentum album that apothecaries make.'

The spicers and the pepperers were nearly all Italians
in the fourteenth century, and the apothecary was necessarily a member of one of these gilds, or he could not ply
his trade. There is a curious passage in one of Arderne's
works which shows that these Italians were already assum-
ing to themselves certain humble medical duties, for he
says, in speaking of clysters and their uses, 'I have gotten
an hundred times gret honour with lucre in diverse places.
ffor why, at London when Lumbardez oft-times ministered
clisteries on their manner to colic men and other men con-
stipate, ne might not availe, I forsooth, with the aforesaid
manner of clystering at the first time within the space of
a forlong or two I delivered the patient for certayne, our
Lord being mene.' The passage is interesting apart from
the reference to the Lombards as specialists in the administration of enemata, because it shows how prevalent
constipation must have been when living was high, people
were sedentary, and purgatives were few. The estimation
of the action of clysters in terms of distance rather than of
time seems to be wholly original. So far as I remember,
however, the apothecaries never came into serious conflict
with the surgeons or with the barbers of London in the
exercise of their occupation. They were soon merged into
the great Company of Grocers and developed into ordinary
shopkeepers as retail sellers of drugs and spices. It was
only when they were formed into a separate body as the
Society of Apothecaries that they became a thorn in the side
of the physicians, but this was more than 250 years later.

The Hospitals

The hospitals in the fourteenth century formed a special
branch of charitable work, just as they do at the present
time. In London they had already existed for nearly 200
years. They were religious institutions nursed by mem-

bers of the Augustinian order, and provided food, rest, nursing, and religious consolation for those who were acutely ill. There was no separate medical or surgical staff until the sixteenth century, and we have no knowledge as to the nature of the treatment followed. The patients were sick persons found in the streets of the City and all the wounded or injured who chose to apply for relief. Every one was received freely and without question. Special servants of the hospital—the beadles—clothed in a distinctive livery and wearing a badge, were appointed to bring patients into the hospital. At St. Bartholomew's Hospital they still exist, and their sixteenth-century charge ran:

'Ye shall separate and divide yourselves into sundry parts of the city and the liberties thereof, every man taking his several walk. And if in any of your walks ye shall happen to espy any person infected with any lothely grief or disease, which shall fortune to lie in any notable place in the City to the noyance and infection of the passers by and slander of this house ye shall then give knowledge thereof unto the Almoners of this hospital that they may take such order as to them shall be thought meet.'

We also know how such patients were received, for the order runs:

'When the patient arrives he shall be received thus: First, having confessed his sins to the priest he shall be communicated religiously and afterwards be carried to bed and treated there as Our Lord, according to the resources of the house; each day before the repast of the brethren he shall be given food with charity, and each Sunday the epistle and the gospel shall be read with aspersion.'

The patient was looked upon as the direct representative of Christ, and was spoken of as Master or Lord, 'Domini nostri pauperes', 'Les Signors malades', 'Our Lords the Sick', a very different form of address from the brutal terms of the eighteenth century, when they were spoken of officially as 'the miserable objects'.

The hospital consisted of a large hall ornamented with a high-pitched roof, a central louvre, beds in rows down the sides and in the centre, rather overcrowded to our ideas, with an altar raised a few steps at one end so that the patients could see the celebrant. The beds clean and neat, for there is a special order that they should be of sufficient breadth and length, and that the coverlets and sheets should be clean, separated perhaps by curtains, occupied certainly by two patients. This, however, was no hardship, because the proverb that 'Travel makes us acquainted with strange bedfellows' is a remembrance of the time when it was usual for a person to share his bed with a stranger, and readers of literature even as late as the eighteenth century will recall many instances where the hero or the heroine has suffered loss at the inn where they have slept with a stranger who rose early and took the purse or the clothes of the heavier sleeper. Indeed, Sir Sydney Waterlow used to tell us when we were house surgeons and complained of the inadequacy of the accommodation offered us by the hospital, that when he was an apprentice he shared his bed with two others and that he slept in the middle because he was the smallest. The use of wooden bedsteads, which was universal at the time, made the bugcatcher an important and useful person at every hospital. The services of the Church compelled the constant attendance of the religious by night as well as by day, and the sick were therefore never left without supervision.

The food was as good as could be obtained and seems to have been liberally supplied; whilst extras were allowed on a somewhat lavish scale, witness the story that is told of the Knights Hospitalers of St. John of Jerusalem. It is said that Saladin desiring to prove for himself the indulgence of the knights to their patients disguised himself as a pilgrim and was received among the sick at the hospital in Jerusalem. He refused all food, declaring there was only one thing he fancied, and that he knew they would not give him. On being pressed, he confessed that it was one of the feet of the Grand Master's horse. The Grand Master was told, and at once ordered the noble animal to be killed and the sick stranger's desire satisfied. But Saladin thinking the experiment had gone far enough declared himself taken with a repugnance to meat, and the animal was spared.

Conclusion

And thus ends a very short account of an interesting period of medicine in England. It is impossible in the scope of a single lecture to give more than a bare outline of the subject, but it has been my intention to show that there was a blending of the old and new during the fourteenth century. Wort-cunning, which still lingers amongst us at the herbalists, was the older Saxon leechcraft; spells were a reminiscence of the Danish rule; classical medicine was coming into vogue through the Arabic translations, and was brought to England from the schools of Salernum and Montpellier. Side by side with this knowledge, altering, modifying, and even creating, was the sturdy originality of the English mind. I shall have effected a part of my purpose this evening if this lecture induces some of you to go to the British Museum, to the university libraries, and to the cathedral libraries in search of the writings of our early predecessors which have escaped destruction but have never yet been printed. Such writings I believe to be numerous—some in Latin, some in racy translations, some in the original English in which they were written.

III

SOME EPISODES IN THE HISTORY OF ST. BARTHOLOMEW'S [1]

MEMORY and the mind's eye sometimes play strange pranks with those who, like myself, have been long connected with this Hospital and who know something of the history of London.

Often as I walk across the Viaduct on a misty evening in December, I remember why Snow Hill runs round obliquely at Burroughs and Wellcome's corner, for do I not see the City wall with its gates right in front of me? And I know that the bend is made to prevent rushes of an armed crowd who might attack this entrance to the City.

As I turn the corner at St. Sepulchre's Church I walk instinctively in the middle of the road, for I am separated from the City wall by the City ditch which runs where is now the out-patient entrance to the Hospital, through the Post Office courtyard to the City ambulance shed, and so on to the Postman's Park. It is still a filthy bog, for our Sheriff had not yet cleared away the refuse collected since the Roman aedile left it.

On such an evening all the buildings in Smithfield fade away; the Meat Market vanishes, and there is nothing in front of me but the City gallows standing on the high ground at the top of St. John's Street. On my left is Hosier Lane, running down to the Fleet river. The ground over which I am walking is dirty and marshy, whilst against the City wall are stacked the bales which show me that the King's Cloth Market is held here.

A.D. 1120.—*St. Thomas à Becket.*—As I walk a fellow citizen overtakes me, saying, 'Dear eme! heard you the strange dream which came to Gilbert Becket's wife who lives in the Poultry, and was yesterday delivered of a son they have called Thomas?' I answer 'No, tell me'. He

---

[1] Midsessional address delivered before the Abernethian Society at St. Bartholomew's Hospital, on 6 December 1917.

replies, 'They say she dreamed last night that the baby was lying naked in the cradle; she looked upon it and asked "Why is the boy unclothed?" to whom the nurse, "Dear Mistress, you see not aright, for surely never was child so swaddled in purple and fine linen", and in truth it was so, as she saw in her vision, for they unwrapt the purple cloth, and it reached from their house in the Poultry through Cheapside, up Newgate Street, and passing through the New Gate still reached along Giltspur Street until it stopped in Smithfield, and the mother interpreting the dream said: "Doubtless it portends that this child will become a great man, and will attain to high dignity in the Church," but, dear eme the holy man who interprets dreams says: "Not so, the boy will in truth grow up, but the red cloth signifies his blood, which shall be shed and spread through all Christendom; nay, more, that a Hospital shall be founded at that place where the cloth stopped, and there will more blood be shed." '

And so the vision passes.

A.D. 1140.—*Rahere*.—Another time, there has risen just in front of the City wall a Hospital, of many scattered buildings, and by its side the Priory Church with which we are still familiar in part, and I see sitting in the Prior's lodgings two Augustinian canons talking as friends, the one I know to be the Prior Rahere Founder; the other Alfune, his Proctor and our first Hospitaler, who built the Church of St. Giles in Cripplegate.

Alfune is saying to Rahere, 'Father, a miracle happened to me this morning. Early I took my bowl and went amongst the butchers collecting food for the poor in our Hospital. Thou knowest well Goodrich, that surly butcher, who never will give aught to the poor. Him I entreated, but he answered as usual that he would give nought; to whom I said that if he gave somewhat of his store the rest should be bought at a price greater even than he asked. And he, scoffingly, took a piece of the worst meat from the worst beast and threw it into my bowl with curses, and, behold, before I had left his stall there came a citizen running and breathless who took hurriedly the rest of that beast, nor asked the price but threw down money and went away, and ·behold it was more than he demanded, and this was noised abroad, and was much noted by the other butchers.'

And I saw that as Alfune told his tale Rahere turned away his head and smiled. I remembered then that Rahere had been a courtier, and was once famed for his wit and jokes in the royal circle, and methought the miracle might perhaps be explained on natural grounds.

A.D. 1250.—*Our tiger Archbishop.*—Again the vision changes, and I see myself as an apprentice standing in the Hospital gate, for I had heard that Boniface, the Archbishop of Canterbury, was coming to visit our Prior at the church. He speaks no English, and his attendants are all foreigners, so I took a stone and threw it, hitting his servant full in the face. I saw the Archbishop turn in a fury as I shouted 'Truant', but he passed on and entered the church and I followed to see what would happen.

The Canons were in their Stalls, and a service was about to begin. I saw the Archbishop rush into the Choir shouting loudly and ordering them to go to the Chapter House. The Sub-Prior said something which I could not hear, and the Archbishop felled him with a single blow of his fist, for he was a stout and handsome man. He beat him unmercifully, and then ensued such a scene as I hope never again to see in a church. We tore the Archbishop's vestments, and, behold, he was fully clad in armour; but we drove him out by the side of the City wall, and made him take boat at Blackfriars, and so were rid of a very tyrant.

A.D. 1305.—*Sir William Wallace.*—Well do I remember that eve of St. Bartholomew when William Wallace had come before the judges in our new hall at Westminster, for it was the first time that I had seen the horrid doom of one whom they called a traitor. I, for my part, had always looked upon him as a true patriot, for never had I heard any one say that he had sworn fealty to our King Edward. But they must have settled his doom beforehand, for preparations had been made at our gallows, though some said he would be executed at Tyburn, but they are wrong, for I saw him dragged at a horse's tail from Aldgate through the City and past our Hospital. I thought at the time that it was a cruel death, but I knew that God was merciful to him, for they had not yet learned to use that ox-hide upon which other traitors were carried to the gallows, and I saw as he passed me that the bumping over the rough paving of the streets had wellnigh shaken the life out of him, strong man as he was.

At the Elms I heard the herald read the warrant that 'for your robberies, homicides, and felonies in England and Scotland you shall be hanged and drawn and as an outlaw beheaded. And afterwards, for your burning churches and relics, your heart, liver, lungs, and entrails, from which your wicked thoughts came, shall be burned, and finally, because your sedition, depredations, fires, and homicides were not only against the King but against the people of England and Scotland, your head shall be placed on London Bridge in sight both of land and water travellers, and your quarters hung on the gibbets at Newcastle, Berwick, Stirling, and Perth, to the terror of all who pass by.'

A.D. 1381.—*Wat Tyler.*—But perhaps the recollection which comes clearest to my mind was that June day when I, a shaveling—for I had recently taken minor orders, and had now a small tonsure upon my head—was working in that grand old hall where most of our patients lay. Word was brought that the crowd were coming to Smithfield, led by one whom they called Wat the Tyler. I ran to the gate to see those of whom I had heard so much, and, behold, just as I got there, the King with his retinue and the Mayor came riding down Long Lane, and stopped just opposite to where I was standing. Wat and his followers were between Hosier Lane and St. Sepulchre's. The march had been long and dusty, and I heard Wat call for water, which I remember that he drank filthily, gargling his throat with a horrid noise and spitting nearly over the

King, whom he shook by the hand and called Richard. Then he shouted for a mug of beer, and as he shouted I heard the Constable of Rochester say that he knew Wat for the biggest rogue unhanged in Kent, and that made Wat furious and he would have killed him in the King's presence. Our Mayor stopped him as he drew his sword with a sounding blow on the head, whereupon Wat furiously struck the Mayor with his dagger, but hurt him not by reason he was well armed. Our Mayor, having received his stroke, drew his blade and grievously wounded Wat in the neck, and withal gave him a great blow on his head. In the which conflict an esquire of the King's house, called John Cavendish, drew his sword and wounded Wat twice or thrice even to the death, and Wat, spurring his horse, cried to the commons to avenge him; the horse bare him about eighty feet from the place, and there he fell down half dead just at my feet. By and by they which attended on the King environed him about so as he was not seen of his company, and many of them thrust him in divers places of his body. I, seeing this, dragged him in through the gate of the Hospital and shouted to have it closed. The King, I saw, turned to the crowd and was speaking to them, and the Mayor was galloping back through Long Lane to the Guildhall. But I had no time to attend to such things. Wat was stunned and bleeding, so four of us carried him to the master's lodging and staunched his wounds. Half an hour passed and we heard the Mayor thundering at the gate demanding admission for himself and his brethren the Aldermen; they rushed in, dragged Wat out, and without more ado chopped off his head just in that space which still remains vacant between the porter's lodge and the Hospital chapel. Many have told me that Walworth, our Mayor, was knighted, and that the King added a dagger to the arms of the City in memory of this day. But I know this to be untrue, for our City arms carried the sword of St. Paul for many a long day before his mayoralty, though Walworth's dagger is still preserved at the Fishmongers' Hall.

But all my memories of Smithfield are not so sombre, for have I not often seen it filled with youth and beauty and nobles of England and many other countries of Christendom.

A.D. 1362.—*Jousts.*—Five days in one May did I not see jousts held, the King and the Queen being themselves there, and nearly all the chivalry of England and of France, of Spain and Cyprus and Armenia holding their own against all pagan comers? Then, again, did I not see Dame Alice Perrers (the King's concubine) as Lady of the Sun riding through Cheap accompanied by many lords and ladies? Every lady leading a lord by horse-bridle till they came into Smithfield, and there began that great joust which lasted no less than seven days.

And once again, was the like riding from the Tower to Westminster, but now every lord led a lady's horse-bridle, and on the morrow began the joust in Smithfield which lasted two days, and there bare them well Henry of Derby, the Duke of Lancaster's son, the Lord Beaumont, Sir Simon Burley, and Sir Paris Courtney. And yet once again in the fourteenth year, when Richard II was King, royal jousts and tournaments were proclaimed to be done in Smithfield, to begin on Sunday next after the Feast of St. Michael.

Many strangers came forth of other countries, namely, Valarin, Earl of St. Paul, that had married our King's sister, the Lady Maud Courtney, and William, the young Earl of Ostervant, son to Albert of Baviere, Earl of Holland and Henault. On that day there issued forth of the Tower, about the third hour, sixty coursers apparelled for the joust, and upon every one an esquire of honour riding a soft pace; then came forth sixty ladies of honour mounted upon palfreys riding on the one side richly apparelled, and every lady led a knight with a chain of gold. These knights being of the King's party had their harness and apparel garnished with white harts and crowns of gold about the harts' necks, for was not the white hind his mother's badge, who was known to us as the Fair Maid of Kent.

And so they came riding through the streets of London to Smithfield with a great number of trumpets and other instruments of music before them. The King and Queen came from the Bishop's Palace of London with many great estates and were placed in chambers to see the jousts. And the ladies that led the knights were taken down from their palfreys and went up to chambers prepared for them.

Then alighted the squires of honour from their coursers and the knights in good order mounted upon them, and after their helmets were set upon their heads, and being ready in all points, a proclamation made by the heralds, the jousts began and many commendable courses were run, to the great delight of us standing by to see them.

A.D. 1393.—Many accidents came to us of these jousts, but none so fell as when those lords of Scotland came into England to get worship by force of arms. On that day the Earl of Mar challenged the Earl of Nottingham to joust with him, and so they rode together certain courses, but not the full challenge, for the Earl of Mar was overborne horse and man and two of his ribs were broken with the fall. And so coming to the Hospital we bound up his hurt and set him on his way towards Scotland. But letters came to us afterwards, saying that he died of his hurt, so we had done well had we kept him with us.

For my part what I saw was mostly done in fair fight, but foul deeds were sometimes done in anger.

A.D. 1442.—One winter's day at the end of January a challenge was done in Smithfield within the lists before our gracious King, Harry VI, there being Sir Philip la Beaufe, of Aragon, Knight, the other an Esquire of the King's house, called John Ansley.

They came to the field all armed, the Knight with his sword drawn, the Esquire with his spear, which spear he cast against the Knight, but the Knight avoided it with his sword, and cast it to the ground.

Then the Esquire took his axe and smote many blows on the Knight and made him let fall his axe and brake up his visor three times, and would have smote him on the face with his dagger for to have slain him, but that the King cried 'Hold', and so they were departed.

A.D. 1446.—And yet other times have I seen the wager of battle essayed in front of our gate, nor did he who was in the right always win, for I mind me of the time when John David appeached his master, Will Catur, of treason, and a day was assigned to them to fight in Smithfield.

The master, being all well beloved and known to every one of us, was so cherished by his friends and plyed with wine that, being therewith overcome, he was unluckily slain by his servant.

But that false servant (for he falsely accused his master) lived not long unpunished, for I with many others followed to see him hanged at Tyburn, for a felony by him committed.

Let such false accusers note this for example, and look for no better end without speedy repentance.

A.D. 1467.—And yet once again there were great days for us when the Bastard of Burgoyne challenged the Lord Scales, brother to the Queen of our noble King Edward IV to fight with him both on horseback and on foot.

The King therefore caused lists to be prepared in Smithfield, the length of 120 tailors' yards and 10 feet, and in breadth 80 yards and 20 feet, double-barred were they, 5 feet between the bars, the timber work whereof cost two hundred marks, besides the fair and costly galleries prepared for the ladies and others; at the which martial enterprise the King and nobility were present.

The first day they ran together with spears, and departed with equal honour. The next day they tourneyed on horseback, the Lord Scales' horse having on his chafron a long spear pike of steel, and when the two champions coped together the same horse thrust his pike into the nostrils of the Bastard's horse. So that for very pain he mounted so high that he fell on the one side with his master, and the Lord Scales rode about him with his sword drawn till the King commanded the Marshal to help up the Bastard, who said: 'I cannot hold me by the clouds, for though my horse fail me I will not fail an encounter companion'; but the King would not suffer them to do any more that day.

The next morning they came into the lists on foot with two pole-axes and fought valiantly, but at the last the point of the pole-axe of the Lord Scales entered into the side of the Bastard's helm and by force made him place him on his knees, but the King cast down his warder and the Marshal severed them. The Bastard required that he might perform his enterprise, but the King gave judgement and the Bastard relinquished his challenge.

And I remember well the courtly ending of these joyous days in early spring. How, when the joust was over there came forth a lady chosen by all the other ladies and gentlewomen and he would give a diamond to the best jouster, saying to him: 'Sir, these ladies and gentlewomen thank you for your desport and your great labour that you have this day undergone in their presence, and the said ladies and gentlewomen sayen that ye have best jousted this day, therefore the said ladies and gentlewomen give you this diamond and send you much worship and joy of your lady.' Thus was done also with the ruby and the sapphire unto the other two next best jousters. Then the Herald of Arms would stand above all on high and cry with a loud voice: 'John hath well jousted, Richard hath jousted better, and Thomas hath jousted best of all.' Then he that had the diamond took a lady by the hand and began to dance, and when the ladies had danced as long as it pleased them, then spices and wine and drink and afterwards an interval.

A.D.1539.—These joyous days soon passed. The clouds came thick upon us and we were reduced to the lowest ebb of poverty and distress. Our Hospital was separated from the Priory, with which we had always been associated in so friendly and helpful a spirit. Our revenues were taken by the King and we were left with but two or three beds. Our Mayor and the Recorder petitioned that the Hospital

might be given to the City, but, alas, for five years no
answer was received and we lived as best we might and in
the most dire despair. At last we were granted a new corporation. A priest for master and four chaplains, to whom
were given the site, the buildings, and church of the old
Hospital of St. Bartholomew's the Less, which we had
loved so well and where we had worked so hard, with all
its goods, jewels, and chattels, but without any other endowment. It soon appeared how bad was the management
of the master and chaplains, for they sold our property,
destroyed our library, and removed so much of the furniture as hardly to leave sufficient accommodation for
three poor harlots great with child. Then it was that the
great City, of which we are proud to be members, came
to the rescue.

A.D. 1547.—The Hospital and its endowments were
vested in the Lord Mayor, Commonalty, and Citizens of
London, because 'of the miserable state of the poore, aged,
sick, low, and impotent people, as well men as women,
lying and going about begging in the common streets of
the said City and the suburbs of the same to the great paine
and sorrowe of the same poore, aged, sicke, and impotent
people, and to the great infection, hurt, and annoyance of
His Grace's loving subjects, which must of necessity goe
and passe by the same poore, sick, low, and impotent
people, being infected with divers great and horrible sick-
nesses and diseases,' so ran the Letters Patent, and with
them came an endowment of 500 marks per annum on
condition that the citizens should rise annually a like sum
to secure a total revenue of 1,000 marks, or £666 13s. 4d.
This they did gladly and quickly, and we started work
again with 100 beds all allotted to surgical cases. I
remember that we had three surgeons to attend upon
them, but there was no physician for the next fourteen
years, and then he had but eight out-patients under his
care.

A.D. 1555.—But if things went badly within the Hospital, they were much worse outside, and I look back with

horror, and even with terror, to that stake set up between
our gate and the gate of the Priory Church, where so many
martyrs testified to the constancy of their faith. Of those
scenes I often dream and wake shuddering to find that in
our spacious times they can never be repeated. The first
I saw was that of our meek pastor of St. Sepulchre's,
Master John Rogers, of the University of Cambridge,
Artium Magister, the friend of Tindall and Miles Cover-
dale. Him the Bishop of London had given a Prebend in
Paul's, and the Dean and Chapter there chose him to read
the divinity lecture, in which place he remained till the
time of Queene Marie. In the morning of the fourth of
February, Anno 1555,—I tell the story as it is told by my
colleague, Dr. Timothy Bright, who dwells with me in the
Hospital, and has invented that short method of writing
which is called stenography; he is a better story-teller
than I am,—'Being munday hee was warned sodainely by
the keeper's wife of Newgate to prepare himself to the fire
(who, then being sounde asleep, scarce with much shog-
ging could bee awaked), and being bid to make haste;
then, said hee, "If it be so, I shall not need to tye my
poyntes." And so was he had downe first to Boner to be
disgraded; that done, he craved Bishop Boner that he
might talke a few wordes with his wife before his death.
This Boner would not suffer: So was hee brought into
Smithfield by Master Chester and Master Woodrofe, then
Sheriffes of London, and cheerefully ended his martirdome
in the fire; washing his handes in the flame as he was in
burning. His pardon was brought him at the stake if he
would have recanted; but hee utterly refused it, and was
the first martyr of Queene Marie's daies.'

The fires thus lighted seemed unquenchable, for, again
in May, on the 30th day, there suffered together in Smithfield John Cardmaker, the preacher, Prebendary of the
Church of Wells, and John Warne, upholsterer, of the
parish of St. John in Walbrook, who was of the age of 29
years. And when they came to the stake, first the Sheriffs
called Cardmaker aside and talked with him secretly so

long that in the meantime Warne had made his prayers, was chained to the stake, and had wood and reed set about him, so that nothing wanted but the string, but still abode Cardmaker talking with the sheriffs. And we onlookers, having heard before that Cardmaker would recant and beholding this manner of doing, were in a marvellous dump and sadness, thinking, indeed, that Cardmaker should now recant at the burning of Warne. At length Cardmaker departed from the sheriffs, and came towards the stake (and in his garments as he was) kneeled down, and made a long prayer in silence to himself; yet the people confirmed themselves in their fantasie of recanting seeing him in his garments, praying secretly, and no semblance of any burning.

His prayers being ended, he rose up, put off his clothes unto his shirt, went with bold courage to the stake and kissed it sweetly: he took Warne by the hand and comforted him heartily, and so gave himself also to be bound to the stake most gladly. We, seeing this so suddenly done contrary to our fearful expectation as men delivered out of a great doubt, cried out for joy (with so great a shout as hath not lightly been heard a greater), saying: 'God be praised, the Lord strengthen thee, Cardmaker, the Lord Jesus receive thy spirit.' And this continued while the executioner put fire to them, and they both passed through the fire to the blessed rest and peace among God's holy saints and martyrs.

And the fires being lighted by that most wicked Bishop, he was no longer content to burn one at a time, but sent whole companies—men and women alike—and together to undergo that most cruel fate. And most I pitied that worthy martyr and servant of God, Master John Bradford, so learned and godly a man that he had the accounts of John Harrington when he was the King's Treasurer at Bulougne, and had been given a Fellowship at Pembroke College in the University of Cambridge. Him with John Leafe, an apprentice to Humphrey Gawdy, the tallow-chandler—our neighbour in the parish of Christ's Church

—they brought to Smithfield in the month of July 1555. And first, when they came to the stake to be burned, Master Bradford lying prostrate on one side of the stake and the young man, John Leafe, on the other side, they flat on their faces praying to themselves the space of a minute of an hour. Then one of the sheriffs said to Master Bradford: 'Arise, and make an end; for the press of people is great.'

And at that word they both stood upon their feet, and then Master Bradford took a faggot in his hand and kissed it, and so likewise the stake. And when he had so done, he desired of the sheriff that his servant might have his raiment. 'For,' said he, 'I have nothing else to give him; and, besides that, he is a poor man.' And the sheriff said he should have it. And so forthwith Master Bradford did put off his raiment and went to the stake, and, holding up his hands and casting his countenance to heaven, he said thus: 'O, England, England, repent thee of thy sins, beware of idolatory, beware of false anti-christs, take heed they do not deceive you.' And, as he was speaking these words, the sheriff bade tie his hands, if he would not be quiet. 'O, Master Sheriff,' said Master Bradford, 'I am quiet; God forgive you this, Master Sheriff.' And one of the officers which made the fire, hearing Master Bradford so speaking to the sheriff, said: 'If you have no better learning, but that you are but a fool, and were best hold your peace.' To the which words Master Bradford gave no answer; but asked all the world forgiveness, and forgave all the world, and prayed the people to pray for him, and turned his head to the young man that suffered with him, and said: 'Be of good comfort, brother, for we shall have a merry supper with the Lord this night.' And so spake no more words that any man did hear; but, embracing the reeds, said thus: 'Strait is the way and narrow is the gate that leadeth to eternal salvation, and few there be that find it.'

And thus they ended their mortal lives most like two lambs, without any alteration of their countenance, being void of all fear, and hoping to obtain the price of the game that they had long run at.

I mind me that it was reported that the surly Sheriff Woodroffe soon came by his own. He it was that when Master Rogers was in the cart going towards Smithfield, and on the way his wife and children would have spoken with him—eleven children there were and one sucking at her breast—the people making a lane for them to come to him, that most wicked sheriff, I say, bade the carman's head should be broken for staying his cart; nor would he suffer Master Bradford to make an end of his prayers. But what happened? He was not come out of his office the space of a year but he was stricken by the sudden hand of God, the one half of his body in such sort that he lay benumbed and bedridden, not able to move himself, but as he was lifted of other, and so continued in that infirmity the space of eight or ten years till his dying day.

A.D. 1565.—Brighter times came when our good Elizabeth was Queen. We had pageants again, the Hospital throve and did much good. But our surgeons were rough, and I often had much ado to keep the peace between them. Master Clowes in particular—good surgeon as he was—had a very rough side to his tongue, and I have known him come to our Company's Hall in Monkwell Street—where it still stands—and not only miscall those who were unfriendly to him but actually stand in our midst and with scoffing words and jests attack each of us in turn sitting there in our fur gowns, a very reverend assembly, calling us great bugbears, stinging gnats, venomous wasps, and counterfeit crocodiles. Indeed, no longer ago than 1577, on the 25th of March, which some used to call our Lady's Day, he and George Baker, contrary to order and to the good and wholesome rules of our house, misused each other and fought together with their fists in the fields, though both were surgeons to the Queen's Highness. Which I hearing of as Master of the Company, or as you would now say President of the College of Surgeons, did cause them to be brought before me, but I pardoned them this their great offence in hope of amendment and wishing that they might be and continue loving brothers together.

But if our surgeons were rough in their manners they were absolutely honest of purpose and sought in all things to make us from a trade into a profession and to scotch quackery. Have I not heard Master Gale say, 'I did see in the two Hospitals of London called St. Thomas's and St. Bartholomew's no longer ago than in the year 1562 to the number of 300 and odd poor people that were diseased of sore legs, sore arms, feet and hands with other parts of the body so sore infected that 120 of them could never be recovered without loss of a leg or an arm, a foot or a hand, fingers or toes, or else their limbs crooked so that they were either maimed or undone for ever. All these were brought to this mischief by witches, by women, by counterfeit javils, that took upon them to use the art, not only robbing them of their money but of their limbs and perpetual health. And I with certain others diligently examining these poor people, how they came by these grievous hurts and who were their chirurgeons that looked upon them and they confessed that they were either witches, which did promise by charms to make them whole, or else some women which would make them whole with herbs and such like things, or else some vagabond javil which runneth from one county to another promising them health only to deceive them of their money. This fault and crime of the undoing of this people were laid unto the chirurgeons—I will not say by part of those who were masters of the same hospitals—but it was said that carpenters, women, weavers, cobblers, and tinkers did cure more poeple than the chirurgeons. But what manner of cures they did I have said, such cures as all the world may wonder at, such cures as maketh the devil in hell to dance for joy to see the poor members of Jesus Christ so miserably tormented.'

At this time too, I remember we got our lay sisters and

nurses under a matron instead of those meek sisters who used to be directed by the Mother Superior as to what they might and might not do. The work of nursing was a new thing to our lay sisters, and it was necessary to keep them a little more strictly than is now the case. They came not out of the ward every night after the hour of seven o'clock in the winter and after nine o'clock in the summer except some great and special cause befell—as the present danger of death or the needful succour of some poor person. They washed and purged the unclean clothes of the patients and other things and, in their spare time when they were not occupied about the poor, they were set to spinning the flax provided by the governors of the Hospital, or to such other manner of work that may avoid idleness and be profitable to the poor of the house. Knitting and crochet work have now replaced the more useful spinning. Above all things they were told to abhor and detest scolding as a most pestilent and filthy vice. Money perhaps went farther in those days but the sisters were no more overpaid then than they are now.

A.D. 1747.—They acquired in time a right to certain small perquisites of which our governors found it hard to deprive them. Thus the matron had an old and accustomed fee of one shilling for the use of a pall to cover the coffin of every patient buried from the Hospital, whilst the sisters did demand and take of the patients and their friends one shilling for earthenware and other necessaries and the nurses likewise sixpence. The nursing staff in the wards devoted to the reception of patients to be cut for the stone had a special allowance, the sister half a crown for each operation and the nurse or helper there one shilling. In the two fluxing wards or foul wards for the reception of the class of patients which is now admitted to the 'Shelter' in Golden Lane the Sister received six shillings and sixpence for every patient who was salivated, but in return she had to provide flannels and other necessaries and pay her nurses one shilling.

A.D. 1821.—There were 24 wards in the Hospital

nursed by a staff of 24 sisters, 48 nurses and 26 night nurses. The salaries of the sisters ranged from fourteen to twenty-seven shillings a week, whilst the nurses received seven shillings a week, and the night nurses ninepence a night. It is not surprising if the women who were tempted by these wages should sometimes develop into the proto-types of Mrs. Gamp, Betsy Prig, and Mrs. Harris. They were, however, the exceptions, for I know that a searching investigation was made into every department of the Hos-pital, and it was reported that 'there was no complaint of any misbehaviour of the sisters or nurses of this Hospital, and the committee is of opinion that the sisters and nurses have done their duty'. The predecessors of our present magnificent nursing staff, uneducated as they were, could still have taught us much that is valuable in the art of practical nursing and the handling of sick men and women. Indeed, I often think as I watch our present sisters and nurses going so deftly about their work that much of what they do is based upon the tradition handed down from these women and is the accumulated experience of nearly 400 years.

Our Hospital increased steadily in reputation under the guidance and fostering care of the great business men of the City, who have never spared time or money in making it second to none. The medical and surgical staff became known throughout the world. William Harvey shed the lustre of his name over us; Percivall Pott, famous amongst the great teaching surgeons of Europe, instructed John Hunter and was thus associated with the first great revolu-tion in modern surgery. But ever as we became a great school of medicine and surgery we became more and more self-centred and our immediate surroundings became more squalid.

The butchers, as always from the foundation of the Hospital, were our immediate neighbours, and in time Smithfield, that open place for jousts and meetings and burnings, was occupied by live cattle, an unclean place, noisy with shouts of drovers, the lowing of cattle and the bleating of sheep. Dangerous at all times and actually impassable at Bartholomewtide when the fair was held, it is no wonder, therefore, if it was rarely visited except by those whose business or needs brought them to the Hospital. Bartholomew Fair was abolished [A.D. 1855] before my time, but I well remember as a small boy the perilous passage of the Smithfield cattle market when we went to tea with my father's friend who afterwards became my own Master—[Sir] William Savory—then living in Charterhouse Square.

And thus my visions end, and I come into the recollections of my own life. How, when I came to this school fresh from Oxford just forty years ago, I found myself amongst an indulgent body who at once appointed me a teacher, invited me to their Christmas dinner and told me that they had given me the opportunity of winning my spurs should I be so inclined. The whole staff of the Hospital then numbered twenty-eight. Doubtless they had their rivalries and little jealousies, but I was too young to be interested in them, and to me every one proved a good friend.

Gradually as I have watched it the school has grown, both as regards the numbers of the personnel and the buildings wherein they are housed. First, the anatomical rooms and these lecture theatres, then the library and museum block, afterwards the out-patient block with its magnificent accommodation for the special departments and the apothecary's shop; still more recently, and within the memory of many of you, the pathological block has been built.

I have to-night told you many visions of things past: there remains one of a thing to come. I have a vision of a time when the present nurses' home shall have been swept away and in its place there has arisen in Little Britain a fine building with a good lounge, a pleasant drawing-room, a well-equipped library, fine baths, plenty of hot and cold water, a separate little bedroom for each, a lift for tired nurses, and an infirmary on the topmost floor made as little like a hospital ward as possible. Such a building has been long overdue but it must come, for our present arrangements are disgraceful and are a standing reproach to the great city of which we have formed an integral part for nearly a thousand years.

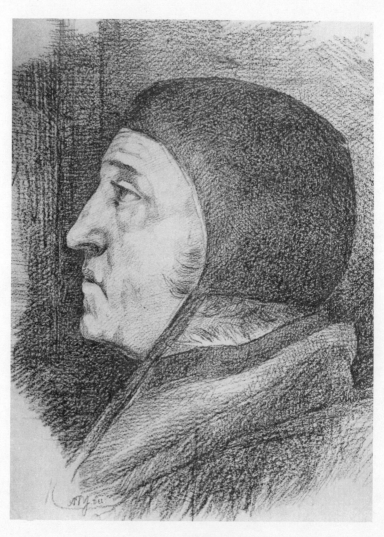

VIII. Thomas Vicary

IV

THE EDUCATION OF A SURGEON UNDER THOMAS VICARY [1]

Mr. President, Master of the Worshipful Company of Barbers, Ladies and Gentlemen,

It is a function of history to correct the errors into which we are betrayed by mere forgetfulness. Generation succeeds generation until we are apt to think that our fathers were less skilful, or were less alive to their surroundings, than ourselves. I have chosen 'The Education of a Surgeon under Thomas Vicary' as the subject of the second historical lecture at this College to combat this thought. We owe the lectureship itself to the goodwill of the Barbers' Company, once our competitors, then our allies, and now our very good friends.

I do not know who decided that the historical lecture should be called The Vicary Lecture, but it was a wise choice, because Vicary, in virtue of his age and position, was foremost amongst that band of pioneer surgeons who, in the reign of Henry VIII, desired to see their calling advanced from a trade to a profession. Their work was not crowned with complete success, but to their labours the surgeon owes in part his present social position in this country.

During the whole of Vicary's life medical education was undergoing changes analogous to those now occurring to which the term reconstruction is applied, and for similar reasons. In many ways the fifteenth century resembled the present time. The Wars of the Roses practically destroyed the old nobility, for attainders and executions altered the ownership of land throughout the country, whilst crushing taxation and the general insecurity hampered trade and materially reduced the wealth of the citizens. It was impossible to do business in London when such thousands

[1] The Second Vicary Historical Lecture, delivered at the Royal College of Surgeons of England on 11 November 1920.

of troops were quartered in the neighbourhood or were actually billeted on the citizens, that 'the Mayor rode daily about the city and the circuit of Holborn and Fleet Street, accompanied by five thousand craftsmen or thereabout, well and sensibly arrayed', to maintain order and prevent looting. From 1450 to 1485 English surgery suffered in the general dislocation of affairs, and no advance was made. The death of Richard on the field of Bosworth, the succession of the Earl of Richmond as King Henry VII, and his marriage with the Lady Elizabeth of York a year later, gave peace to the realm. Then, as now, the surviving generation turned for a time to religion rather than to secular matters. There was a period of church building, church restoration, and the foundation of chantries, in the same spirit which is now leading to the erection of crosses and memorials in churches and villages throughout the country.

Surgeons undoubtedly felt the lean time. London had always supported a small body of surgeons independently of the barbers. These men performed the same duties as ourselves. They undertook the more difficult operations, were called in consultation to obscure cases, and generally considered themselves to be on a higher plane than the barbers. Their practice, however, was somewhat different from our own, for they were itinerant; that is to say, when they undertook an operation they stayed with the patient until he was cured, and they seem for the most part to have been attached to the persons of the higher nobility. They charged large fees, because they could only undertake a single case at a time, and might be months before they were released from their attendance. When their lord was called out in the course of war they accompanied him, and thus saw much military service.

During the Hundred Years' War with France, and during the Lancastrian and Yorkist wars in England, surgeons no doubt made a good but precarious living. With the reign of Henry VII began a long and settled peace, which obliged the surgeons to reconsider their position.

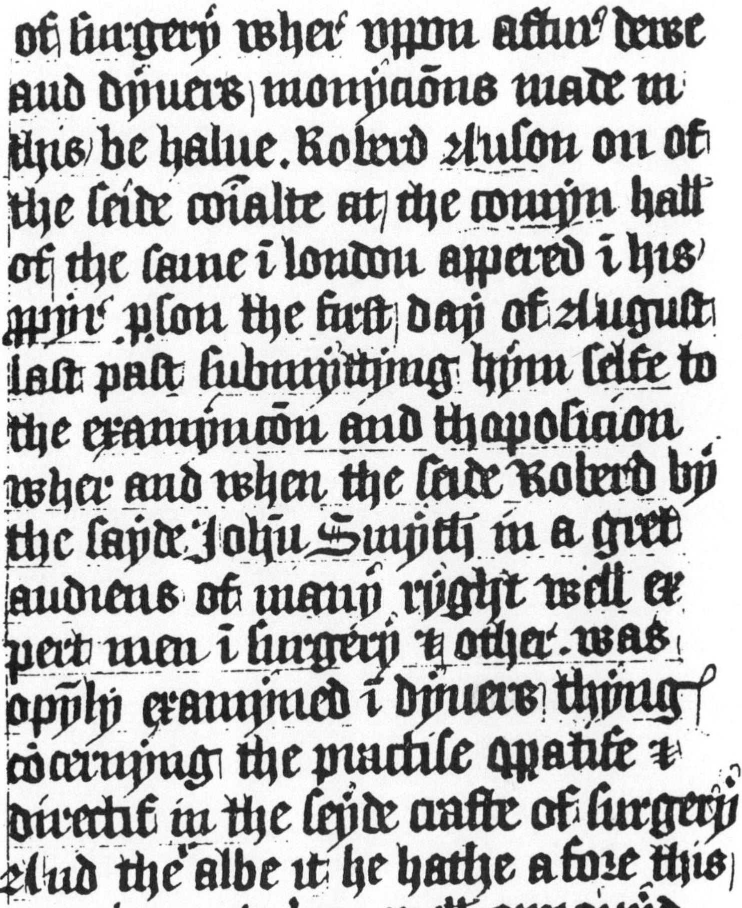

of surgery wher vpou aftur dere
and diuers monyaons made in
this be halue. Robert Ahufon on of
the seide coialte at the counyn hall
of the same i loudou appered i his
apur plou the first day of August
last past submyttyng hym selfe to
the examynaon and thapolicaon
wher and when the seide Robert by
the sayde John Smyth in a gret
audiens of many ryght well ex
pert men i surgery & other was
oppyly examyned i diuers thyng
coernyng the practise qpatife &
directif in the seide crafte of surgery
Alud the albe it he hathe a fore this
many tymys ben well approuyd
yet now he is newly haleyd be
the seide doctour and felyship and

Fig. 1. A page of Robert Anson's 'Licence', 1497.

The old and wealthy nobility had been destroyed, and they were compelled to turn their attention to the newly formed middle class as it was represented by the citizens. For this purpose they entered into an agreement with the Barbers' Company in 1493—the eighth year of the reign of King Henry VII—and in this agreement there is a special clause dealing with the examination of surgeons. The licence of Robert Anson is still in existence, and is dated 8 August 1497. It states (Fig. 1) that he was examined by 'Master John Smyth Doctour in Phesik, Instructour & examenar of the feliship . . . in a gret audiens of many ryght well expert men in surgery & others'. Even at this early period, therefore, a special examiner had been appointed to conduct a public examination in surgery. Examination of surgeons, however, was no new thing in the fraternity of surgeons, for it was proposed in the abortive scheme of 1423, which aimed at uniting surgeons and physicians, as well as in the ordinances of 1435, which regulated the gild for many years. It seems, therefore, that the fraternity of surgeons dealt more with the practising surgeon than with the apprentice. It desired to ascertain what a man knew rather than how he had gained his knowledge—in other words, whether he was a reasonably safe practitioner—before he was allowed to practise in the area over which it ruled.

The Company of Barbers, on the other hand, dealt more with the apprentice, for the London gilds, even before they became chartered companies, had always taken an interest in the education of their members, and had endeavoured by a system of apprenticeship to provide satisfactory craftsmen. Provision for teaching and evidence of professional knowledge, both before and after admission to the freedom, had always been made by the Company of Barbers in London. Elsewhere in England the custom varied. Education was insisted upon when the gild consisted of barbers united with surgeons, as at Norwich, Bristol, and Edinburgh, and when the barber surgeons and physicians worked together, as at York. There was no such demand when the mystery of surgery and barbery was a mere trade, as at Oxford where it was associated with the waferers and makers of singing-bread, or at Newcastle where it was combined with the wax chandlers; but even in these gilds there is evidence that a minimum of professional knowledge was demanded of applicants for the freedom on the surgical side.

The Company of Barbers was formally united with the fraternity of surgeons by the Act of Parliament which received the royal assent on 25 July 1540. Vicary was elected Master of the United Company at the end of John Pen's term of office, and acted in this capacity from September 1541 to the usual date of election in September 1542. The Union is commemorated in the well-known picture by Holbein, which has fortunately preserved for us portraits of the chief actors.

The United Company immediately proceeded to consider the state of the profession, and found that there were two problems to be solved—the one internal, the other external. The internal problem was itself twofold, and concerned the better education of the profession; the external problem was the better education of the public to appreciate the proper treatment of surgical disease. The internal problem had already been partially answered, and by combining the customs of the barbers in regard to their apprentices with the regulations of the surgeons in dealing with those licensed to practise, a fairly adequate system of surgical education was evolved. No complete medical education, however, could be given so long as the surgeon was subordinate to the physician. This subordination remained for many years, and the second part of the internal problem could not therefore be solved.

Apprentices

Very few lists of apprentices to barbers have been published, but it is clear from a study of such of them as exist that the boys were drawn from the lower classes, as the occupation of the father is frequently given as a 'labourer'.

There is no evidence to show that the surgeons' apprentices came from a much higher class. A successful surgeon sometimes took his son as apprentice, as in the case of Thomas Gale and his son William Gale; William Clowes and William Clowes junior. The Arris family, to whom we owe the Arris bequest, lasted through three generations. Jasper Arris was a barber as well as a surgeon; Mr. Alderman Edward Arris, his son, was a surgeon and did no barbery; his eldest son Robert followed the grandfather and father as a surgeon, whilst the second son became a doctor of medicine, a Fellow of the Royal College of Physicians, and a Member of Parliament; but then Mr. Alderman Arris was the father of twenty-three children, so he could well afford to give two to the profession of medicine. As a rule, however, the surgical apprentices were drawn from the humblest ranks, and owed any position to which they attained entirely to their own talents. Thomas Gale says in *An Institution of a Chirurgion*, 'Few that have wel brought up their sonne will put him to the arte, bicause it is accounted so beggerly and vile'. Similar testimony is borne by Sir Humphrey Gilbert as late as 1570 in that curious tract[1] which foreshadows the present University of London. Writing to Queen Elizabeth about 'The erection of an Achademy in London for educacion of her Maiestes Wardes and others the youth of nobility and gentlemen', he says, 'The Phisition shall practize to reade Chirurgerie, becawse thorough wante of learning therein we haue verie few good Chirurgions yf any at all. By reason that Chirurgerie is not now to be learned in any other place than in a Barbors shoppe.' Here, too, is the story of Mr. Thomas Hollier, who was Master of the Company in 1673. He was surgeon at St. Thomas's Hospital, and cut Mr. Pepys for the stone. Indeed, he was so lucky a lithotomist that he cut no less than thirty persons for the stone in one year without a single death. Mr. Pepys was fortunate in coming under him at this time, for his instruments afterwards became septic, and

---

[1] Brit. Mus. Lansdowne MS. 98.

many of the rest of his patients died. I have only lately discovered this contemporary story of his rise. It is told by the Rev. John Ward, Vicar of Stratford-on-Avon, whose commonplace books I am slowly transcribing. He says:

'Mr. Holliard, the great Chirurgion in Warwick Lane, was a poor boy in Coventrie, his father was a cobbler, or at best but a poor shoemaker in Coventrie, and one Dr. Mathias (I think he was Queen Anne's Dr.)[1] about that time frequently coming to Combe Abbey and using Coventrie much spoke to Abraham Ashby an Apotecarie there to help him to a boy to dresse his horses and ride along with him; and Mr. Ashby spoke to Mr. White the School-master who told him he could help him to one, but his father was a foxing, drunken fellow, and the boy that he helped him to was this Mr. Holliard, the Chirurgion; and afterwards Dr. Mathias died and Mr. Holliard got himself a little money and put himself prentice to Mr. Mullins his father of Shooe Lane and now he comes to what he is.'

The Mullins, father and son, were surgeons to St. Thomas's Hospital and were also eminent lithotomists.

Apprenticeship

The first step in the life of an apprentice was the sealing of his indentures and their enrolment at Barber Surgeons' Hall in Monkwell Street and at the Guildhall. For this purpose the boy had to appear before the Court or governing body of the Company to show that he was not deformed or suffering from any chronic disease, for it was a tradition handed down from the earliest days of the gilds that the apprentices should be healthy, and free from blemish or from spot. The opportunity was taken to ascertain that he could at least read and write, and it was hoped that he might have some knowledge of Latin. Latin was taught at this time as a living language in the grammar schools throughout the country, so that a smattering of it might reasonably be expected, and a boy who knew no Latin must have been very badly educated indeed. Ac-

[1] Anne of Denmark, married to James the First of England and Sixth of Scotland.

cordingly, in 1556, an ordinance was issued that no surgeon should take as an apprentice 'but that he can skill of the Latten tongue and understand of the same', under penalty of a fine of forty shillings. It seems, however, to have been impossible to maintain the rule, for it was rescinded the following year, and in 1563 Thomas Gale, dedicating his *Enchiridion of Surgery* 'unto the young men of his Companie, students in the noble art of Chirurgerie', says that he wrote in English 'because the books you should use are written in a tongue which the most of you understand not'.

At this time the boy was about 14 years old, and if he passed before the Court and his indentures were registered his period of servitude began. It usually lasted for seven years, in which case he would be made free of the Company and could practise on his own account by the time he was twenty-one. The period of apprenticeship, however, might be prolonged for eight or even nine years. The fee paid to the master was at first merely sufficient to cover the expense of clothing and feeding the boy in return for his services. In later years—when apprenticeship carried with it valuable reversions, as in the case of those who were bound to hospital surgeons like Hunter, Abernethy, and Astley Cooper—fees of £500 to £1,000, which were then thought to be enormous, were readily paid.

Each master was allowed to take three or four apprentices according to his position in the Company, and if he died the apprentice was 'turned over' to another master or to the widow for the remainder of the term for which he was bound.

The average number of apprentices presented annually at the Barbers' Hall was 150, so that if the indentures lasted seven years there were always about 1,000 apprentices belonging to the Barber Surgeons alone, and the other City companies had them in proportion. They were all strong and lusty young men, and a tight hand had to be kept over them. The Barber Surgeons fortunately had ample disciplinary powers over their apprentices, for they

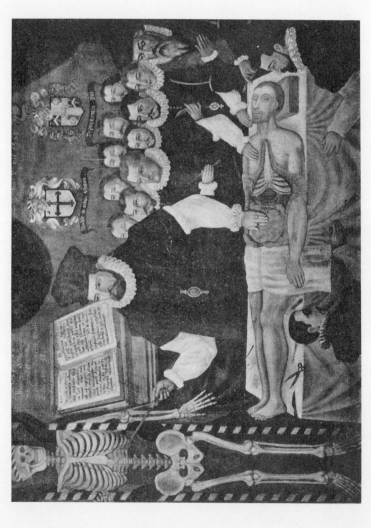

IX. John Banester delivering the Visceral Lecture at the Barber-Surgeons' Hall, London, in 1581

By permission of the Wellcome Historical Medical Museum

could whip or imprison them, or suit the penalty to the crime, as when they ordered a young dandy's head to be shaved when it was fashionable to wear the hair long.

Surgical Education

As soon as the United Company had obtained the Act of Parliament in 1540, arrangements were made to provide an improved system of surgical education. Some machinery already existed for the purpose, as the Gild of Surgeons had always taught both its members and apprentices by a system of lectures. Each member of the gild was pledged under a fine of twenty shillings, either to lecture himself or provide an efficient substitute. The lectures must have been oral and, so far as I know, there are no manuscripts or students' copies of them in existence at the present time. Morested, Bradwardyn, Ferris, Keble, and other great surgeons of the fifteenth and sixteenth centuries are thus nothing more than names to us, for they have left no literary remains, though we know from the evidence of their pupils that they exercised a great influence in promoting a higher standard of surgical teaching and ethics. It is probable that their lectures dealt largely with their own experience and with the remedies they found most serviceable.

Anatomy

Anatomy had always been taught, for it was the basis of surgery, but some far-seeing members of the gild got its teaching regularized by the introduction of the following clause in the Act of 1540:

'That the sayd maysters or gouernours of the mistery and comminaltie of barbours and surgeons of London, and their successours yerely for euer after their sa[i]d discrecions at their free liberte and pleasure shal and maie haue and take without contradiction foure persons condempned adiudged and put to deathe for feloni by the due order of the kynges lawe of thys realme for anatomies without any further sute or labour to be made to the kyngs highnes his heyres or successours for the same. And to make incision of the same deade bodies or otherwyse to order the same after their said discrecions at their pleasures for their further and better knowlage instruction insight learnyng and experience in the sayd scyence or facultie of surgery.'

A supply of bodies was thus insured and the Company at once elaborated a system for putting them to the best use. They appointed a lecturer with the title of Reader of Anatomy, and four stewards or, as they would now be called, demonstrators under him. The Reader of Anatomy seems at first to have held office for an indefinite period, but he was afterwards appointed for terms of three to five years. The stewards acted for four years; during the first two they learnt their duties, and during the last two they executed them under the direction of the Reader, and were called Masters of Anatomy. Unfortunately there are no extant records of the first few years of the Company's existence, so that it is impossible to discover who was appointed the first Reader of Anatomy. I believe, personally, that it was Master Vicary himself, and that he lectured on the old lines. My predecessors, the surgeons of St. Bartholomew's Hospital, published *The Englishemans Treasure. With the true Anatomye of Mans Body*, after his death. It is a worthless treatise on anatomy based upon the teaching of Lanfranc and Henri de Mondeville, but it shows that Vicary was looked upon as an anatomist by his contemporaries, and the edition of 1548 may have been the text from which he had lectured. Be this as it may, a vacancy for a Reader of Anatomy occurred about 1546, and the Company adopted the wise policy of choosing the best possible man for the post. They elected, no doubt by the advice of Vicary and on the recommendation of Dr. Butts, Dr. John Caius, a Cambridge graduate, aged 36. Caius had lately returned from Italy, where he had been a fellow lodger with Vesalius at Padua and an acquaintance of Realdus Columbus, the two great anatomists of their age. He was also a competent Greek scholar, and had made a special study of Galen, hunting through the great libraries of Italy for accurate texts. In 1544 he issued his edition of the *De Medendi Methodo* and other works of Galen which had not previously been published. No better choice could have been made by a young and virile society which included a large uncultured element amongst its members. Caius was a grave and learned man, a stickler for etiquette, and a bachelor. He lived in the immediate neighbourhood of the Barber Surgeons' Hall in Monkwell Street, for he had a house in St. Bartholomew's Hospital, and could thus devote sufficient time and energy to his work. He held office until 1563, and was succeeded by Dr. Cunningham. His long tenure of the lectureship left a permanent mark upon the teaching. The Reader of the Anatomy was ever afterwards a young university graduate. The post was well paid, and many of its holders subsequently achieved fame. The Anatomy of Realdus Columbus was long a recognized text-book, and some work of Galen, either the *De Methodo* or the *Therapeuticon*, with a slight knowledge of Hippocrates, was required of every apprentice or surgeon before he was granted the licence of the Company.

It is easy to reconstruct the manner in which anatomy was taught in the sixteenth century, for Plate IX is a faithful representation of such a lecture as it was given in the anatomical theatre at the Barber Surgeons' Hall. It shows John Banester delivering the visceral lecture in the year 1581. The two Masters of Anatomy with a probe and scalpel stand beside him, whilst the two stewards are on the opposite side of the table. The minute accuracy of detail is shown by the *vade mecum* which is being used as the text of the lecture, and it will be noticed that the skeleton is supported and crowned with the colours of the Barber Surgeons' arms, whilst a wreath of the same colours surmounts the helmet in Banester's arms. The book on the reading desk is Realdus Columbus, and from its size I thought it must be the folio edition printed at Venice in 1559. Reference to this edition, however, shows that the passage at which the book is open occurs on folios 227 and 228. The picture gives the pages 419 and 420. Looking about for another edition, I found the octavo published at Paris in 1572, and turning to Chapter 5 of Book XI, I discovered the latter part of the passage quoted occurring just as the painter saw it on pages 419 and 420. It shows that Banester had not only chosen the last edition of his text-book to lecture from, but for the convenience of the students he had selected the cheaper and more portable book. Time has dealt gently with Banester, for in addition to the picture of his lecture, there exists in the University Library at Cambridge a casket of wood and leather ornamented with gold and blind tooling, containing the anatomical figure of a man and an ivory skeleton. The inscription on the box (Plate X) reads

Iohannes Banister Medicus
Londinensis, & Anatomicus insignis, Academiae
Cantabrigiensi dono dedit cistellulam hanc, unà-
cum artificioso Sceleto, & exteriorum musculo-
rum humani corporis Icone, affabrè factis, & in
eadem contentis. Anno Dom. 1591.

The casket is too fragile to travel, but Dr. Jenkinson, the University Librarian, has kindly allowed me to have it and its contents photographed (Plates X and XI).

The subjects were probably chosen with considerable care during their life, as the executions were so numerous that a selection could be made. The material was of the best, as very little physical damage was done at the hanging. The medical students in Vicary's time, therefore, were in a much better position than their successors two hundred years later, who had to resurrect the body, and, in consequence, rarely had an opportunity of seeing the muscles and tissues of the neck, which were always lacerated in the process of exhumation, or by the violence of the long drop. Indeed, so slight was the injury inflicted at Tyburn, and the subjects so often recovered when they were brought to the Hall, that the following order was made on 13 July 1587:

'Item yt ys agreed That yf any bodie wch shall at anie tyme here-

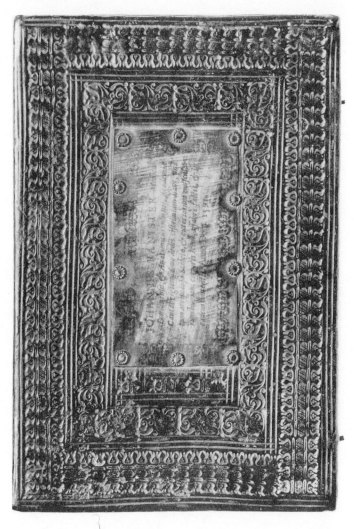

X. The lid of John Banester's casket in the University Library, Cambridge

after happen to be brought to oᵗ Hall for the intent to be wrought
uppon by Thanatomistes of oᵗ Companie shall revyve or come to
lyfe agayne as of late hathe ben seene The charges aboute the same
bodie so reviving shall be borne levied and susteyned by such person
or persons who shall so happen to bringe home the Bodie. And
further shall abide suche order or ffyne as this Howse shall Awarde.'

After this the subjects do not appear to have come to life
again. There was no difficulty at first in obtaining the
bodies, but in later years the Company had sometimes to
be assisted by a military guard, so fierce was the resistance
offered by the mob at the place of execution.

Bodies being relatively plentiful, they were dissected by
systems rather than by regions, a plan which is still customary in the veterinary schools of this country. The
viscera were considered first, as being the most perishable,
the muscles and arteries next, the bones, ligaments, and
joints last. Different benefactors endowed different lectureships for this purpose, and thus arose a visceral lecture,
a muscular lecture, and an osteological lecture. Of these
lectureships vestigia still remain in our Arris and Gale
lectureship; the Arris bequest being originally devoted to
a muscular, and the Gale to an osteological lectureship.

The anatomical teaching was long kept in the hands of
the Barbers and Surgeons' Company as a strict monopoly,
and no body could be dissected by any of its members
without leave from the Company. Such leave, however,
was not unduly withheld when application was made in
a proper manner. Thus there arose two classes of anatomy.
The one, called the public anatomy, was the formal dissection of the bodies of the four criminals. It soon became
one of the sights of London, and involved the United
Company in some expense to provide proper accommodation for the crowds who attended. The second class consisted of private anatomies held as opportunity occurred,
or as occasion required, by those who were devoting themselves to anatomy as a study.

Each of the public anatomies lasted for three days, after
which for another three days the masters of the anatomy

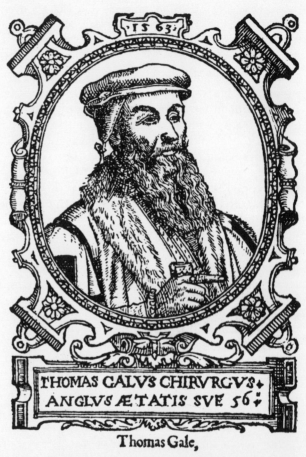

THOMAS GALVS CHIRVRGVS
ANGLVS AETATIS SVE 56

Thomas Gale,

Fig. 2. From his 'Certaine Workes of Chirurgerie', 1563.

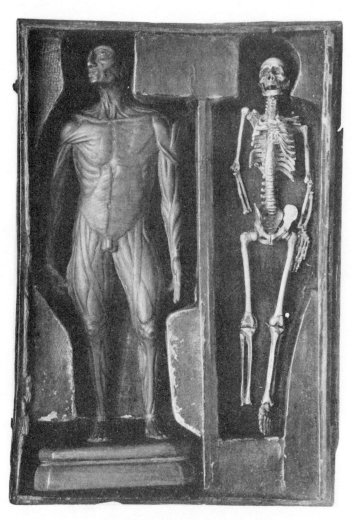

XI. The contents of John Banester's casket

were allowed to teach their pupils, the whole business being ended with a feast, and it was the duty of the two junior stewards of anatomy to see that the tables were properly furnished. The more distinguished visitors attending the dissection were invited to the banquet, and to this hospitality on the part of the Company we are indebted for the account left us by Mr. Pepys, on 27 February 1662–3, of Dr. Scarborough's demonstration of the parts concerned in vesical calculus. For each of the public anatomies the lecturer received £10 and the masters of anatomy £3 each, the total expense being £22 14s. 6d.

Surgery

Surgery was taught by a compulsory lecture given every Tuesday afternoon throughout the year; Tuesday being chosen because it was the day on which the Court of Assistants, or, as we should say, the Council, held its ordinary meeting. The earlier apprentices and surgeons of the United Company were fortunate in their teachers. Caius was the lecturer on anatomy; Gale (Fig. 2), Clowes, Halle (Fig. 3), and Balthrop taught surgery. Rough men, of uncertain temper and with much mother wit, they had been trained in the wars, were attached to large hospitals, and had the chief surgical practice in London. They quarrelled violently, fought each other with their fists, and sometimes promised to cure patients who were incurable, for which they were duly reprimanded by the Company and made to refund the fee. But in their writings at any rate they speak kindly of each other, and wrote verses to recommend each other's books. They were in truth a band united, as I shall show presently, with the common object of raising the status of surgery.

The lectures were arranged in courses, each course being given in turn, the 'auncientist Surgeon' beginning, and the others in due order following. As in the case of anatomy, the lectures took the form of a running commentary upon a text-book, the text-book being either one in traditional use, like Guydo's *Questions*, which had been

translated into English, or the *Surgery* of Tagaultius,
which was in Latin, or it might be one written by the
lecturer himself. Gui and Tagaultius were respectively the
'Rose and Carless' and the 'Gask and Wilson' of the day.
I have read both. They really contain a great deal of sound
and useful surgery if they are considered in the light of
contemporary knowledge. A part of the course was devoted to bandages, the recognition of surgical instruments,
and the use of such drugs and external applications as were
allowed the surgeons by the physicians.

Lapse of years removed this brilliant band of surgeons,
and no worthy successors were forthcoming. The Company made repeated appeals to the surgical members, and
tried to make them lecture, or in default pay a fine. They
preferred to pay the fine, until, at last, in desperation, a
paid lecturer on surgery was appointed, and the surgeons
were ordered to find his salary of £20 a year out of their
own pockets. I show you here the surgical text-books of
the time. In addition to Gui and Tagaultius, which I have
just mentioned, they are Oribasius; Halle's edition of
Lanfranc; Gale's *Surgery* and translations of Galen; several
works of Clowes; Banester's *Treatise on Ulcers*; Bullen's
Dialogues; Valerius Cordus for drugs; and Realdus Columbus for anatomy.

Pathology

Pathology was sometimes allotted to the lecturer on
anatomy and was sometimes a part of the surgical course.
Inflammation and its results, and the various kinds of
tumours, were common to each course. In the hands of
the anatomist—because he was a physician—various
treatises of Galen and a little Hippocrates were also dwelt
upon; the surgeon, less learned and knowing no Greek,
either had the Latin versions translated into English, or,
as is more likely, curtailed this portion of the course to the
great advantage of his audience, for the matter was both
dry and useless. It is somewhat remarkable that no
attempt was made to teach by clinical examination; indeed,

there is some evidence to show that the introduction of
patients at lectures was definitely forbidden. It was not
until 1602 that a clinical examination was first required,
and then it was in Scotland.

Examination

The United Company elaborated their system of examination with considerable care. No one could practise
surgery in the city of London or within a radius of seven
miles without their licence, and it was decided that
examination was the best means of determining a man's
fitness to practise. Two classes of candidates presented
themselves: (i) their own apprentices, and (ii) surgeons
who had been in practice elsewhere—foreigners as they
were called technically—and who wished to settle in
London. The first step of the United Company, therefore, was to appoint eight examiners, the number being
afterwards increased to ten—freemen of the Company, of
course, but not necessarily of the Assistants or Council.
Four of these examiners undertook the examination of
candidates in the presence of the Master and Wardens of
the Company, who might, of course, be barbers, knowing
nothing of surgery. Upon the report of the examiners the
Master, Wardens, and Court of Assistants granted the
licence, or preferment of grace as it was called.

We have a clear picture of the method of procedure.
As soon as the apprentice was out of his indentures he
presented himself at the Hall in Monkwell Street with a
recommendation from his Master. Ushered into the Hall,
he was asked by the Master and Wardens what he intended to do after he was made free of the Company. If
he replied that he proposed to practise surgery, he was
asked whether he meant to settle in London. If he said,
'That is my intention', he was sent over to the examiners,
of whom four were always present, and they proceeded to
test his knowledge. They asked him in English about
anatomy and surgery; of what parts they consisted; what
were the bones, their number in different parts of the

body, how they were moved; where the large vessels ran; what was the use of the liver, the spleen, and brain; in surgery and pathology what were the tumours *praeter naturam*, how he would treat an apostume or inflammation, what should be done for the bite of a mad dog, what were the causes of blood in the water, what was a struma, and so on. If his answers proved satisfactory—and they did not always prove so—he was licensed to practise surgery for a term of years varying with the knowledge he had shown, and was admitted a freeman of the Company.

In the early days, of which alone I am now speaking, he was advised at the same time to proceed to the higher degree of Master of Anatomy and Surgery—the second preferment of grace—and was told that he could do so either by writing an Epistle, i.e. a thesis to be read before the Company every six months; or, if he were not gifted with the pen of a ready writer, he might be examined half-yearly to determine what improvement he had made in practice. If the candidate were then approved, he was formally admitted a Master of Surgery and Anatomy, which was, a permanent licence to practise, and allowed him to apply to the Bishop of London for the Bishop's licence, which 'is said to be confirmation of a Surgeon'. Few, however, took the second step, and it seems to have quickly fallen into disuse, its place being taken by 'the Great Diploma', granted after a special examination to those who aspired to the highest surgical position. It was somewhat analogous to our Fellowship examination.

The cost of the licence was viii*d*.; the cost of the Mastership was a spoon weighing an ounce of silver, with the applicant's name written upon it, as a present to the Company, and viii*d*. to the clerk for enrolling the name.

Rejections were not infrequent, but it was more usual to grant an ignorant man a temporary licence, either for a short time or on condition that he should call in some more experienced member of the Company whenever he had to treat a patient. Occasionally the candidate was so shockingly bad that the coroner was invited to hear the examination—a good practical way of saving subsequent inquests. Here is an example:

'One John ffoster a poore and unskylfull man of this Company made his appearance before the Mrs. of this Company and was examined concerninge his skyll in the arte of Surgery and was found altogether unskilfull in all the partes thereof. Whereuppon it is ordered that Mr. Wilbraham, Coroner to this Cytie, be warned to be here with the Coroner's Inquest on Thursdaye next by tenne of the clock in the forenoone to be satisfied by their owne hereinge of the unskilfullness of the said ffoster.'

When the apprentice said that he did not intend to practise in London or the suburbs, he was admitted to the freedom of the Company without examination, and went his way to get the licence required in the district where he settled, whilst he had the added dignity of having been educated in London.

It was also possible for a surgeon to obtain a licence to practise even though he had not served an apprenticeship to a freeman of the Company. Such licences were often granted to pleasure some great man and upon his personal application. It was productive of much harm, and detracted from the reputation of the Company when the Master and Wardens were mercenary, or when the Company was in financial straits, as frequently happened, for unworthy men were then admitted. John Read, of Gloucester, took the Company to task for this fault. He says many do

'practise abroad their accustomed deceipts under the colour of admittance from the Hall of London. . . . A thing greatly to be lamented that those which are or should be the fathers of arte and upholders of good artists should so slightly passe their licence to such ignoraunt asses, to maintaine them, not onely in coosening her Majesties subjects of their monie, but oftentimes depriue them of their lims, yea and also their lives. But it is no meruaile for monie is sweete, and what is it but Lucre may doe? for I myselfe, talking with one of the same companie and felowship, complayning uppon the abuses thereof, in passing their licences to such, made me this answere. In deed, quoth he, it is not well, but we were as good to take their monie for they would play the knaves nevertheles . . . I know someone of small learning and lesse knowledge, who hauing trauelled 180 miles to fetch a seale weying fower pound besides the apurtenances therunto belonging, whereby he is growen so farre in love with himself and so undiscretlie doteth ouer his owne doings at his returne that he maketh his travel, and conquest as he thinketh, ordinary table talke, for he walked from Tauerne to Tauerne and from Alehouse to Alehouse with his licence at his girdle closed in a boxe, as though he had been the proctor of some spitell house agrauating the latter so monstrouslie, as if he had endured the verie labours of olde Hercules, and no meruaile, for when he had made his market, and receaued his letters of marke, falling in companie with some others, and grewe in speeches of practise (for there uppon he standeth, but his method is small) did not stick to confirm that Arsenick and rusty Bacon, was a present remedie for wounds made with goon-shot. And being another time demaunded by a learned Doctor in Phisicke how a wound came to be an ulcer was stricken dum. And yet of like he might aunswere his examinations well. For that (as he saith) he was used so familiarly and plast amongest the best. A meane surely to embolden him well for he was but bashfull when he was before the worshipfull Doctor. And yet will not stick to make himselfe comparable to any and will impudentlie cracke, that any man shal neuer attaine to do the like cures as he hath don, with a great deal more of shamles comparisons.'

The possession of a licence did not relieve its holder from what would now be called post-graduate teaching. Under penalty of a fine the members of the Company, including the Master and Wardens, were obliged to attend the demonstrations in anatomy and the lectures on surgery, exemptions being only rarely granted. They had not only to attend, but for the honour of the Company they had to come properly dressed, they were bound to remain the whole time, and were enjoined not to ask questions until the lecture was ended, when they might courteously point out anything which they thought had been taught incorrectly.

Education of the Public to Appreciate Surgery

The education of the public to appreciate the value of better surgical treatment proved to be a more difficult task than the education of the surgeon himself. Surgery had reached a very low ebb at the beginning of the sixteenth century, for in 1511 an Act of Parliament for the appointing of physicians and surgeons recites that

'the science and cunning of Physic and Surgery is daily within this Realm exercised by a great multitude of ignorant persons of whom the greater part have no insight in the same nor in any other kind of learning. Some also can no letters from the Book, so far forth that common Artificers as Smiths, Weavers and Women boldly and accustomably take upon them great Cures . . . to the great infamy of the Faculty and the grievous Hurt, damage and destruction of the King's Liege people most especially of them that cannot discern the uncunning from the cunning.'

This is confirmed by Clowes some years later, who says

'that many in these days do take upon them to intermeddle and practise in this art, wherein they were never trained nor had any experience; of the which a gret number be shameless in countenance, lewd in disposition and brutish in judgement, which do forsake their honest trade whereunto God hath called them and do daily rush into physic and surgery. And some of them be Painters, some Glaziers, some Tailors, some Weavers, some Joiners, some Cutlers, some Cooks, some Bakers and some Chandlers. Yea, now-a-days it is apparent to see how Tinkers, Tooth-drawers, Pedlars, Ostlers, Carters, Porters, Horse-gelders and Horse-leeches, Idiots, Apple-squires, Broom-men, Bawds, Witches, Conjurors, Sooth-sayers, and Sow-gelders, Rogues, Rat-catchers, Runagates and Proctors of Spittle houses with such other like rotten and stinking weeds which do in Town and country, without order, honesty or skill, daily abuse both physic and surgery, having no more per-severance, reason or knowledge in this art than hath a goose, and most commonly useth one remedy for all diseases and one way of curing to all persons both old and young, men, women and children which is as possible to be performed or to be true as for a shoe-maker with one last to make a shoe to fit for every man's foot and this is one principal cause that so many perish.'

Gale complains bitterly of the 'counterfeit javils' whose promises to cure by charms led to later amputations; and it is clear that the whole country was overrun with quacks.

This state of affairs in London is borne out by Clowes, who mentions that he had amputated seven arms and legs in a morning at St. Bartholomew's Hospital. This statement was not made boastingly, but incidentally as showing a part of his routine work.

It was no better in Kent, for Master John Halle (Fig. 3) of Maidstone reports that in 1562 there came

'one William, a shoe-maker, pretending to be very cunning in curing of diseases of the eyes; and being brought to a friend of myne to have his judgement in one eye, whereof the sight was weake; first putting them in much fear of the eye he at length promised to doe great thinges therto. But the friends of the party diseased desired me first to talke with him to understande his cunning; which, at their request, I did at a time appointed and asked him if he understoode what was the cause of her infirmitie. He said he could not tel but he wold heale her he doubted not. Then I asked him whether he were a surgion or a physitien; he ansered no he was a shoe-maker but he could heale all manner of sore eyes. I asked him where he learned that; he sayde that was no matter. Well, sayde I, seyng that you can heale sore eyes what is an eye? Whereof is it made? Of what members or parts is it composed? And he sayde he knewe not that.

'Then I asked hym if he were worthy to be a shoe-maker or to be so called that knewe not howe or wherof a shoe was made? He answered, no, he was not worthy. Then, sayde I, how dare you worke on such a precious and intricate member of man as is the eye, seyng you knowe not the nature therof? and why or by what reason it doth see more than a man's nose or his hand? He answered that though he could not tell this yet could he heale all maner of sore eyes. And that whereas maister Luke of London hath a great name of curyng eyes he coulde do that which maister Luke coulde not doe nor turne his hande to. Thus bragged this proud varlette against and above that reverent man of knowne learning and experience.

'And I sayde, I thought so, for Maister Luke, sayde I, is no shoe-maker. Well, sayde he, I perceive you do but skorne me and flunge out of the doores in a great fume and could not be caused to tary and drynke by any intreaty neither have I since that tyme heard anythyng of hym.'

The same story comes from Gloucester, where, as it was

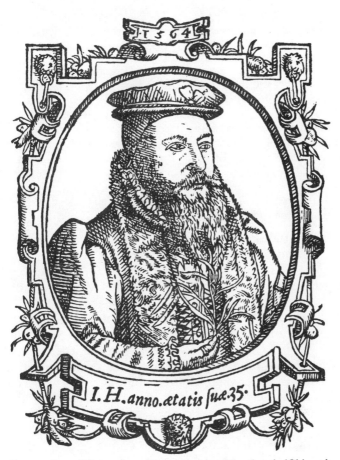

FIG. 3. JOHN HALLE, from his translation of Lanfranc's 'Chirurgia Parva', 1565.

near a seaport, there were foreign, as well as indigenous, rogues to contend with. For example: Read tells us that

'there came a flemming into the cittie of Gloceter named Woolfgange Frolicke, and there hanging forth his picture, his flagges, his instruments and his letters of marte with long labels, great tossels, broad seales closed in boxes, with such counterfeit showes and knackes of knaverie cosening the people of their monie without either learning or knowledge, and yet for money got him a license to practise at Bristowe [Bristol]. But when he came to Glocester & being called before some being in aucthoritie by my selfe & others, he was not able to aunser to any one poynt in Chirurgerie, which being perceived and the man knowen the matter was excused by way of Charitie to be good to straungers.'

This attitude of tolerance towards quacks was the root of the evil, and it was so general that in 1542 (34–35 H. 8. Ch. 8) a Bill was promoted in Parliament 'that persons being no common surgeons may minister Medicines notwithstanding the Statute'. The Bill passed, and it 'ordained, established and enacted that at all time from henceforth it shall be lawful to every person being the King's subject, having knowledge and experience of the nature of herbs, roots and waters by speculation or practise to use and minister them to their cunning'. This opened the door very widely to unlicensed practitioners, for the position of the surgeons was not safeguarded in any way, not even as Guthrie suggested many years later (29 April 1834), that a quack should be allowed to practise if he took out an annual licence, and should be punishable for ignorance as well as negligence, whilst a duly qualified practitioner should not be required to renew his licence annually and should only be punishable for negligence.

Lack of Medical Education

Surgery in England had always been subservient to physic, and in this subordinate position it was destined to remain until our own times. The physicians, oppressed by the weight of tradition, were bound by the fetters of the various sects which arose successively in medicine.

They only made very slow advances in practice, and their progress was actually retarded by the interposition of the apothecaries between themselves and their patients.

The surgeons, on the other hand, were necessarily brought face to face with the same problems which confront us to-day. When should wounds be closed? When must they be left open? Was it safe to leave a head injury untreated, or should it be operated upon? What was best to be done for the injuries which daily presented themselves as a result of trade accidents, or the disputes which were of constant occurrence in medieval towns where every one went armed and passions were easily inflamed. Readiness of resource, mother-wit, and a fair average of manipulative skill were characteristics of the Tudor surgeon, and he trepanned the head, opened the chest, cut for stone, and amputated with remarkable success. He also had some knowledge of herbs and simples, and there had been handed down to him an antidotary or collection of prescriptions which had proved useful to his predecessors. But of medicine he had no knowledge. All that he did was empirical, and he was in complete ignorance of what would now be called the Institutes of Medicine even as they were then understood.

The result is interesting. There arose for a generation or two excellent surgeons who wrote well in their native tongue and were able to record their experiences. Their books are still worth reading, but they are one and all records of individual cases. No attempt is made to generalize from the results obtained, even when the writer could collect from his own observation several similar cases or even whole groups of cases. I suppose we have all passed through this stage when, as young men, we were proud to publish a single case in one of the medical journals; but as we gained greater experience we cared less for individual facts and thought more of the conclusions we were able to deduce from the correlation of them.

The Tudor surgeons were arrested at the earlier stage, and it was not until a century later that Wiseman began to generalize on his own experience. The absence of this faculty of generalization was, I think, felt instinctively by the great Elizabethan surgeons. They knew that something was wanting in their education, and they believed that if their pupils could be taught medicine as they had learnt surgery, they would be the better for it. Gale says: 'Young men should take counsel as well of the learned physician as of the learned surgeon, for this art is so joined together that neither may the parts be divided neither yet the instruments without the overthrow and destruction of the whole art.' And in the same way Read says: 'I do withall affirm that all chirurgeons ought to be seen in physic, and chirurgery is divided from physic not without great hurt unto mankind.' I have no doubt that if the physicians had allowed the surgeons to be taught some medicine they would have been the better for it, and their social position would have been improved, but it is very doubtful whether surgery as a whole would have derived any benefit. Medicine itself was nebulous so long as it was based on speculation rather than on observation, and its teaching at this time would probably have reduced surgery from practice to theory. Gale, like Halle and Banester, puts the position quite temperately when he says,

'To counsel with a physician being a grave and learned man in the principles of this art—in matters of weight—I take it to be very necessary; for what is he that is wise that will refuse the counsel of a wise and learned man, and especially of him that possesseth the principles of the same art? For physiologia, whereof the physician taketh his name, is the first and chiefest part which he that worketh in the art of medicine doth prove for that it doth consist in the knowledge of the several natural things, and in the residue thereto appertaining. But yet this doth not follow that a learned and expert chirurgeon should not use diet and purgations and other inward medicines at all times when need doth require.'

John Banester writes in the same strain but somewhat more rhetorically:

'Some of late more precise than wise have fondly affirmed, foolishly feigned and frantically faced, that the chirurgeon hath not to deal in physic. Small courtesy is it to break faithful friendship or at-one-ment, but it is mad dotage to part that which cannot be separated. How can physic be praised and surgery discommended? Can any man despise surgery and not defame physic? No, sure, he that speaketh evil of the one slaundereth both, and he that robbeth the one spoileth the other. For though they be at this time made two distinct arts and the artists severally named, yet sure the one cannot work without some aid from the other, nor the other practise without the aid of both.'

So, again, John Read—a much younger man and John Banester's son-in-law—claimed that

'Chirurgery is maimed and utterly unperfect without the help of those other parts—which consisteth of prescribing inward medicines and convenient diet, and is so near linked with these in alliance that no man deserves to be called a chirurgeon that is ignorant in physic . . . and I do withal affirm that chirurgeons ought to be seen [i.e. examined] in physic, and that the Barber's craft ought not to be termed chirurgery.'

Nothing, however, came of this well-intentioned advice. The surgeons remained on a lower plane, and when the reformers died—first Read, then Gale, followed in due course by Clowes and Banester—no successors, with the exception of Woodall, carried on their work in England under James and Charles.

Thus ends the second Vicary Historical Lecture. I have tried to show how much the education of a surgeon owes to the wise counsel of a few great men in those critical times, when the fraternity of surgeons could no longer continue along the traditional lines and there was a real danger of surgery passing into the hands of a trade gild. The example set in London was quickly followed in the provinces, and, within a few years of the establishment of the United Company of Barbers and Surgeons, the large towns of England had remodelled their Barbers' Gilds, and had often followed the example of the United Company in the most minute detail. In due course surgery outgrew the need for a union with the barbers, and in

1745 a dissolution of the partnership took place. The disastrous history of the Surgeons' Company showed how useful the alliance with the barbers had been to the surgeons. The barbers were business men, the surgeons were thoroughly unbusinesslike. The Clerk of the Surgeons' Company defaulted and left the Company penniless; their building became ruinous; their library contained no books; and, finally, by sheer ignorance of their own Constitution, the Company destroyed itself after an inglorious career of forty years. By its supineness and by its tactless methods a host of enemies had been raised up—and it became impossible to establish the bankrupt Company on the old lines. The present College rose, indeed, upon its ruins; but, because we are now flourishing, do not let us forget how much we owe to the Company of Barbers, our business partners for more than two hundred years, and we shall then understand that the Union of Barbers and Surgeons was not so incongruous or so useless as it at first sight appears.

V

THE FEES OF OUR ANCESTORS

THE question of fees is one of perennial interest to every practitioner in medicine, although the medical profession from the earliest times has been eminently philanthropic and has given its services freely and without thought of gain in suitable cases. SS. Cosmas and Damian have been the patron saints of medicine throughout the civilized world from the earliest Christian times. It is told of them that they ministered to the wants of all who sought their help and steadfastly refused payment for their services, exercising their art only for the love of God and for charity, so that they earned for themselves the title of ἀνάργυροι or the moneyless because they took no fees. Indeed, it is recorded of a later and degenerate Cosmas and Damian, the sons of Theodotus, that a woman named Palladia once gave Damian three eggs as a reward for a cure, a gift which so enraged Cosmas that he forbade his neighbours to bury his brother with him in the same tomb. But after the death of the brothers and while they were debating what should be done with the corpse, a camel, which had been cured by the saints, spoke and absolved Damian, saying that he had been compelled by a vow to take the eggs and that they were not in the nature of a fee. It is evident, therefore, that Cosmas was irritated by the mere acceptance of the eggs and not, as might otherwise have been suggested, by its paltriness.

Fees were small during the Arabic period of medicine which dated from A.D. 640 to 1400. Dr. Chatard [1] says that in the days of Avicenna (A.D. 980–1037)

'The teachers as a rule were well paid, some receiving over 200 dollars [£40] a month; . . . the medical fees of those days were small, except among the most famous men. The following schedule of fees is rather interesting: A. The poor must be treated gratui-

[1] 'Avicenna and Arabian Medicine'. *Bulletin of the Johns Hopkins Hospital*, June 1908, xix, 158.

tously. B. The Physician must visit his patient at least twice each day, and if requested by the latter, once also at night. For this he received for every day of treatment: (*a*) In the city or at his residence half a tarenus or $0.14 [which was about sevenpence]. (*b*) Away from his residence, when (1) The patient paid his travelling expenses three tareni or $0.85 [equivalent to three shillings and sixpence], (2) The doctor paid his travelling expenses four tareni or $1.17 [which is about five shillings and eightpence in English money]. The fee was usually stipulated in advance or during the course of the disease, as one writer says: "Make it high (the fee), as, after recovery, recollection of the services rendered declines rapidly".'

One of the earliest records of fees in England is that given by John of Arderne [who had treated the Black Prince and had received from him a grant of land in Connaught] (fl. 1370) in his treatise of the fistula, and as it gives an excellent account of the method of bargaining with patients I quote it in detail, copying from a translation of the Latin original made in the early part of the fifteenth century. The spelling is modernized:

'If the leech will favour to any man's asking, make he covenant with him for his travail and take it beforehand. But advise the leech himself well that he give no certain answer in any cause but he see first the sickness and the manner of it; and when he hath seen and assayed it, although him seem that the sick may be healed, nevertheless he shall make prognostication to the patient of the perils to come if the cure be deferred. And if he see the patient perceive [watch] busily the cure, than after the state of the patient, ask he boldly more or less but ever be wary of scarce asking for over scarce asking setteth at nought both the market and the thing. Therefore, for the cure of a fistula in ano, when it is curable, ask he competently of a worthy man and a great, an hundred marks or forty pounds, with robes and fees of an hundred shillings term of life by year. Of less men forty pounds or forty marks, ask he, without fees. And take he not less than an hundred shillings; for never, in all my life took I less than an hundred shillings for cure of that sickness. Nevertheless, do another man, as him think better and more speedful.'

This means that when John Arderne charged his highest

fee for the cure of a fistula he got forty pounds down with
a suit of clothes annually and an annuity of a hundred
shillings a year so long as his patient lived. This custom
of paying an annuity for a successful surgical operation
lingered for a long time in England, for Richard Wiseman
(1621–76), in speaking of a patient says: 'This person
retired into the Country afterwards and returned to
London at the end of two years and acknowledged to me
his Cure by settling Thirty pounds a year upon me during
his life and paid me sixty pounds for the two years passed.'
Readers of French history know that Louis XIV paid
Dr. François Felix the sum of one hundred and fifty
pounds, and settled a farm upon him in 1686 for curing
him of a fistula.

The same method of payment was adopted in Ireland,
where the amount of a leech's remuneration depended
partly on his own eminence and partly upon the status of
the king or chief to whose household he was attached.
The stipend generally consisted of a tract of land and a
residence in the neighbourhood, held free of all tithe and
tribute, together with certain allowances and perquisites;
the physician was also allowed to practise outside his
patron's household. The usual allowance of land was five
hundred acres, and some of these estates—now ordinary
town lands—retain the family name to this day. Thus
Ferrancassidy in Fermanagh was the ferran or land belonging to the O'Cassidys who were the family physicians
to the Maguires of Fermanagh.

The household physician to a king in Ireland held a very
dignified position. He lived like a prince with a household
and dependants of his own. He was always amongst the
king's immediate retinue and he was entitled to a distinguished place at his table. When a wound had been
treated a certain time was always allowed to test the cure.
If it broke out afresh before the end of this period of probation the cure was regarded as unsuccessful and the leech
had to return the fee and pay a fine. Moreover, if he and
his pupil had lived in the patient's house during the treat-

ment, the cost of maintenance had also to be refunded. The testing time for a wound of the arm or hand was one year; for a wound of the leg a little longer; for a wound of the head, probably a fractured skull, three years. When the testing time was ended the physician and the wounded man were alike exempt from any further claim, no matter what happened.

In 1415 Henry V crossed the Channel to engage in the campaign which ended so gloriously for England at the field of Agincourt. A record of the medical arrangements for the army during this campaign is preserved in the indentures between the King and his physician, Nicholas Colnet, and his surgeon, Thomas Morstede. The agreement is dated 29 April 1415 and is to the effect that Nicholas Colnet was to accompany the King for a year as physician to the forces in Guienne and France. He was to be attended by three archers as a guard, each archer receiving sixpence a day, whilst Colnet drew twelvepence for his own pay. Thomas Morstede, the surgeon, had also three archers assigned to him for protection, and he, too, received twelvepence a day in addition to the usual allowance of one hundred marks (£66 13s. 4d.) a quarter, the pay, it is stated, of thirty men-at-arms, with a share of the plunder. Morestede was also directed to take with him twelve of his own craft, each subordinate surgeon to receive the pay of an archer—sixpence a day. As a pledge for the punctual payment of the daily and quarterly allowances Colnet and Morestede were permitted to take certain jewels belonging to the King.

The scale of pay seems liberal. The ordinary labourer at this time was receiving a penny a day as wages. Each archer and each surgeon, therefore, was considered to be worth the wages of six day-labourers, and the two chiefs double their assistants. Nowadays a labourer in London earns at least a guinea a week or three shillings a day, so that the surgeons and archers, if paid on the same scale, would receive eighteen shillings a day, and the heads of departments thirty-six shillings a day. But at the present time a surgeon on probation in the army only receives eight shillings, and he has to serve for ten years before his pay is increased to fifteen shillings a day.

The retaining fee and the booty must have been welcome additions to the pay. The King took a third of the plunder with all the precious stones, gold, and silver when the value amounted to six pounds and upwards, but the King's share was always badly collected and the surgeons were probably not unduly officious in declaring their gains. But in addition to the regular payments there were other means of obtaining money at the wars. When armour was worn and tournaments were frequent the leaders suffered much more than the rank and file who could run away when they were hard pressed. The surgeon, therefore, treated the nobility and gentry in the army at least as often as the common men, and for this he was paid separately and often in kind, for money was scarce. Ambroise Paré received at different times a cask of wine, fifty double ducats and a horse, a diamond, a collection of crowns and half-crowns from the ranks, and other honourable presents of great value; from the King himself 300 crowns and a promise that he would never let him want; another diamond —this time (says Mr. Stephen Paget) from the finger of a duchess—and a soldier once offered him a bag of gold.

In Elizabethan times each cure was a separate bargain and the average fee was perhaps a mark (13s. 4d.), but this sum might not be all in money. Here is an instance from the Records of the Barber Surgeons of London:

'2nd October 1576. Here was likewise a complaint against one Thomas Adams against John Paradice for that the said John had received certain money in hand and a gown in pawn for the remainder to cure the daughter of the said Thomas which daughter died and the poor man made request for the gown again and so the Master and Governors [of the Barber Surgeons of London] awarded that the said John Paradice should re-deliver the gown next Tuesday and that the said Thomas Adams should give unto the said John Paradice towards his boat hire, spent in going to the maid at Putney, five shillings.'

Sometimes the bargain was for a certain sum of money down and the balance when the cure was ended.

'1st March 1648. Henry Ivatt complained against Anthony Mold for his evil practice on the wife of the said Ivatt who being afflicted with the King's Evil whereof he undertook to cure her. And for that purpose did receive of the said Ivatt thirty shillings in hand and was to have forty shillings more when she was cured; both parties referred themselves to this Court, whereupon this Court doth order that the said Mold do restore twenty shillings back again to the said Ivatt, which he promised to pay accordingly and so all differences between the said parties by their own consent to cease and determine.

'In like manner on 19th April 1569. Here was the wife of Richard Selby of London, Ironmonger, plaintiff against William Wyse for that he cured not her husband's leg as he promised he would have done. And it was ordered that William Wyse shall repay again of the money which he received in part of the bargain made between them and there was in the presence of this Court paid unto Agnes the wife of the abovesaid Richard Selby six shillings and eightpence and so William Wyse is clearly discharged of patient and all.'

The following extract from the *Annals of the Barber Surgeons*, by Mr. Sidney Young, F.S.A., may also be quoted because it shows that the Barber Surgeons' Company was no respecter of persons. William Clowes was Serjeant Surgeon to Queen Elizabeth and was one of the most renowned practitioners of his age, especially in the treatment of syphilis.

'2nd February 1575. Here came one William Goodnep and complained of William Clowes for not curing his said wife *de morbo gallico* and it was awarded that the said Clowes should either give the said Goodnep twenty shillings or else cure his said wife, which Clowes agreed to pay the twenty shillings and so they were agreed and each of them made acquittance to the other.'

The *Levamen Infirmi*, published in 1700, makes the following statement about the fees of doctors:

'To a graduate in physic, his due is about ten shillings, though he commonly expects or demands twenty. Those that are only licensed physicians, their due is no more than six shillings and eight-pence, though they commonly demand ten shillings. A surgeon's fee is twelvepence a mile, be his journey far or near; ten groats (3s. 4d.) to set a bone broke or out of joint; and for letting of blood one shilling; the cutting off or amputation of any limb is five pounds but there is no settled price for the cure.'

This points to the fact that the noble, and afterwards the angel, each worth from six shillings and eightpence to ten shillings, was looked upon as the customary fee during the seventeenth century. At the Restoration in 1660 a new coin—the guinea—came into use, and the opportunity seems to have been taken to raise the doctor's fee. The guinea was equivalent at first to twenty shillings, but its value rose to thirty shillings, and for many years it was never worth less than twenty-one shillings and sixpence. It ceased to be coined in 1813, and although non-existent it is still used by barristers, doctors, and horse-dealers at its nominal value of twenty-one shillings.

Dr. Radcliffe (1650–1714) charged patients one guinea, but he wrote prescriptions for apothecaries at half a guinea when they came to him at the coffee-house in the evening and did not ask him to see the patient. His fee for a con-sultation at Bow when he was living in Bloomsbury Square was five guineas. Dr. Mead (1673–1754), like Radcliffe, charged the apothecaries who waited on him at his coffee-houses half a guinea for prescriptions written without seeing the patient. His evening coffee-house was Batson's, whilst in the forenoon he was to be found at Tom's in Russell Street, Covent Garden. When Dr. Freind was obliged to give over business on account of his politics Dr. Mead supplied his place among his patients, and when his Jacobite tendencies were forgiven Mead presented him with a purse containing 11,400 guineas, 'which', said he, 'I have received as your deputy'. The guinea thus became the regular consultation fee until about the year 1870, when it became usual to give two guineas on the occasion of the first visit and one guinea afterwards. When the physician or surgeon was called upon to make a journey he charged his patient one guinea a mile in addition to his consultation fee, but about 1845, when he was able to take advantage of the new method of locomotion by railway, the charge was reduced to two guineas for three miles, and it still remains at this rate.

The country practitioner fared much worse than his brother in town. He charged for the medicine which he supplied and not for the advice tendered. The more medicine the patient could be induced to take the larger became the bill, and for many years the patient's account was 'Bleeding one shilling and sixpence; bolus one shilling and sixpence; iter [a journey to his house] one shilling and sixpence'. Many medical men made up the medicine in the form of single doses, each in its own bottle. These draughts were sent out in packets of a dozen at a time with an appropriate pill in a small box balanced on the cork of each bottle. The charge for the draught and pill being one shilling and ninepence apiece. The Poor Law appointment in 1845 was generally about £20 a year for each parish, midwifery being paid ten shillings a case extra with an additional two shillings and sixpence when the patient lived more than three miles away.

VI

NOTES ON THE BIBLIOGRAPHY OF THREE SIXTEENTH-CENTURY ENGLISH BOOKS CONNECTED WITH LONDON HOSPITALS[1]

THE middle of the sixteenth century witnessed a revolution in the treatment of the sick poor in London, and produced a number of books written by men who had the interest of surgery at heart, and who strove to raise their calling from a trade to a profession. Vicary, Gale, Clowes, Banester, Read, and Maister Peter Lowe wrote books which are still a joy to read. Their language is charming, their invective is fierce, their poetry is vile, but they give so lively a picture of the times in which they lived that many a profitable hour may still be spent in their company.

The object of the Bibliographical Society, however, is Bibliography, so I leave this band of writers and will ask you to consider three books whose history has not yet been completely elucidated.

(i) 'The Order of the Hospitalls'

I will begin with this little duodecimo, the title-page of which is reproduced in Fig. 4. The book is in black letter and has neither the name nor the place of the printer. The copy here shown has been re-backed and re-labelled, but the leather covering the sides is original. The edges of the leaves and the edges of the leather binding are gilded, and there is marbled paper at each end of the volume.

The book itself consists of 57 leaves and 113 pages. The paper is of good quality, but it is badly discoloured throughout. Written in the bold hand of a clerk on the reverse of the title-page is the inscription: 'To the Right Worp[ll]. S[r]. Humphry Edwin Kn[t]. and Alderman, Governor of Christ's Hosp[ll].' The book was also in the possession of a Governor of St. Bartholomew's Hospital

---

[1] Read before the Bibliographical Society of London, 21 March 1921.

The Order

Of the

Hospitalls of K. Henry the vijth and K. Edward the vith,

viz. {
St. Bartholomew's.
Christ's.
Bridewell.
St Thomas's.
}

By the Maior, Cominaltie, and Citizens of London, Governours of the Possessions, Revenues and Goods of the sayd Hospitalls,

1557.

Fig. 4.

in 1809. It contains his summons to attend at the Blue-coat School on St. Matthew's Day and go 'from thence to Christ Church to hear a sermon and afterwards to hear the Oration in the great Hall according to ancient Custom.

'NB. It is particularly requested that you take a Green Staff, as a Governor of this Hospital, upon entering the Great Hall.'

In spite of the date and the type I have always thought there was something wrong about the book. I have brought it here this afternoon for your inspection, with such facts as I have been able to gather, that you may sit in judgement upon it, and, I fear, damn it as an impostor.

The book contains the rules which the citizens of London desired should govern the Charities which had been placed under their control after the upheaval in the middle of the sixteenth century. It declares how many governors shall be elected; the manner in which they shall be chosen; the length of time they shall serve and the charge to be given to them; the manner of conducting the Courts and of appointing the Officers; the duties of the Officers, and many other details, serviceable and necessary at the time, but of no interest to us at present.

The first notice of the Orders occurs in the Repertories at the Guildhall, where, under the date 1557, 28 Sept., 4 & 5 Ph. & Mary, it appears that the 'Court of Aldermen agreed that all the articles and ordinances then read concerning the government and ordering of the Poor in West Smithfield and the hospitals of the City, lately devised by S[i]r Martin Bowes and S[i]r Rowland Hill, knights, and diverse other aldermen and commoners of this city being Governours and Surveyors at that present of the said house should be entered of record and from thenceforth put in due execution'.

The Order is headed 'Offley, Maior', and Sir Thomas Offley was Mayor in 1556–7.

The *Memoranda, References, and Documents relating to The Royal Hospitals of the City of London*, compiled by Mr. James Francis Firth, the Town Clerk, and issued by the Court of Common Council in 1836, state that 'these articles and ordinances do not appear to be entered of record but were printed in 1557 under the title "The Order of the Hospitalls", etc.' There is no doubt that the Orders were duly made in 1557, and it is a little remarkable that they should never have been transcribed in the archives of the City. They were certainly circulated to the four Royal Hospitals, for there is plenty of evidence to show that they were known to, and acted on, by the governing bodies of these charities.

The next notice of the Orders is in Strype's edition of Stow's *Survey*,[1] where it is stated that the Orders 'were printed in a little book in the time of Mr. Goodfellow, Towne Clerk'. This is amplified by Gough[2] as follows: 'the Order of the Hospitalls, etc., since reprinted in the old character and size at the expence of Mr. Secretary Pepys. O.' Mr. Bernard Kettle, of the Guildhall Library, tells me that O. is William Oldys, the antiquary (1696–1761). The statement that a reprint was made at the expense of Mr. Secretary Pepys is repeated by Ames in Herbert's edition (p. 1596), and by Lowndes (p. 1124). I also find in Lowndes that the book has fetched the following prices at sales: Nassau, pt. i, 2469, £1 18s.; Strettell, 1057, 5s.; Towneley, pt. i, 563, 7s. 6d.; Inglis, 1076, 8s.

It is generally assumed, therefore, that there are two editions of the Orders, the one printed in 1557; the other, a facsimile, printed at a much later date. I have examined the various copies of the book which are accessible to see in what respects they agree or differ, taking my own as a standard. The British Museum and the Bodleian Libraries have each two copies; the Guildhall Library, the Society of Antiquaries, Christ's Hospital, the Pepysian Library at Cambridge, the Medico-Chirurgical Society at Bristol, and the Surgeon-General's Library at Washington have one copy apiece. Sir William Osler's library has this copy, which Lady Osler kindly allows me to show you, and I

---

[1] Lond. 1754, i. 195.
[2] *British Topography*, Lond. 1780, i. 639.

have a copy. Twelve copies of the book are thus available for comparison, and I have particulars of all of them. They are printed on similar paper, and in every case the paper is discoloured as it is in these two copies. In each case there are three vertical chain lines on a page, but it is only in my own copy and in the two copies in the Bodleian that there is any watermark. In my own copy there is a device on the third fly-leaf in front and on the last fly-leaf at the end. It is in the nature of a shield with a double border. Miss Anderson has kindly examined the two copies in the Bodleian and she writes:

'The volumes seem to me to agree in watermarks. On one page I think I trace COME, and in the corresponding leaf of the gathering NY, the intermediate letters are in the binding and I could not distinguish them. The more common watermark is something like a horn on an ornamental shield but, as it is everywhere close in to the binding, and besides cut at the top, it is not very easy to be definite. Ordinarily the pages have three vertical lines each. 8° Rawl. 586* has on the second flyleaf at the beginning as watermark a portion of a fleur-de-lys enclosed in a shield—the upper portion is cut away; the end flyleaf has as watermark a crown over a shield, but the shield is almost entirely cut away as is also part of the crown.

'8° Rawl. 586** has, on flyleaf two, what seems to be the remains of ⓖ but the top line of the T is cut away. All the watermarks are close into the binding and have been cut by the binder.'

None of the other copies that I have examined have any watermarks.

Nearly every copy has an inscription similar to the one I show you. It is written in a bold text hand, is on the reverse of the title-page, and states that the book has been presented to an alderman or Governor of Christ's Hospital about the end of the seventeenth century.

All the copies that I have seen appear to me to be part of one issue, which was put into circulation at the end of the seventeenth century. It is probable, therefore, that they are all examples of what Oldys called the Pepys reprint.

I have not found a single example of any earlier edition. It seems almost certain that no edition was printed in 1557, but that the Christ's Hospital authorities printed directly from a manuscript copy, possibly, as tradition states, at the expense of Mr. Samuel Pepys. Moreover, the manuscript from which the book was printed had only recently come into the possession of the Blue-coat School, for the Order beginning 'Offley, Maior', is signed 'Goodfellow', whereas if it had been printed from the original it would have been signed 'Blackwell'. William Blackwell was Town Clerk from 1541 to 1570; John Goodfellow was Town Clerk from 1690 to 1700. The book was printed, therefore, between 1690 and 1700. This is corroborated by the inscription in my copy, which shows that it belonged to Sir Humphry Edwin. Edwin was a Skinner and a Barber-Surgeon who was alderman of the Tower Ward. He was Master of the Barber-Surgeons Company in 1686, and served the office of Sheriff in the same year. He was knighted in 1687 and was Mayor in 1697.

Having thus fixed the approximate date I set to work to discover whether there was any special reason for printing *The Order of the Hospitalls* at the end of the seventeenth century when they had remained so long in manuscript. I found that in 1681 the Court of Aldermen made a determined effort to regain their ancient jurisdiction over the four Royal Hospitals, which had practically lapsed from disuse. On 14 February 1681 'a reference was made to the presidents of the four hospitals and four aldermen to inquire into and examine the ancient method of managing the hospitals and appointing governors'. The result of the inquiry was to show conclusively that the Court of Aldermen had jurisdiction over the Hospitals, but it was found difficult to enforce it—St. Bartholomew's Hospital proving especially refractory—and the dispute dragged on for several years.

On 28 October 1690

'the Clerk of Christ's Hospital was ordered by that day seven-night to deliver an account in writing how, and in what manner, the

Governors of that Hospital were anciently nominated and appointed, and when and how the same came to be altered'.

On 10 March 1690–1, the Committee reported that

'by an act of Common Council 5th of August, 4th and 5th Ph. & Mar. it was ordained that the Lord Mayor for the time being and such of the Aldermen, commonalty and citizens as should be appointed by the Mayor and Court of Aldermen for the time being to be governors of the possessions, etc., and their successors for evermore (and gave authority to them to make statutes and ordinances for well governing the hospitals, and to nominate, appoint, make, create, and ordain such and so many officers, ministers, and governors under them in the said hospitals as shall be thought meet by their discretions, to the intent the poor therein may be well and honestly provided for).

'That pursuant to that act certain ordinances were made by the Court of Aldermen for the government of the hospitals and how the governors should be chosen . . . according to which Order the new governors were presented to and approved by the Court of Aldermen till the year 1615. That although the entry of confirmation of new governors by the Court of Aldermen was omitted for many years . . . the Mayor and Aldermen were summoned.'

The result of the inquiry which evidently turned upon the consideration of *The Order of the Hospitalls* was satisfactory, for 'The Committee did not find any authority for altering the way of election or for electing other than citizens for the presidents and governors of the hospitals or any or either of them. The report was well liked, approved and ordered to be entered on the Repertory'. This appears to have settled the matter, for the Court of Aldermen resumed its authority and the hospitals acquiesced.

The printing of *The Order of the Hospitalls* seems to be the immediate outcome of this struggle. It must have been necessary for all the governors of the hospitals who took an active interest in them to study the Orders, which had hitherto existed only in manuscript. A new copy was therefore obtained from the Guildhall and its authenticity was guaranteed by the signature of the Town Clerk. It was printed and a sufficient number of copies were struck off for the use of the governors. The edition was of a considerable size. It was not put on sale, but a copy was probably given to each governor and to each member of the Court of Aldermen.

The conditions which led to the active interference of Mr. Pepys in the affairs of the Blue-coat School at the end of the seventeenth century are well known, and are clearly set out by the [late] Bishop of Worcester in his *Annals of Christ's Hospital*. The school passed through a difficult period during the Treasurership of Nathaniel Hawes from 1683 to 1699, when there was a general relaxation of discipline. Mr. Pepys, with his accustomed energy, set himself to improve the administration, having already obtained a voice in the management by securing a grant of public money for the newly established Mathematical School. This school was originally intended to train officers for the King's ships and, as Secretary of the Admiralty, Pepys was directly interested in its success. It is quite possible, therefore, that Pepys paid for the printing of *The Order of the Hospitalls*, though I am informed that there is no documentary evidence of the fact in the Christ's Hospital records.

The name of the printer is not given, but a few years later Mr. Edward Brewster bought and gave to the use of the Blue-coat School a book called *Synopsis Algebraica*. In 1708 it was reported that, the first impression being now almost spent, the Committee of Christ's Hospital ordered Mr. Newton and Mr. Dutton, the master of the new Mathematical School, to revise and correct the book, and translate it into English, in order to have the same reprinted and made of more general and public use. It was hoped that 'the advantage arising therefrom may defray the charge of the impression'.

The Committee ordered 750 copies in Latin and 1,000 in English. Samuel Cobb, the undermaster, received ten guineas for his translation, and it was arranged to sell the book to three specified booksellers at 2s. 6d. a copy in sheets.

I thought that this information might help to elucidate the publisher of *The Order of the Hospitalls*, so I visited the British Museum and obtained 'A Synopsis of Algebra being the posthumous work of Joannes Alexander of Bern in Swisserland to which is added an Appendix by Humphry Dutton. For the use of the two mathematicall Schools in Christ's Hospital, London. Done from the Latin by Samm. Cobb M.A. London. Printed for the Hospital by J. Barber and are to be sold by S. Keble and D. Tooke in Fleet St. and D. Midwinter in St. Paul's Churchyard. MDCCIX.'

The Appendix has on the title-page: 'London, Printed by J. Barber, Printer to the said Hospital. MDCCIX.' It appears from this that the Blue-coat School had its own printer twenty years after the publication of *The Order of the Hospitalls*. I looked through the volume, but could find no paper mark, and I am not sufficiently skilled to say whether the type used in printing *The Order of the Hospitalls* bears any relation to that used by J. Barber.

The Order of the Hospitalls is reprinted in full both in the 1836 and 1863 editions of *Memoranda, References, and Documents relating to The Royal Hospitals*: it is summarized in Sir Norman Moore's *History of St. Bartholomew's Hospital*.

(ii) *Vicary's 'Anatomy of Man'*

The second book to which I wish to draw your attention is Vicary's *Anatomy of Man*, as there is also a little bibliographical difficulty connected with it. The first edition of which we have certain knowledge is a 12mo which was entered at Stationers' Hall in 1577 with the following heading:

Tricesimo die Januarii (1577)

Henry Bamforde ⎰ Lycensed unto him. 'A briefe Traytise of the Anatomye of Man's Bodye.' xiid and a copie. . .

The title-page (Fig. 5) makes two definite statements: first, that the book was compiled, not written by Thomas

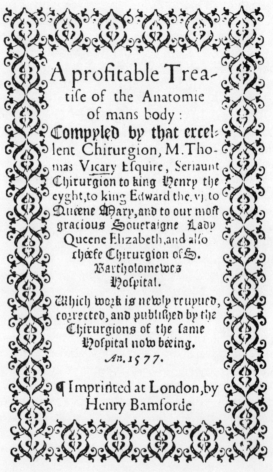

A profitable Trea-
tife of the Anatomie
of mans body :
Compyled by that excel-
lent Chirurgion, M. Tho-
mas Vicary Esquire , Seriaunt
Chirurgion to king Henry the
eyght, to king Edward the. vj. to
Quæne Mary, and to our most
gracious Soueraigne Lady
Queene Elizabeth, and also
chæfe Chirurgion of S.
Bartholomewes
Hospital.

Which work is newly reuyued,
coyrected, and published by the
Chirurgions of the same
Hospital now bæing.
An. 1577.

¶ Imprinted at London, by
Henry Bamforde

Fig. 5.

Vicary; secondly, that it was revived, i.e. revised, after his death by the surgeons who had been his colleagues at St. Bartholomew's Hospital. Clearly, therefore, the book was attributed to Vicary by those who had first-hand knowledge of his work. There must have been some previous copy from which this edition was revised, and Aikin, in his *Biographical Memoirs of Medicine in Great Britain*, published in 1780, says of Vicary: 'the name of this person deserves recording as the author of the first anatomical work written in the English language. . . . The title of his work is "A Treasure for Englishmen containing the Anatomie of Man's Body", printed London 1548'. No trace of this book has been found in spite of a diligent search by many persons extending over many years.

Dr. Frank Payne made a critical examination of the book as it was revised in 1577,[1] and showed conclusively that it was an abridgement of a manuscript which was then in his possession, and which I have seen, the work of an English surgeon whose personality is clearly displayed though his name is not given, and it is in the English language. The date of composition is given in the text as the year of our Lord 1392, but the manuscript itself was probably written about a century later. Vicary's *Anatomy* is practically a compilation from this manuscript. He omits a great deal and abbreviates a great deal, for his treatise is not more than half as long as his copy. The quotations from ancient writers are given very loosely and inaccurately by Vicary, but they are the same as those given fully in the manuscript. Dr. Payne therefore came to the conclusion that Vicary was in possession of a copy of this treatise, of which he made an abridgement, using the same words, sometimes not understanding them, and brought it out as his own; or alternatively, as one does not like to think of Vicary as an actual literary impostor and there is another possibility, that Vicary did not profess to be the author.

[1] *Brit. M. J.*, 1896, i, 200.

'The only authentically known printed edition was brought out,' says Dr. Payne, 'fifteen years after his death by his colleagues at St. Bartholomew's Hospital, and they may have found a manuscript tract which they regarded as Vicary's, though he had never laid claim to it or published it as his. In any case the real author or compiler was our anonymous friend of the fourteenth century, about whom I wish I knew more. His book is, I think, interesting as an example of the medical language of the time. Vicary's book is not really an example of the language of his time, his nomenclature being quite out of date, though the spelling and diction are modernized.'

I am glad to be able to take the matter a step backwards and so clear my predecessor, Vicary, of the suspicion of literary forgery, and, at the same time, show that there is some truth in both Dr. Payne's hypotheses.

John Halle, a distinguished surgeon, who lived at Maidstone from his birth in 1529 to his death in 1568, was a younger contemporary of Vicary and one of his personal friends. In 1565 Halle produced an edition of Lanfranc's Surgery, and he thus describes his treatment of the work of that great Italian surgeon, who died in 1306:

'I dedicate this excellent compendious worke, called "Chirurgia parua Lanfranci", . . . which was translated out of Frenche into the olde Saxony englishe, about twoo hundred yeres past. Which I haue nowe not only reduced to our vsuall speache, by changyng or newe translating suche wordes, as nowe be inueterate, and growne out of knowledge by processe of tyme, but also conferred my labours in this behalf with other copies both in Frenche and latin; namely with maister Bacter, for his latine copie and Symon Hudie for his french copie, and other English copies; of the which I had one of John Chamber, and another of John Yates both very auncient, with other mo: whose good helpe hath not a little farthered me in these things, to the intent that it might perfectly come forth to a publique profite which to doe I was constreigned, not only because I would not truste too muche to myne owne rude iudgement: but also that by the authoritie of dyuers men of knowledge, this excellent worke (as it is worthy) may the more effectually be alowed and accepted.'

Halle also takes back the story of Vicary's *Anatomy* to a time antecedent to the edition of 1577, for he says in the prologue to his first treatise of Anatomy, which is dated 1565, that he is somewhat encouraged to publish it 'by the example of good maister Vicarie, late Sargeante chyrurgien to the queenes highness; who was the firste that euer wrote a treatyse of Anatomye in English (to the profite of his brethren chirurgiens and the helpe of younge studientes) as farre as I can learne'.

In 1588 John Read, an energetic surgeon living at Gloucester, published a treatise on Fistula which had been written by John of Arderne in 1376, and, as in the case of Vicary and Halle, he used a fifteenth-century English translation, though he also had an earlier Latin version before him, because he inserts a few lines which had been accidentally omitted in the English version.

Several deductions can be made from these facts. There is no doubt that Vicary compiled his treatise on anatomy and issued it with the full knowledge that it was already out of date, because he thought it would be useful to the students of the United Company of Barbers and Surgeons, which had been founded in 1540. There is little doubt that he pursued and perhaps originated the plan which Halle imitated. He borrowed a manuscript and copied it with such alterations as his limited knowledge of anatomy allowed. He did not know, or did not think it worth while to incorporate, the work of Vesalius or even of Geminus, who was one of his colleagues, as surgeon to King Edward the Sixth. Halle did his compilation more thoroughly, for he compared several manuscripts; Vicary condensed and compiled from a single manuscript; Read merely copied his original without change. The surgeons at this time seemed to have been in the same frame of mind as the Oxford graduates in the early Tractarian days, when Pusey and Newman set their pupils to work to edit the Fathers of the Church.

Vicary's *Anatomy*, however, served its purpose, for it

remained in print until 1651, and the following editions appeared:

Edition.			Publisher or Printer.
(1) During the lifetime of Vicary .			? Publisher.
(2) 1577 in 12mo .	.	.	Henry Bamforde.
(3) 1586 ,, 4to .	.	.	John Windet for John Perin.
(4) 1587 ,, ,, .	.	.	George Robinson for John Perin.
(5) 1596 ,, ,, .	.	.	T. Creede.
(6) 1599 ,, ,, .	.	.	T. Creede.
(7) 1613 ,, ,, Called 6thly		.	Thomas Creede.
(8) 1626 ,, ,, ,, 7thly		.	B. Alsop and T. Fauucet.
(9) 1633 ,, ,, ,, 8thly		.	Bar. Alsop & Tho. Fawcet.
(10) 1641 ,, ,, ,, 9thly		.	B. Alsop and T. Fawcet.
(11) 1651 ,, 12mo .	.	.	T. Fawcet. Sold by J. Nuthall.
(12) 1888 ,, 8vo .	.	.	N. Truebner & Co.

The title-page of the 1586 edition (Fig. 6)—except for the change of the printer's name and the date—remained until the 1613 edition, when a section was added of 'Oynments and Plaisters; | with especiall and approved remedies for the Plague, and | Pestilent Fever, which never came to light before this | present; By W. B. Practitioner in Physicke | and Chyrurgerie'.

W. B. was W. Boraston of Salop. This edition was further enriched by a whole plate engraving of a skeleton moralizing, with a tomb in the background, and 'Sic transit gloria Mundi' as a legend. The 1641 edition also has a plate of the distribution of the veins.

The book had really fulfilled its purpose, but it was thought worth while to publish it once again in a smaller form and with an altered title. Accordingly in 1651 this 12mo appeared with the title-page in red and black inside a ruled border (Fig. 7).

The edition of 1888 is published by the Early English Text Society, and was edited by Dr. F. J. Furnivall and his son Percy Furnivall, using the text of the 1577 edition.

The Englishemans Treasure thus had a long career, but it probably owed its sale to the number of receipts it contained and not to the *Anatomy*, which was long out of date when the book first appeared. Indeed, as showing how

THE ENGLISHE-MANS TREASVRE,

OR TREASOR FOR ENGLISHMEN:

VVith the true Anatomye of Mans
Body, Compiled by that excellent
chirurgion Maifter Thomas Vicary
Efquire Sergeant Chirurgion to King
Henry the 8. To King Edward the 6.
To Queene Mary. And to our
Soueraigne Lady Queene
Elizabeth.

And alfo cheefe Chirurgion to S. Bartholomewes hofpit all.

Wherunto are annexed many fecrets appertaining to Chirurgery, *with diuers excellent approued Remedies for all difeafes* the
which are in man or woman, with emplafters of fpeciall cure
with other potions and drinkes approued in Phifike.

Alfo the rare treafor of the Englifh Bathes, Written by
William Turner, Doctor in Phificke.

Gathered and fet forth for the benefit of his friendes and
countrimen in England by *William Bremer* Practitioner in Phificke and Chirurgery.

AT LONDON,
¶ Imprinted by Iohn VVindet for Iohn Perin
dwelling in Paules Church-yard at the figne of the Angell,
and are there to be fold. 1586.

Fig. 6.

THE
SURGIONS
DIRECTORIE,
FOR
Young Practitioners,

In Anatomie Wounds, and Cures, &c.

SHEWING,

The Excellencie of divers Secrets
belonging to that noble Art and
Mysterie.

Very usefull in these Times upon any
sodaine Accidents.

And may well serve,

*As a noble Exercise for Gentle-
women,* and others ; who desire Science in
Medicine and Surgery, for a
generall Good.

Divided into X. *Parts.*
(Whose Contents follow in the next Page.)

Written by *T. Vicary* Esquire, Chyrurgion
to *Hen.* 8. *Edw.* 6. *Q. Mary. Q. Eliz.*

LONDON,

Printed by *T. Fawcet* dwelling in *Shoo-
Lane,* at the Signe of the *Dolphin.* 1651.
And are to be sold by *F. Nuthall,* at his Shop in
Fleetstreet at the signe of *Hercules* Pillers.

FIG. 7.

little attention was paid by the successive editors, it may be noted that the mistranslation which appears on page 44 of the 1586 edition is unchanged in the 1651 edition [p. 66]. The passage runs: 'The seconde portion of the guttes is called jejunium, for he is evermore emptie, for to him lyeth evermore the chest of the Gal beating him sore, and draweth forth of him al the drosse, and cleanseth him cleane.' This is a misreading of the manuscript, which has 'Biting him sore', referring to the supposed irritant properties of the bile.

I feel that I have done my duty to Thomas Vicary by showing that he was not a purloiner of other men's brains, but that the *Anatomy* was issued originally as part of a scheme to go back to old writers at a time when surgery was just beginning to take a new lease of life after the dead period of the Wars of the Roses.

(iii) *'The Ordre of the Hospital of S. Bartholomewes in West-Smythfielde in London'*

The third book I wish to speak about is a small book of Orders issued in 1552 for the government of St. Bartholomew's Hospital (Fig. 8). It presents few points of bibliographical interest, but, such as they are, it is as well to place them on record. The colophon of the 1552 edition states that the book was 'imprinted at London by Ry|charde Grafton, Printer to the | Kynges maiestie. | Cum priuilegio ad imprimen-|dum solum'. Bound up with it is a pamphlet containing the 'Orders taken and Enacted for Orphans with their porcions. Anno. MDLI'; an Order about Carts, and another on Dues for Tythes.

Strype, in his edition of Stow, says that it was reprinted in 1580, but this appears to be an error. It was certainly reprinted as a quarto in 1652 under the title 'Orders and Ordinances for the better government of the Hospitall of Bartholomew the lesse'. 'As also Orders enacted for Orphans and their portions MDLXXX. Together with a Briefe Discourse of the laudable Customes of London. London, Printed by James Flesher, Printer to that

The ordre of the hospital of .S. Bar-tholomewes in west-smythfielde in London.

¶ I. Epist. Jhon. ij. Chap.

He that sayeth he walketh in the lyght, and hateth his
brother, came neuer as yeat in the lyght. But
he that loueth his brother, he dwel-
leth in the lyght.

LONDINI,
ANNO
1552.

Fig. 8.

Honourable City 1652.' This reprint is abridged, as the prayers are omitted, since the Church of England was in abeyance during the Commonwealth. The abridged reprint appears in full in Strype's edition of Stow.[1] In 1884 Mr. Morrant Baker—a surgeon to St. Bartholomew's Hospital—reprinted the 1652 edition with a prefatory note in *Saint Bartholomew's Hospital Reports*.[2] In 1885 he caused some separate copies to be struck off in quarto and prefixed a typo-etching of an engraving of the Hospital in 1720. This reprint is in special type, and has the ornaments copied from the 1652 edition. The ornament on page 35 has been inadvertently transposed by the printer. In 1885 Mr. Morrant Baker issued privately an abstract of *The Orders and Ordinances* in a quarto volume with the heading 'The Two foundations of St. Bartholomew's Hospital A.D. 1123 and A.D. 1546'. This volume has an engraving of Rahere's tomb, copied from that in the *Vetusta Monumenta*, and bears the imprint of Smith, Elder & Co. Fourteen copies were struck off in folio size.

The 1552 edition was reprinted in full by Dr. F. J. Furnivall and Mr. Percy Furnivall as an appendix to their edition of Vicary's *Anatomy* in the Early English Text Society's Publications, London, 1888. An abstract of the 1552 edition is also given by Sir Norman Moore in his *History of St. Bartholomew's Hospital*.[3] The copy of this little book now in the British Museum belonged, says Sir Norman Moore, to King Edward VI. It is mentioned by J. G. Nichols, *Literary Remains of King Edward VI*, Roxburghe Club, 1857. The volume, when Mr. Nichols wrote, seems to have had its original binding stamped with 'E. vi. R.' and roses and crowns. This was no doubt decayed, as the book now has a modern binding. Sir Norman Moore further notes that 'on the title-page of "The Ordre" is written Y. 24. 2, which may perhaps be the pressmark of the Royal Library'.

The preface of the 1552 edition gives the following

[1] Lond. 1720. Vol. ii, Book 6, Appendix, p. 51.
[2] *St. Barth. Hosp. Rep.*, 1884, xx.   [3] 1918, ii. 164.

account of the genesis of the book. It states that in five years, after the foundation of the Hospital, 'there haue bene healed of the Pocques, Fistules, filthie Blaynes and Sores, to the nombre of .viij. hundred, and thence saufe deliuered, that other hauyng nede myghte entre in their roume; Beside eyght skore and .xii. that haue there forsaken this life, in their intollerable miseries and griefes, whiche elles might haue died, and stoncke in the iyes & noses of the Citie, if thys place had not vouchedsaufe to become a poompe alone, to ease a commune abhorryng'. The citizens that had the care of the Hospital were exclaimed against even in the pulpits, as if they had wronged this charity by the mistaken supposition that this Hospital should have made a general sweep of all the poor and afflicted, and so for their care the governors were rewarded with nothing but open detraction.

Upon this slander so widely spread, 'It is thought good to the Lord Mayour of thys Citie of London, as chief patrone and gouvernour of this Hospitall, in the name of the Citie, to publishe at this present the officiers and ordres by hym appoincted and from time to tyme practysed and vsed by twelue of the Citizeins moste auncient, in their courses, . . . partly for the staye and redresse of such slaundre and partly for that it myght be an open wytness, and knowledge vnto all men, howe thynges are administred there & by whom', and likewise to excite all well-disposed persons more and more to bestow their charity here.

The Orders are quite interesting and must have been extremely well thought out, for with a few minor changes and necessary additions they regulate the working of the Hospital to this day. Each officer of the Hospital still receives a Charge or definition of his duties when he is first appointed, and each Charge, in the case of the subordinate officials, concludes with the words: 'This is your charge and office with the which ye have to do and not with any other thing, neither with any other office in this house. But if you shall perceive at any time any thing done

by any officer or other person of this house that shall be
unprofitable thereunto, or that may be occasion of any dis-
order, or shall engender slander to the same that ye then
declare it to the Treasurer or Almoners or to one of them
and no farther to meddle therein.' I received this injunction so frequently in the course of my service at the Hospital that I was quite pleased to be told, when I reached
the highest ranks, that it was part of my duty to see that
the affairs of the Hospital were well ordered and managed.

The 1552 edition of the Orders contains the daily service, which is omitted in all the reissues except Dr. Furnivall's. The regulations order

'A daily seruice for the poore. At the Houre of eyght of the Clocke
in the mornyng, and .iiij. of the clock at the afternoone, throughout
the whole yeare, there shal a bel be rong the space of halfe a quarter
of an houre, and immediately upon the seassyng of the bell, (the
poore liyng in their beddes that cannot aryse; & kneling on their
knees that can aryse in euery warde, as their beddes stande,) they
shal by course, as many as can rede, begyn these praiers folowyng.
And after that the partie, whose course it shalbe, hath begon, all
the rest in the warde shal folow and aunswere, vpon paine to be
dismissed out of the house. And thryse in the weke, that is to saie,
Sondaie, Wedensdaie and Fridaie, they shal saie the letany in maner
and forme as it is [at] thende of this booke. The minister shal
begyn and the rest shal folowe.'

The morning service was of considerable length. It
began with the Lord's Prayer and responses; two psalms;
an anthem; a third psalm; the lesson; the Benedicite; the
Kyrie; the Creed; more responses and prayers for the
King, the Governors of the Hospital, and the sick poor
themselves.

The afternoon prayers were no shorter; they consisted
of the Lord's Prayer and responses; the 86th and the 96th
psalm; the lesson and the 57th psalm with the Kyrie and
'all the suffrages and Collectes vsed in the mornyng
praier'. There was also 'The Euensong praier at .vii. of
the clock at nyght', consisting of the Lord's Prayer, responses, the 121st psalm, and a collect. The day's prayers

ended with the words: 'God saue our souereigne lorde the kyng, al the Gouernours of this house & the holie chirche vniversal and graunt vs peace in Christ and grace for euer. Amen!'

These prayers must have taken up a considerable portion of each day, and the minister and his staff were not overpaid, as appears from the entry, 'To the ministers of the churche within the Hospitall that is to saie to a Vicare, a clerck & a sextein . . . xxiii.l. vi.s. viii.d.' Although the prayers were omitted in editions subsequent to the original, all the reissues contain a passport which was in common form and was given to every patient of the Hospital who came from a distance to enable him to get home safely and without molestation from the authorities. It runs:

'A PASSEPORT to be deliuered to the Poore. To all Maiours, Bailiefs, Constables &c. Know ye, that A.B., taileur, borne in the towne of S.T. in the countie of Northampton, beyng cured of his disease in the Hospital of St. Bartholomews in West smithfield in London, and from thence deliured the .xiii. daie of August, in the syxt yeare of the Reigne, &c. hath charge by vs, A.B.C. the gouernours of the same, to repaire within   days next ensuyng the date herof, to his sayd place of natiuitie, or to Westhandfield the place of his last abode, and there to exhibite this present passeport to the head officer, or officers, in either of the places appointed, that they maie take further order for his demeanour.'

Sir Norman Moore [1] says 'the carriers to Northamptonshire started from the Ram in Smithfield and the proximity of this Inn to the Hospital gate may explain why that county chances to be mentioned in the passport'.

There is one Order which is of especial interest, for to it we owe the unbroken series of records which are in the possession of the Hospital. It is:

'An Order for the saufe kepyng of the euidences and writeinges apperteining to the Hospitall. There shall one fayre and substanciall chest be prouided and the same be set in the moste conuenient and surest place of the house the which shal haue .iii. seuerall lockes and iii keyes, whereof the President alwaies to haue one, & the

---

[1] Op. cit., ii, 182.

Treasourer one and a Commoner appointed by the whole house to haue the thirde. And it shal not be laufull to any of the Gouernours to haue any specialtie, euidence or writyng out of the said chest, neither any other persone, to cary any of them out of the house (no, though it be for the affaires of the said house) but onlie a copie therof which shalbe taken in the presence of the .iii. persones aboue named, that haue the keyes & the original forthwith to be locked up agayne.'

The books were ordered to be kept by 'The Renter Clerk'. They were a Repertory, a book of Survey, a book of Accounts, and a Journal.

'And first you shall note that before euery of these Bookes ye must haue a Calendre, into the whiche ye may entre, by order of letters of the A.B.C. all proper names & matters that shall be conteyned in every of them. And for the better accomplishyng hereof, ye shall, with your penne, in the heade of the lefe, nombre the pages of euery lefe, in euery of these bookes, and then addyng in your Calendre the nombre of the page where the name or matter is entred in your boke, the reader without any difficultie may tourne to the same.

'The Vse of the first boke called a Repertory. Into this booke shall ye first entre the foundacion of this Hospital, and also al dedes, obligacions, acquitaunces and other specialties; vsyng alwaies in the margent of the sayde booke to note in a fewe Englyshe wordes, the somme and content of euerye article of these wrytynges that shall appiere noteworthie; and the same notes particularly to enter into their seueral and propre places of your calendre, accordyng to the order of the A.B.C.'

In the book of the Survey were to be entered all matters connected with the property of the Hospital, and the cost of repairs, &c.

'The Vse of the third booke, called a Booke of Accomptes, was to contain all the Accomptes (being allowed by the auditours). And for the ready fyndyng of euery matter conteined in euery accompt, ye shal in the margent of this boke, vse as is aforesaid, to note dyuers generall wordes, *Accomptes, prouisions, liueries, giftes, legacies, revuardes, agreementes, Surrenders, Bargaynes, Sutes, recoueries, pencions, Fees,* &c. Addyng to euery of these, beyng placed in your calender, the lefe wher euery of them is mencioned in any of the accomptes conteined in this booke, that at a woorde may be sene what hath bene done in all these thynges, from the first Treasaurour to the last. And in the ende ye shall manifestly declare the names and sirenames of so many diseased persones as that yeare haue bene cured and deliuered out of this house, and also the names and sirenames of so many as that yeare haue died in the house. The names and sirenames also of as many as then shall remaine sycke and diseased in thys house together with the name of the shier where-in eche was borne & their faculties, exercise, or occupacions.

'The Use of the .iiii. boke called a Iournall. This Booke must also haue a Calender; & it shal alwaies be brought furthe at suche tyme as the President and moste parte of the Gouernours shall sit within this Hospitall for the generall affaires of the same. And into this booke shall ye entre all suche orders & decrees, as from tyme to tyme shall by the sayde Gouernours or greatest part of them be decreed and ordeined. And in the margent thereof ye shall do as before is assigned . . . in few words set furth the somme of euery decree, order &c. conteyned therein. And chiefely ye shall vse the generall woordes before described in the booke of accomptes, that by the enteraunce of them into your calender euery matter may easilie and readylie be founde. And ye shall not fayle, but in fyue dayes next after the enteraunce of any thyng into this booke, to enter the same by a generall worde in to the Calendre, that as wel when you are absent, as present, the gouernours may without difficultie be satisfied of that they seke for therein.'

These admirable orders were carried out by the successive Clerks to the Hospital, with the result that Sir Norman Moore was able to write a very complete history of the Hospital.

VII

DR. WILLIAM HARVEY AND ST. BARTHOLO-MEW'S HOSPITAL

SIR JAMES PAGET, in his *Records of Harvey*, and
Sir Norman Moore, in his *History of St. Bartholomew's
Hospital*, have gathered all that is known about Dr. William Harvey from the Journals and Minute books of the
Hospital. I can do little more, therefore, than blend what
they have written.

I have long wished to know why Harvey did not go
back to Cambridge on his return from Padua in 1602,
and why he attached himself to our hospital rather than
to St. Thomas's, which, being then on the Surrey side of
London Bridge, was a little nearer to his home at Folkestone; at that time every additional mile on a journey was
a serious consideration. At the beginning of his career
Harvey was more engaged in the study of anatomy and
experimental physiology than upon clinical medicine, and
such work could have been done as well, or perhaps better,
at Cambridge than in London. His energy may have told
him that he was unsuited for college life, and that he
needed the larger sphere of action open to him in London.
How great was his energy was shown more than thirty
years later, when the Earl of Arundel wrote to the Rev.
William Petty from Ratisbon, saying, 'I hope I shall see
that little perpetual movement called Dr. Harvey here
before my going'.

I should like to think that Inigo Jones was the cause of
Harvey's coming to us. We know that the great architect
and the great physiologist were friends in later life, because
in 1655, three years after the death of Inigo Jones, John
Webb published *Stonehenge Restored*, at 'the instigation of
Harvey and Selden', a work which Jones had left unfinished; but there is nothing to show when the friendship
began.

Inigo Jones was five years older than Harvey. He was

the son of a cloth-worker and, although a Roman Catholic, was baptized in the Church of St. Bartholomew-the-Less on 6 July 1573. His parents, therefore, must have been living within the hospital precincts, though they moved afterwards to a house in Paul's Wharf, close to where St. Paul's Station now stands.

Inigo Jones was sent to Italy in 1597 to study painting and architecture at the expense of William Herbert, third Earl of Pembroke, his father dying shortly before he went abroad. Inigo never married, but left his three sisters— Joan, Judith, and Mary—to take care of the house whilst he was away and, as they were a very affectionate family, it remained his home as long as he lived. He returned to London in 1604, after visiting Denmark; Harvey returned from Italy two years earlier.

Europe was comparatively safe for travellers before the outbreak of the Thirty Years' War in 1618, if they chose to travel with an armed retinue, as was then the custom. Spa and Padua were the chief continental resorts of wealthy Englishmen. Both had baths where a cure could be taken, and Padua had the additional advantage of a University within easy reach of Genoa, Venice, Florence, and Milan. It was unsafe to travel further south, and no wise Protestant visited Rome, except as a passing traveller, lest he should excite suspicion of his orthodoxy when he returned home. He might stay as long as he liked at Padua and Venice, where he was a welcome visitor. It thus happened that both these towns had a colony of influential and art-loving Englishmen, and we are not justified in thinking of Padua merely as a University town where the best of the rising generation of English physicians received a part of their medical education. Inigo Jones spent the greater part of his time at Venice, Harvey at Padua; and I should like to think that the two young geniuses began their friendship at this period. Harvey may even have prescribed for those 'sharp vomitings' from which Inigo Jones suffered during the greater part of his life, and which he attributed 'to the spleen and vomiting

melancholy', though it would now be called migraine or
sick headache. Harvey certainly treated him later in life,
but without much effect, although the attacks were becoming less frequent and were not so severe. Harvey, too,
had more than a general knowledge of the fine arts, for he
was selected by the Earl of Arundel—one of the greatest
collectors of art treasures at a time when such collectors
were at their zenith—to accompany him to the Palatinate
in 1636, whence he was sent to Venice to buy pictures for
King Charles I, himself a connoisseur.

Now when Harvey came back to London he may have
brought an introduction from Inigo Jones to his three
sisters at their house in Paul's Wharf, with instructions
to tell them of their brother's work and plans. The girls
had early memories of the hospital, within whose gates
they had been born, and they, in turn, may have introduced the lively young doctor, newly arrived from Italy,
to the hospital authorities and to Dr. Lancelot Browne,
whose daughter Elizabeth he married at St. Sepulchre's
on 24 November 1604.

But this is all guesswork, and the first documentary
evidence of Harvey's connexion with St. Bartholomew's
Hospital exists in the minute dated Saturday, 25 February
1608–9, when at a Court of Governors, with Sir John
Spencer, President, in the chair, and in the presence of
twelve other Governors,

'Mr. William Harvey, doctor of physic, made suit for the reversion
of the office of physician of this house when the same shall be next
void and brought the King's Majestie his letters directed to the
Governors of this house in his behalf and shewed forth a testimony
of his sufficiency for the same place under the hand of Mr. Dr.
Adkyns, president of the College of the Physicians & divers other
doctors of the ancientest of the said College. It is granted at the
contemplation of his Majestie's letters that the said Mr. Harvey
shall have the said office next after the decease or other departure
of Mr. Dr. Wilkenson who now holdeth the same with the yearly
fee and duties thereunto belonging, So that then he be not found
to be otherwise employed that may let and hinder the charge of the
same office which belongeth thereunto.'

This method of reversionary appointment put the person appointed in a position somewhat similar to that now occupied by an assistant physician, for he was expected to perform the duties of the holder of the office when he was absent from any cause, but without payment. It lasted from 1547 until Dr. John Clarke was appointed assistant physician to Harvey in 1634.

Dr. Wilkenson must have been ill when Harvey was appointed to the reversion of his office, because on 28 August of the same year

'Mr. William Harvey, doctor of physic, came before the Governors beforenamed [i.e. Mr. Gayus Newman, Mr. Shawe, Mr. Bewblock, Mr. Ireland, Mr. Aungell, and Mr. Woodforde] and is contented to execute the office of physician of this house until Michaelmas next without any recompense for his pains therein; which office Mr. Dr. Wilkenson late deceased held. And Mr. Doctor Harvey being asked whether he is not otherwise employed in any other place which may let or hinder the execution of the office of the physician towarde the poor of this hospital; hath answered that he is not, wherefore it is thought fit by the said Governors that he supply the same office until the next Court, And then Mr. Doctor Harvey to be a suitor for his admittance to the said place according to a grant thereof to him heretofore made.'

Accordingly on Saturday, 14 October 1609, in the presence of Sir John Spencer, the President, and fifteen other Governors, 'Mr. William Harvey, doctor of physic, is admitted to the office of physician to this hospital, which Mr. Doctor Wilkenson deceased late held according to a former grant to him made and the charge of the said office has been read unto him'.

The charge directed him to 'attend one day in the week at least or oftener as need shall require and cause the Hospitaler, Matron or Porter to call before you in the Hall of this hospital such and so many of the poor harboured in this hospital as shall need the counsel and advice of the physician'. It was also told him that 'you shall not for favour, lucre or gain appoint or write anything for the poor but such good and wholesome things as you shall think fit with your best advice will do the poor good without any affection or respect to be had to the apothecary'.

The office of physician carried with it the right to rent a house within the hospital, but as Harvey was living at the time in Knightrider Street, and none of the houses in the hospital were vacant, he did not claim the privilege until 28 July 1614, when

'it is thought meet by this Court that Mr. Doctor Harvey or his successor physician for this hospital shall have the houses now or late in the tenures of Mistress Gardner and Dr. Bonham with a parcel of the garden now in the tenure of William Allen in West Smithfield after the expiration of the lease sometime granted to Robert Chidley gent, which the said William Allen now holdeth. And the same then to be divided and laid forth at the discretion of the Governors of this house for so long time as he shall be Doctor to this house for such yearly rent and upon such conditions as this Court shall think fit.'

The hospital did not come into possession until twelve years later, for it was not until 31 March 1626, when Sir Thomas Bennett was President, that

'Mr. Doctor Harvey, physician to this hospital, made suit to have the house in West Smithfield late in the tenure of Widow Allen deceased according to a former grant. It is ordered that if he will sufficiently repair the same in all manner of reparations to the contentment of the Governors and give the yearly rent of £13.6.8; or otherwise pay the yearly rent of £20 and the said house to be repaired at the charge of this hospital, Then he to hold the same so long as he shall be Doctor to this hospital and shall inhabit the same and shall give his personal attendance for the visitation of the poor of this hospital. And Mr. Treasurer, Mr. Pallmer, Mr. Hill, Mr. Strangwayes and such other of the Governors as shall meet on Monday next to confer with him accordingly.'

It appears that Harvey took some time to consider the Governors' offer, and he probably took the advice of his younger brothers, who were all good business men, for it was agreed on 9 June

'that forasmuch as Mr. Doctor Harvey, physician of this hospital, hath been warned to this Court to give his answer whether he will accept of the offer made to him at the last Court of a Messuage or Tenement in Smithfield late in the tenure of Sara Allen widow deceased according to an order then set down who hath refused to take the same accordingly. It is therefore thought good for the benefit of the poor of this hospital that if he shall not accept thereof before the 19th day of this instant month, Then it is granted that John Meredith Skynner shall have a lease of the same tenement for 31 years if he and Elizabeth his now wife shall so long live, for the fine of £100 to be paid at the sealing and the yearly rent of £4 and he to bestow in and upon the same tenement in needful reparations within one year next following the sum of £100 and to be bound to all reparations.'

The incident is closed with the minute on 7 July 1626, that 'it is granted that Mr. Doctor Harvey, physician, shall have his stipend being £25 per annum augmented to the sum of £33 6s. 8d. in consideration that he do relinquish all his claim of any former grant of a house in Smithfield late in the tenure of Widow Allen which was ordered for him, who hath refused to take the same upon such conditions as this Court hath thought fit'.

It thus happened that Harvey never lived within our gates.

It will be remembered that Dr. John Caius, afterwards the founder of Caius College, Cambridge, lived for many years in a house just inside and on the right of the entrance gate from Smithfield when he was teaching anatomy at the Barbers and Surgeons' Hall in Monkwell Street. He was a solitary man who never married, and the inventory taken after his death—for he returned to it to die—states that there was a hall containing most of the chairs and the table; a bedchamber and a room over the bedchamber; a chamber over the hall; a garret and a kitchen where the servant probably slept, because it contained a bed. He led the life of a recluse, for Parkhurst, who was afterwards Bishop of Norwich, wrote to his friend Conrad Gesner, the Professor of Natural History at Zürich, on 21 May 1559, a few months after Caius had been elected Master of the newly-founded College:

'As soon as I came to London I sought out your friend Caius that I might give him your letter; and, as he was from home I delivered it to his maid servant for he has no wife nor ever had one. Not a week passes in which I do not go to his house two or three times. I knock at the door, a girl answers the knock but without opening the door and peeping through the crevice asks me what I want. I ask in reply, where is her master? whether he is ever at home, or means to be? she always denies him to be in the house. He seems to be everywhere and nowhere and is now abroad; so that I do not know what to write about him. I shall certainly tell him something to his face whenever I do chance to meet him, and he shall know what kind of man he has to deal with.'

Caius was never attached to the hospital but rented the house from 1551, paying a rent of £4 a year until 1567, when he was granted a lease for twenty years at an annual rent of £2 13s. 4d. He died on 29 July 1573.

The hospital records appear to contain no further allusion to Harvey until 21 January 1629–30, when he appeared before the Court of Governors and declared

'that he is commanded by the King's most excellent Majesty to attend the illustrious Prince the now Duke of Lenox in his travels beyond the seas and therefore desireth that this Court would allow of (Edmund) Smith, doctor in physic, for his deputy in performance of the office of physician for the poor of this hospital during his absence. It is thought fit that the Governors of this hospital have further knowledge and satisfaction of the sufficiency of the said Mr. Smith, Then they to make their choice either of him or some other whom they shall think meet for the execution of the same place during the absence of the said Dr. Harvey.'

The Duke of Lenox was James Stewart, afterwards first Duke of Richmond, a staunch adherent of King Charles I. He was at this time a young man of twenty-one, who had just left Cambridge and was about to make the grand tour through France, Spain, and Italy. The details of Harvey's movements during this tour have not yet been completely unravelled, although sufficient material exists for doing so, and it was probably during this period that he revisited Italy.

For some reason Dr. Smith was not a *persona grata*, and on 25 April 1631, at a meeting of the Governors held at the Mansion House in the presence of Sir Robert Ducie, Lord Mayor, President, 'it is granted that Richard Andrewes, doctor in physic, shall have the reversion next avoidance and place of physician to this hospital after the death, resignation or other departure of Dr. Harvey now physician to this hospital late sworn physician in ordinary for His Majesty's household with a yearly stipend thereunto now belonging'. Harvey's attendance on the King led him to be so frequently absent from the hospital that on 19 January 1632–3,

'it hath been thought convenient upon the complaint of some of the chirurgeons of this hospital that whereas Doctor Harvey, physician for the poor of the said hospital, by reason of his attendance on the King's Majesty cannot so constantly be present with the poor as heretofore he hath been, but sometimes doth appoint his deputy for the same, That therefore Dr. Andrewes, physician in reversion of the same place to this hospital, in the absence of Dr. Harvey do supply the same place whereby the said poor may be more respected and Dr. Andrewes the better acquainted to perform the same office when it shall fall, and in the meantime to be recompensed by this Court yearly as shall be thought fit. This order not to prejudice Dr. Harvey in his yearly fee or in any other respect than aforesaid.'

A few months later, on 13 May 1633,

'this day came into this Compting House Dr. Smith, physician, by the appointment of Dr. Harvey, physician to this hospital, who is to attend the King's Majesty into Scotland and tendered his service to Mr. Treasurer and other the Governors for the poor in the behalf and absence of Doctor Harvey. Answer was made by Mr. Treasurer that Dr. Andrewes, physician in reversion to this house, was by the Court ordered to attend the occasions of this house in the absence of Doctor Harvey and to have allowance from this house accordingly. Nevertheless if Doctor Smith pleased to accompany Doctor Andrewes in the business, this house would be very well content, under which Doctor Smith replied that if Doctor Andrewes were appointed and did perform accordingly; There is no need of two.'

In spite of this Dr. Smith appears to have taken a part in the work of the hospital during the absence of Harvey in Scotland. On 15 October 1633, 'on the motion of Dr. Harvey it is granted that Mr. Treasurer shall pay unto Dr. Smith who is the deputy of Dr. Harvey and by him appointed in his absence to visit the poor of this hospital the sum of £10 in gratuity from this Court and he is thereupon entreated in respect that the hospital hath now two physicians that he do not henceforth trouble himself any more to visit or prescribe to the poor of this hospital'. Dr. Smith, who lived in Shoe Lane, was a graduate of Caius College, and was a lifelong friend of Harvey. He was a staunch Royalist, and was later with the King at Oxford. He survived only a fortnight the opening of the Harveian Museum in 1653, of which he and Dr. Prujean were such active promoters that his name appeared upon the frieze outside the building, which ran in letters three inches long, 'Suasu et curâ Fran. Prujeani, praesidis et Edmundi Smith, elect: inchoata et perfecta est haec fabrica An. Mdcliii'. [This building was begun and finished in the year 1653, at the suggestion and under the eye of Francis Prujean, the President, and Edmund Smith, an Elect.] Dr. Richard Andrewes, on the other hand, was a graduate of St. John's College, Oxford. He was educated at Merchant Taylors' School, and probably had the active support of the Merchant Taylors' Company, which would account for his being preferred to Dr. Smith.

It was during this visit to Scotland that Charles was crowned at Holyrood, and Harvey took the opportunity to visit the Bass Rock, of which he gives such an interesting description in the eleventh essay of his treatise *De Generatione*. Harvey was in London again in October 1633, for on the 5th day of this month, 'upon the motion of Dr. Harvey, physician to this house, It is thought fit that Tuesday senight in the afternoon be the time that the Governors shall hear himself and the Chirurgions upon some particulars concerning the good of the poor of this house and reformation of some orders conceived to be in this house, And the Chirurgions and the Apothecary to be warned to meet accordingly. And Mr. Alderman Mowlson, Sir Maurice Abbott, Mr. Alderman Perry and others the Governors here present are entreated to meet at the compting house to hear and determine the same'. Accordingly, on the 15th of October, A. D. 1633, in the presence of Sir Robert Ducie, Knight and Baronet, President, and others of the Governors,

'this day Dr. Harvey, physician to this hospital, presented to this Court certain articles for the good and benefit of the poor of this house, which the Governors have taken into their considerations and do allow and order them to be put in practice. And all defaults in the not performance of any of the said articles to be corrected and amended by the Governors as they in their discretions shall think fit and convenient.

'Forasmuch as the poor of this house are increased to a greater number than formerly have been to the great charge of this hospital and to the greater labour and more necessary attendance of a physician; and being much more also than is conceived one physician may conveniently perform.

'And Forasmuch as Dr. Harvey the now physician to this hospital is also chosen to be physician to His Majesty and thereby tied to daily service and attendance on His Majesty,

'It hath been thought fit and so ordered that there shall be for this present occasion two physicians for this hospital, and Dr. Andrewes physician in reversion be now admitted to be also an immediate physician to this hospital, And to have the salary or yearly fee of £23 6s. 8d. for his pains henceforth during the pleasure of this court.

'And this court for the long service of the said Dr. Harvey to this hospital and in consideration that he is physician to his Majesty do give and allow him leave and liberty to dispose of himself and time and to visit the poor no oftener than he in his discretion shall think fit.

'And it is ordred that Mr. Treasurer shall also pay unto the said Dr. Andrewes the sum of £20 for his pains taken in visiting and prescribing for the poor of this house for this year last past by the direction and at the request of the Governors of this house.'

On the same day Dr. Harvey,

'physician to this hospital presented to this court certain orders or articles by him thought fit to be observed and put in practice—viz.:

'1. That none be taken into the hospital but such as be curable or but a certain number of such as are incurable. Allowed.

'2. That those that shall be taken in for a certain time be discharged at that time by the hospitaler unless they obtain a longer time; And to be discharged at the end of that time also. In use.

'3. That all such as are certified by the doctor uncurable and scandalous or infectious shall be put out of the said house or to be sent to an out-house.[1] And in case of sudden inconvenience this to be done by the doctor or Apothecary. Allowed.

'4. That none be taken into any out-house on the charge of this hospital but such as are sent from hence. Allowed.

'5. That no chirurgion, to save himself labour, take in or present any for the doctor; otherwise the charge of the apothecary's shop will be so great and the success so little as it will be scandalous to the house. Allowed.

'6. That none lurk here for relief only or for slight causes. Allowed.

'7. That if any refuse to take their physic they may be discharged by the doctor or apothecary or punished by some order. Allowed.

'8. That the chirurgions in all difficult cases or where inward physic may be necessary shall consult with the doctor at the times he sitteth once in a week, and then the Master himself relate to the doctor what he conceiveth of the cure and what he hath done therein, And in a decent and orderly manner proceed by the doctor's directions for the good of the poor and credit of the house. Agreed unto.

'9. That no chirurgion or his man do trepan the head, pierce the body, dismember or do any great operation on the body of any but with the approbation and by the direction of the doctor (when conveniently it may be had) and the chirurgions shall think it needful to require. Agreed unto.

[1] The two institutions known as the Out-houses date back to very ancient times, and had probably been used as leper hospitals. They were originally six in number, and were situated at Mile End, Hammersmith, Highgate, Kingsland, Knightsbridge, and Old Kent Road. They gradually disappeared until only two remained—'the Out-house' in Kingsland Road which was appropriated to women suffering from venereal disease, and the 'Lock' in the Old Kent Road for men. The two junior assistant surgeons were appointed 'guides', or surgeons in charge of these out-houses, which were placed under the care of 'keepers', who were allowed fourpence a day for the diet of each patient. They retained to the end a certain religious character.

'10. That no chirurgion or his man practise by giving inward physic to the poor without the approbation of the doctor. Allowed.

'11. That no chirurgion be suffered to perform the cures in this house by his Boy or servant without his own oversight or care. Allowed.

'12. That every chirurgion shall show and declare unto the doctor, whensoever he shall in the presence of the patient require him, what he findeth and what he useth to every external malady; that so the doctor being informed may better with judgement order his prescriptions. The chirurgions protest against this.

'13. That every chirurgion shall follow the directions of the doctor in outward operations for inward causes for recovery of every patient under their several cures and to this end shall once in a week attend the doctor at the set hour he sitteth to give directions for the poor. Agreed by the chirurgions.

'14. That the Apothecary, Matron and Sisters do attend the doctor when he sitteth to give directions and prescriptions that they may fully conceive his directions and what is to be done. Allowed.

'15. That the Matron and Sisters shall signify and complain to the doctor or Apothecary in the doctor's absence if any poor lurk in the house and come not before the doctor when he sitteth, or taketh not his physic but cast it away and abuse it. Allowed.

'16. That the apothecary keep secret and do not disclose what the doctor prescribeth nor the prescriptions he useth but to such as in the doctor's absence may supply his place, and that with the doctor's approbation. Allowed.'

The surgeons at this time were Joseph Fenton, John Woodall, author of *The Surgeon's Mate*, 1617, and Henry Boone, with James Mullins, surgeon for the stone. Richard Eden was 'guide' to the Lock Hospital, and John Topliff was 'guide' at the Kingsland Spittal. Richard Glover was the apothecary, and Frances Worth was curer of scald heads.

On 7 August 1634, 'this day [John] Clarke, doctor in physic, is chosen to be assistant to Dr. Harvey, physician to this hospital, in the room and place of Dr. Andrewes, late deceased. And it is ordered that he have the salary of £33 6s. 8d. yearly paid to him for his pains during the pleasure of the court and the charge of the physician hath been read unto him which he hath promised in all parts faithfully to observe and perform, and this hospital do order that after Dr. Harvey his death or departure there be but one physician forthwards'. Harvey, however, outlived him, for he died on 30 April 1653, his place being taken on 13 May in that year by John Micklethwaite, who had been appointed physician in reversion on 26 May 1648.

Harvey ceased to be a regular attendant at the hospital from the time of Dr. Clarke's appointment. In 1636 he went to the Palatinate in the suite of the Earl of Arundel and visited Venice and Rome. In 1639, 1640, and 1641 he accompanied the King to Scotland on those ill-starred visits which marked the beginning of the Civil War. In August 1642, when the King left London for Nottingham, Harvey was in attendance 'not only with the consent but at the desire of the Parliament'. Previous to this he had official lodgings at Whitehall, and it was during his absence at this time that the mob of citizen soldiers entered his rooms, stole his goods, and scattered his papers. The papers consisted of the records of a large number of postmortem examinations, with his observations on the development of insects and a series of notes on comparative anatomy. How bitterly Harvey regretted the loss of these papers is recorded in his lamentation, 'let gentle minds forgive me, if, recalling the irreparable injuries I have suffered, I here give vent to a sigh. This is the cause of my sorrow;—whilst in attendance on his Majesty the King during our late troubles and more than civil wars not only with the permission but by the command of the Parliament, certain rapacious hands not only stripped my house of all its furniture but, what is a matter of far greater regret to me, my enemies have abstracted from my museum the fruits of many years of toil. Whence it came to pass that many observations, particularly on the generation of insects, have perished with detriment, I venture to say, to the republic of letters'.

Harvey was present at the Battle of Edgehill on 23 October 1642, and was in charge of the two Princes,

boys of ten and twelve years old, who afterwards became
Charles II and James II. All the morning was spent in
collecting the King's troops, and it was not until one
o'clock that the Royal army descended the steep hill leading to the wide plain in which stand the village of Radway
and the little town of Kineton. Harvey and the two
Princes had walked along the brow of the hill from the
inn at Sunrising to the Royalist head-quarters about a mile
further east and, tired of waiting, betook themselves to the
wide ditch at the very edge of the hill, where Harvey took
out a book and began to read. But he had not read very
long before the shot from a great gun grazed the ground
near him and made him move his place. We may feel sure
that this roused him to instant action. He put away his
book and began to attend the wounded, with such success
that, amongst others, he succeeded in reviving Adrian
Scrope, who had been stripped and left for dead on the
field.

After the battle Harvey accompanied the King to Oxford, and resided there until 1646, being incorporated
M.D. in the University on 7 December 1642, and serving
as Warden of Merton College in 1645.

The Treasurer and Governors of the hospital, realizing
that he was unlikely to do any more work for them, made
their last payment to him in 1643. His absence, too, was
noticed in other places, for the *Journal* of the House of
Commons records, under the date 12 February 1643/4:
'a motion this day made for Dr. Micklethwaite to be
recommended to the warden and masters of St. Bartholomew's Hospital to be physician in the place of Dr. Harvey
who hath withdrawn himself from his charge and is retired
to the party in arms against the Parliament.' The hospital
took no action and Dr. Micklethwaite was not formally
elected physician until 13 May 1653.

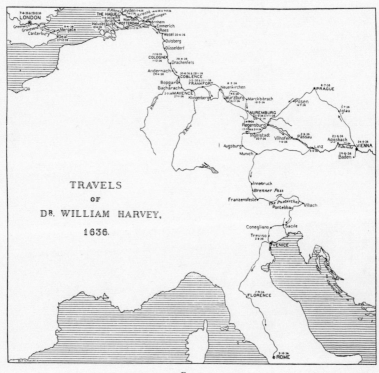

FIG. 9

VIII

A REVISED CHAPTER IN THE LIFE OF
DR. WILLIAM HARVEY, 1636

IT has long been known that Harvey travelled abroad
in the year 1636; that he left England in the train of
Thomas Howard, the second Earl of Arundel—the father
of virtu in England—when that nobleman was sent to
Vienna by King Charles I as Ambassador Extraordinary
to the Emperor Ferdinand II in the final stage of the
Palatinate discussion; that Harvey quitted the Mission at
Ratisbon, travelled to Italy, rejoined the Mission later in
the year, and returned with it to London in December.

It must often have been a matter of surprise to those
who thought about the matter why Harvey should have
been attached to the Mission at all; why, being attached,
he should have left it at a time when travelling was so
perilous, and why—strangest of all—when he visited
Venice, Florence, and Rome, he did not go to Padua,
where he would have been welcomed by some of his old
fellow-students. It is like an Oxford man, who, going to
Banbury and Warwick after an absence of thirty years,
should fail to take his Alma Mater on the way.

Accident has recently led me to read three books which
throw light upon Harvey's movements during the year
1636, and the information I have thus obtained is worthy
of record. The first work is 'A | Trve Relation | of All |
The Remarkable | Places | And | Passages Observed
In | the Travels of the right honourable | Thomas *Lord*
Howard, *Earle* of | Arundell and Surrey, Premer Earle,
and Earle | *Marshall of* England, | Ambassadour Extra-
ordinary to his sacred Majesty | *Ferdinando* the Second,
Emperour of *Germanie*. | *Anno Domini* 1636 | By *William
Crowne*, Gentleman.' It is a quarto pamphlet of 70 pages,
printed in London in 1637, and is the diary of William

Crowne from the day the Embassy left Greenwich on 7 April until it returned safely to Hampton Court on 30 December. It may be noted that Crowne's dates agree exactly with the few dated letters written by Harvey whilst he was abroad.

In 1911 the Historical Manuscripts Commission issued a report on the manuscripts of the Earl of Denbigh, preserved at Newnham Paddox, Warwickshire.[1] Amongst these manuscripts was a packet of letters written by Dr. Harvey to Basil Feilding afterwards the second Earl of Denbigh. The letters were written after Harvey had left England in the train of the Earl of Arundel, and show *inter alia* that he visited Italy with a direct commission from King Charles I. These letters were bought by Sir Thomas Barlow, who generously presented them to the Royal College of Physicians of London.

In 1915 Cecilia, Countess of Denbigh, published an interesting account of the first and second Earls of Denbigh under the title of *Royalist Father and Roundhead Son*. She gives a detailed account of Basil, Lord Feilding, to whom Harvey addressed these letters, and shows that, like the Earl of Arundel, he was a collector of art treasures and more especially of pictures.

It is a little difficult at first sight to explain why Harvey was chosen to accompany the Earl of Arundel, that stately nobleman of whom it was said that he 'resorted sometimes to Court because there only was a man greater than himself and went there the seldomer because there was a greater man than himself'. A little reflection will show that Thomas Parr was in all probability the link between the two men. The Earl had caused the old man to be brought up from Shropshire as a curiosity to show the King, his age being reputed to be 152. He died in London, and Harvey made an examination of his body on 16 May 1635. Harvey thus became known to the Earl, who conceived an affection for him, found that they had some artistic tastes in common, applied to have him

[1] Part v, Lond., 1911 (Cd. 5565).

attached to the Embassy, and eventually submitted to become his patient for the relief of an osteo-arthritis from which he suffered.

The Embassy started from Greenwich by barge at 3 a.m. on Thursday, 7 April 1636, dropped down the river to Gravesend, took coach there, and slept the night at Canterbury.

Leaving Canterbury on Friday, 8 April, they reached Margate in time for dinner, and at 3 p.m. embarked on the King's ship *The Happy Entrance*.

Saturday, 9 April, was spent at sea and a landing was made at Helvoets-sluis in Holland on Sunday morning. No time was lost in getting ashore, and after passing Briel the party crossed the river at Maas-sluis, went on by wagon to Delft and reached The Hague the same evening. The Queen of Bohemia, sister of King Charles I, sent her carriages a mile out of the town to meet the mission as the Earl Marshal was well known to her. He had been sent to The Hague in 1632, just after the death of her husband, to persuade her, but ineffectually, to return and settle in England.

The Embassy remained at The Hague from Sunday to Thursday, the time being spent in a series of visits to the Queen of Bohemia, the Prince of Orange, the States, and to the French, Venetian, and Swedish ambassadors.

The journey was continued on Thursday, 14 April, through Leyden and Woerden to Utrecht, where the night was spent. Harvey, however, was left behind at Leyden to look after Thomas, son of Mr. Secretary Windebank, who had fallen ill. The illness must have proved trivial, for Harvey had rejoined the party at Cologne on 21 April. Lord Arundel speaks of a visit to the Jesuit College and Church on that day, and says 'they received me with all civility', and then adds, jokingly, 'I found in the College honest little Doctor Harvey, who means to convert them'. If Harvey followed the mission from Leyden to Cologne he went to Utrecht, crossed the Rhine at Rhenen, slept at Arnhem, took boat at Emmerich, and slept at Wesel without landing, as the inhabitants were dying of the plague at the rate of thirty a day. He dined the next day at Duisberg, slept at Düsseldorff, and reached Cologne on the Wednesday or Thursday in Easter week. Crowne says of the church: 'The Jesuits have built them a very stately Church and richly adorned it with gildings and erected an Altar, one of the stateliest I ever saw; in the City likewise there is a great Church called the Dome.' The Jesuits' Church is still standing in Cologne. It was built in 1618–29 and, to our taste, the decoration is overdone. The party stopped at Cologne from Friday, 22 April, until Thursday, 28 April, when they proceeded up the Rhine in a boat drawn by nine horses past many villages which had been recently pillaged. The boat anchored the first night off Drachenfels and the party slept on board. On Friday they anchored for the night off Andernach. Saturday proved an eventful day, for the boat was shelled as it passed Coblenz but without injury, and the night was spent at Boppard. The journey was continued on Whit Sunday, 1 May, past Baccarach, 'where the poor people are found dead with grass in their mouths', to Assmannshausen, and on Whit Monday to Mainz, 'where we anchored. Heere likewise the poore people were almost starved, and those that could relieve others before now humbly begged to bee relieved, and after supper all had reliefe sent from the Ship ashore, at the sight of which they strove so violently that some of them fell into the Rhine and were like to have bin drowned'.

The whole journey so far was hazardous, for active hostilities were in progress, and the Ambassador's boats were accompanied at one time by a guard of soldiers on the bank, whilst at another the party went in deadly fear of the enemy's 'outliers', the freebooters of a guerrilla warfare. 'From Collein hither', says the chronicler of the voyage, 'all the Townes, Villages and Castles bee battered, pillaged, or burnt, and every place we lay at on the Rhine on ship-board we watched, taking every man his turne.'

Coryat has left some interesting particulars of the Rhine

journey in the seventeenth century.[1] 'All barkes or boates that come downe do goe very easily, because it is with the streame; which is the reason that all passengers which descend do pay but a small price for their passage: but on the contrary side all that doe ascend strive very painfully against the streame. So that all their vessels are drawen by horses with great might and maine. For this cause all passengers that ascend into the higher parts of Germany doe pay much more for their carriage than those that descend.'

The stopping-places, too, for each night were not arbitrary, but were governed by the position of the town where toll had to be paid. Coryat[2] says, 'I observed many custome towns between Mentz and Colen, which are in number eleven. They belong to divers Princes Spirituall and Temporall, who receive a great yearlie revenue by them. All passengers, whatsoever they are, noble or ignoble, must arrive in each of these places and stay awhile till the boatman hath paid custome for his passage. To the passenger it is no charge at all, but only to the master of the boate. If any should dare in a resolute and wilfull humour to passe by any of these places, and not pay the stinted summe of money, the Publicans that sit at the receipt of custome will presently discharge a peece of Ordnance at them and make them an example to all after-commers.'

The Main was reached on Thursday, 3 May, and Frankfort the same day, 'in much anxiety all the way "from freebooters", which are commonly called the Boores (a name that is given unto the lewd murdering villaines of the country that live by robbing and spoyling of travellers, being called Freebooters because they have their booties and prey from passengers free, paying nothing for them except they are taken), do commit many notorious robberies near the Rhene who are such cruell and bloody horseleaches (the very hyenae Lycanthropi of Germany) that they seldom robbe any man but forthwith they cut his throat. And some of them doe afterward escape by

---

[1] *Crudities*, ed. 1905, ii. 361.   [2] *Ibid.*, ii. 295.

reason of the woodes nere at hande in which they shelter themselves free from danger'.[1]

Hollar, the engraver, probably referred to this part of the journey when he told Aubrey that 'Dr. Harvey would still be making observations of strange trees and plants, earths, &c., and sometimes he was like to be lost, so that my Lord Ambassador would be really angry with him for there was not only a danger of thieves but also of wild beasts'. It will be remembered that the Earl of Arundel brought Hollar back with him to England and married him at Arundel House to 'my ladie's wayting maid, Mistress Tracy, by whom he had a daughter that was one of the greatest beauties I have seen,' says Aubrey, 'his son by her dyed in the plague, an ingeniose youth; drew delicately'.

The party rested at Frankfort from 3 May to 8 May. A fresh start was then made past Klingenberg to Neuenkirchen, 'guarded by a company of musketiers, but even then the whole night was spent in walking up and down in feare with carabines in our hands'.

Würzburg was reached on the following day, Monday, 9 May. The accommodation was so bad at Marckbibrach [Markt-Bibart] on 10 May that the night was spent 'on the plancher, for the village was pillaged but the day before'. It was no doubt unpleasant to have to sleep on the floor, but later in the journey as the party travelled into Austria it became a common experience. 'Earely the next morning wee went away and passed through Neustadt, which hath beene a faire City, though now pillaged and burnt miserably, heere we saw poore children sitting at their doores almost starv'd to death, to whom his Excellency gave order for to relieve them with meat and money to their Parents.'

Nuremberg was reached on Wednesday, 11 May, and the party remained there until Sunday, 22 May, to refresh themselves after the fatigues of the journey, and to see the many objects of interest in the town.

[1] *Crudities*, ii. 308.

Harvey wrote from Nuremberg to Caspar Hoffmann, dating his letter 20 May 1636. I quote Dr. Willis's translation:

'Your opinion of me, my most learned Hofmann, so candidly given, and of the motion and circulation of the blood, is extremely gratifying to me; and I rejoice that I have been permitted to see and to converse with a man so learned as yourself, whose friendship I as readily embrace as I cordially return it. But I find that you have been pleased first elaborately to inculpate me and then to make me pay the penalty, as having seemed to you, "to have impeached and condemned Nature of folly and error; and to have imputed to her the character of a most clumsy and inefficient artificer, in suffering the blood to become recrudescent and making it return again and again to the heart in order to be reconcocted, to grow effete as often in the general system; thus uselessly spoiling the perfectly made blood, merely to find her in something to do". But where or when anything of the kind was ever said, or even imagined, by me—by me, who on the contrary, have never lost an opportunity of expressing my admiration of the wisdom and aptness and industry of Nature—as you do not say, I am not a little disturbed to find such things charged upon me by a man of sober judgement like yourself. In my printed book I do, indeed, assert that the blood is incessantly moving out from the heart by the arteries to the general system, and returning from this by the veins back to the heart, and with such ebb and flow, in such mass and quantity that it must necessarily move in some way in a circuit. But if you will be kind enough to refer to my eighth and ninth chapters you will find it stated in so many words that I have purposely omitted to speak of the concoction of the blood and of the causes of this motion and circulation, especially of the final cause. So much I have been anxious to say that I might purge myself in the eyes of a learned and much respected man, that I might feel absolved of the infamy of meriting such censure. And I beg you to observe my learned, my impartial friend, if you would see with your own eyes the thing I affirm in respect of the circulation—and this is the course which most beseems an anatomist—that I engage to comply with your wishes, whenever a fit opportunity is afforded; but if you either decline this, or care not by dissection to investigate the subject for your self, let me beseech you, I say, not to vilipend the industry of other, nor charge it to them as a crime; do not derogate from the faith of an honest man, not altogether foolish or insane, who has had experience in such matters for a long series of years.

'Farewell and beware! and act by me as I have done by you; for what you have written I receive as uttered in all candour and kindness. Be sure in writing to me in return, that you are animated by the same sentiments.'

Caspar Hoffmann (1572–1648) had been a fellow-student with Harvey at Padua and was Professor of Medicine at Nuremberg. He had already interested himself in the anatomy of the heart, for he acknowledged the passage of the blood by the pulmonary artery and veins from the right to the left side of the heart instead of by the septum, and modified the idea of the mere to-and-fro motion of the blood in its respective vessels, by likening it to what we see in a lake ruffled by the wind. The veins, however, in conformity with the physiological views of the day, he still held to be the special conduits of the nutrient blood; the arteries the channels of the vital spirits.[1]

As the Embassy left Nuremberg on Sunday and the letter was written on Saturday, it does not seem likely that the promised demonstration was given at this time. I believe that it took place during the homeward journey in November, when the Mission stayed at Nuremberg from 10 November to 13 November. The most likely days are Saturday, 12 November, or Sunday, 13 November, when the rest of the party were engaged in sight-seeing. Tradition says that the demonstration was given in public and proved satisfactory to every one except to Hoffmann himself. The old man—already past the grand climacteric, with hardened arteries and about to suffer from the stroke which paralysed him for several years before his death—remained unconvinced, and, as he continued to urge objections, Harvey at last threw down his knife and walked out of the theatre.

Leaving Nuremberg for Regensburg on Sunday, 22 May, the party slept at Neumark on Monday, and at Hemmaw on Tuesday. Hemmaw had been pillaged

[1] Willis's *Harvey*, p. 214.

twenty-eight times in two years and twice in one day. Regensburg (Ratisbon) was reached the next day— 24 May—and the Mission remained there until 28 May, when they started off again and were received at a Jesuits' monastery, where they stayed until Tuesday, 31 May. On this day they travelled down the Danube in four boats, sleeping at Straubingen and arriving at Vilhofen on 1 June. 'The next morning as his Excellency was taking Boate he spied a poore Boy standing among other poore people begging for reliefe, who looked very strangely and could neither speake nor heare but a little at his mouth and nose, having neither eares nor passage to heare with, and his face very thin & drawne aside, yet when one hallowed hee heard and answered againe with a noise. There was with him his sister, a pretty girle who, when one spoke to him, made him understand by signes. These two his Excellency tooke along with him in his Boate to a City called Passaw, seated on the right side of the Danuby, where we landed & lay, and there commanded to have new clothese made for them & gave them monie and sent them home to their friends.'

Passau was reached on 2 June, and after three days' rest the journey was continued until Linz was reached on Sunday, 5 June.

The Mission remained at Linz until 25 June and the Earl was received several times in audience by the Emperor and Empress.

Harvey wrote twice to Basil Feilding from Linz, once on 9 June and a second time on 16 June. The first letter runs as follows: [1]

DR. WILLIAM HARVEY *to* LORD FEILDING

[1636,] June 9/19. Lintz.—'Right honourable, My sweete Lord, Soe much the more I now condemn my self (having att this hower receyved such sweete and loving lines from you) in that I did not send those letters I intended by the bearer hereof. His suddayne and unexpected departure was the cause that from Nurem-

[1] *Hist. MSS. Commission,* p. 28.

berg I did not by writing present my humble service, which I beseech you to accept in excuse, and not lay on me soe fowle a fault as neglect of one soe extreamely well desearving, and to me ever soe kind and frendly.

'I thank your honor that you vouchsafe to advertize me of one whome I hard before would write agaynst me, butt till now never heard he did, or ever yett saw that book. We are heare lately arrived thorowgh that ruined desolat country of Germany into Austria, and att Lintz have had only twise audience. Our bysenes, to expecte the delivery of the Palatinate, is not unknown to your Excelency. My lord will omitt noe dilligens or labour to effect it. This day sum of us accompanyed his Majesty the Emperor a huonting, which was thé killing of too deere encompassed by a toyle in a little wood, and soe putt forth for the Emperor and Empres to shoote with carabines, which they performe with greate dexterity.

'The post stayeth for this letter upon thornes, and therfore I must deferr any farther untill the next occasion. Yf ever I have done and may be able to doe service to you, ther is nothing wilbe more comfort and joy unto me, wheare all good endeavours bring forth soe much good frute, and all service is soe plentifully acknowledged.

'I should be glad of any occasion to see Venis once more, soe much the rather to have the happiness of your conversation, untill which time I will live in hope to see your Ecellent lordship, and in certenty ever to remayne your Excellent lordships humble at command, Will. Harvey.'

Postscript.—'Your letter receyved by James Quirke.' 1 *p.*

The second letter is also dated from Linz a few days later:

DR. WILLIAM HARVEY *to* LORD FEILDING

1636, June 16/26. Lintz.—'Not to lett slipp any occasion of presenting my service and thanks to your Excellency for your letters, att this time I am bould to write, and to congratulate with your Excellency of the honorable fame and esteme of your dispatches and abilityes, whereof I heare in that honorable employment you are in, with the expectation of your future increase and perfection therein, as wilbe to our Master and the Kingdom of greate and beneficiall use, and to your self honnour.

'My lord here hath not yett had answeare. We hope it wilbe good and satisfactory, though we are not out of feare of delayes. Our greatest certenty groweth from the necessity they have here of

making peace on any condition, wheare ther is noe more meanes
of making warr or scarce of subsistence; and this warfare in Germany without pay is rather a licence to prey and of oppression, and
threateneth in the ende anarchy and confusion, then a just and
laudable warr to establish peace and justice. I have been twise or
thrise a hunting with the Emperor, who certenly in his owne disposition is a pious good man, desierous of all love, quietnes, peace
and justise. How the concurrents and interests of the times will
permitt him I know not.

'Yesterday my lord was feasted by the nobility att the house of
the Count of Melan, the cheife major-domo of his Majestie. We
drunke hard, and had many expressions and many good wishes.
What will succeed is of noe less expectation and consequences then
our desiers are to know it.

'We heare from Ingland the plauge increaseth not much, yet is
soe feared as the tearme is for that cause put off. James Querck
earnestly desiers to have his service remembered to your Excellency,
and hath done well, though he lost his *fede*. My sweete lord, with
all the commendation I can, I desier to remain your Eccellencys
humbly at command, Will. Harvey.' 1 *p. Seal* [*with interlaced
triangles*].

Neither of these letters wants much comment. The
audiences mentioned were those given by the Emperor
and Empress to the Earl of Arundel as Ambassador from
the Court of St. James's. The first audience was granted
on Monday, 6 June, and the second on Wednesday,
8 June, the day before Harvey wrote the first letter. The
banquet, as Harvey states, was given on Wednesday,
15 June, when 'we were nobly entertained at the Count
Megaw's'. Perhaps the second letter was written on
Thursday, 16 June, to while away the time because 'as
we were at dinner there came a mightie clap of thunder
and lightning which burnt downe three houses presently,
being not above an English mile off, on the other side of
the water, . . . and about foure of the clocke in the afternoone, his Excellence had audience the third time and we
all invited to a Balto by the Empresses command, to the
Count Slavataes, who is Chancellour of Prague, where all
the Ladies assembled and there spent the time in dancing'.

Of the *fede* or bill of health needed as a passport, Harvey still had much to learn as will be gathered presently.

The letters are addressed to Basil, Lord Feilding, who had been created a Viscount at the coronation of King Charles I. He was the eldest son of the first Earl of Denbigh by Susan, sister of George Villiers, the first Duke of Buckingham. Basil Feilding, after acting as Master of the Robes and Gentleman of the Bedchamber to the King, was sent to Venice in 1634, ostensibly as Ambassador but really to collect art treasures in Italy. Lady Denbigh (op. cit., p. 108) quotes a letter from Mr. Secretary Windebank, dated from Westminster, April 1635, in which, after some general instructions, he adds: 'I am likewise commanded by His Majesty to let you know that whereas Daniel Niz, a merchant, has a cabinet of curiosities of great value, at Venice deposited with certain merchants of Holland whose names are Vlop and van Noodon that you do your best with that state, that the cabinet be not opened but reserved closed till the return of Daniel Niz, His Majesty intending to buy it off him for his own use.' In like manner Lord Arundel and Surrey writes to Feilding from Arundel House in November 1635: 'Noble Lord, I am glad to find my Lord Hamilton and others of our country incline so much to make collections of matters of art, to which it would give so propitious a help and I shall be the more glad to see England increase in them, because I grow so lame that I may have more use of my eyes though I shall have less of my feet.' Lord Feilding appears to have been a very lovable person if we may judge from the letters written to him by his mother and his wives. He held high rank in the Parliamentary army during the Civil War, whilst his father and mother remained staunch Royalists. He died at Dunstable in 1675. The exact year of his birth is unknown, but it was before 1608. He was, therefore, aged about 28 when these letters were written and Harvey was aged 58. The Court Medical Department—physicians, surgeons, and barbers—formed a part of the Wardrobe, and Harvey would thus have been brought into touch with Lord Feilding when he was Master of the Robes.

The Mission left Linz on Thursday, 23 June, going down the Danube by boat and sleeping the night at 'a little poore Dorp called Aspagh', probably Aggsbach. Vienna was reached on the following day and the party remained there until Friday, 1 July, when the journey to Prague was commenced. Harvey made use of the time by visiting Baden, situated seventeen miles from Vienna on the Schwechat. It is beautifully placed, and is still a favourite resort on account of the warm sulphur springs. He wrote the following letter from Baden to Lord Feilding. The date given as 9 July should be 29 June, Wednesday:

DR. HARVEY *to* LORD FEILDING

1636, July 9. Baden.—'So greate is my desier to doe your Excellency all service as I cannot lett slip any occasion whereby I may give any testimoney thereof. This gentilman, whoe is now comming for Venise, although I love, yett I a little envey, that he should enjoye the happines of that place and your Excellencys sweete conversation and that I cannot. My lord embassador, heare now att Vienna, did receyve att Lintz such an answeare to his demands as caused him to send an express to Ingland, before whose retorne I thinke we shale not see the Emperor agayne. Yesterday we visited at Vienna the Queene of Hungary and the Archduke, and too very fine little babyes her children. To-morrow my lord intendeth to retorne by Prage in Bohemia to Ratisbone, wheare is expected the diett wilbe; wee finde heare great expressions and many wishes for the success of my lord his embassadg; how the effects will prove we hope well, butt cannot certeynly assure our selves. I thinke the miserable condition of Germany doth more then requier it. I am this night heare by chance with this gentleman, to see these bathes, wheare such is my bad pen and inke and the shortnes of my time as I am humbly to intreat your Excellency his pardon for this hasty and rude scribblinge and soe, your Excellency his assuredly devoted servant, Will. Harvey.' 1 *p.* *Seal of arms [but not his own]*.

The Earl did not start from Vienna on Thursday, as he had intended, but on Friday, 1 July, the party took the road to Prague in wagons, and spent the first night at Holebrun, 'a poore village, where we lay all night on the

straw, having travelled seven Dutch miles, and every
Dutch mile is foure English. The next day early from
hence . . . to Swamb, a prettie town where we dined,
having past that fore-noon in danger neere a great company of Crabats, who were thereabouts, who frighted the
towne, for when his Excellencies harbenger entered the
gates an hour before us, they were all shutting up of their
shops and running out to defend the towne. . . . After
dinner wee came to Bodewich, a poore village, where we
lay on the plancher, and travelled that day seven Dutch
miles'. Bodewich is Maihaich-Budwitz, close to Brunn,
where the Abbé Mendel recently did such good work in
furthering Darwin's theory of Variation. The journey was
continued through 'a part of a wood called Hertz-waldt
. . . to Iglo, a beautifull built towne seated on a little hill,
where we lay that night. Earely the next morning . . .
thorow Haybeireitz, a village, in which an Oast killed at
several times of his guests ninetie men and made meat of
them . . . to Holebrum, where we lay that night on the
plancher, which was a most fearful night of thunder and
lightning, having travelled seven Dutch miles. The next
morning wee departed . . . past a silver mine of the Kinge
of Hungaries, which was by the way side on a little hill,
into which wee entered to see their works, the oare being
two hundred and fiftie fathom deep . . . and thence to
Colen, two English miles off, where we dined, and so to
Bemishbrade, where wee lay on the plancher againe. The
next morning earely being the sixth of July, from thence
to Prague to dinner, being five Dutch miles'. In the afternoon a Rabbi circumcised a child, and no doubt Harvey
was present at the ceremony. The party remained at
Prague until 13 July, the time being spent in seeing the
numerous sights for which the town was celebrated. A
masque was performed at the Jesuits' College, over which
an Irishman was presiding.

The return journey to Regensburg was begun on
Wednesday, 13 July. The party left in wagons, and slept
the first night at Beroum, the second night at Pilsen, the

third night at Bishopsteine, having travelled only four Dutch miles as the road lay over the Böhmerwald mountains. Redtz was reached the following night, and the party was safely back at Regensburg on Sunday, 17 July.

The Embassy remained at Regensburg until 21 July, when his Excellency determined to visit Augusta (Augsburg), where there were many art treasures, in order to kill time, as the Emperor had not yet arrived at Regensburg. The first night was spent at Neustadt. 'My Lady Abbesse gave his Excellence a banquet' the next day at Bezanzon [? Münchsmünster]. The night was spent at Palermo [? Ingolstadt], and Augsburg was reached the following day, Saturday, 23 July.

Harvey left the main party at Augsburg, and travelled into Italy to see Lord Feilding at Venice, and 'execute a commission for the King', he says in his letters. The nature of the commission is explained in a letter written from Ratisbon by one of the Embassy, which says, 'Honest little Harvey whom the Earl is sending to Italy about some pictures for his Majesty'. The distance from Augsburg to Venice is about 460 miles, and the journey was made on horseback with one or two attendants. There is no indication as to the route followed from Augsburg to Villach, but it is probable that he went from Augsburg to Münich (67 miles), from Münich to Innsbruck (105 miles), from Innsbruck to Franzensfeste, over the Brenner pass (49 miles), from Franzensfeste to Villach (13 miles). The letters show that he travelled from Villach to Pontebba (30 miles), from Pontebba to Sacile, from Sacile to Conegliano (9 miles), and from Conegliano to Treviso (17 miles). At Treviso he was only 18 miles from Venice, and must have thought his journey ended, only to be woefully disappointed. His first letter from Treviso is dated Wednesday, 3 August, and if he left Augsburg as soon as the Earl of Arundel arrived there on 23 July, he covered the whole distance at an average rate of 40 miles a day. The only news of him during these ten days is contained in a letter from Sir Thomas Roe to the Queen of Hungary saying that Dr. Harvey assured his private friends of great hopes of justice and equity from the Emperor, but he believes the Doctor judges by symptoms like a physician.

At Treviso he met with a serious check, which, for a time, spoilt both his health and his temper. His own letters tell the tale.

DR. HARVEY *to* LORD FEILDING

1636, Aug. 3/13. Treviso.—'My sweete lord, I came this morning to the gates of Treviso with greate joy, and hoped this night to have had the happines to have beene with you att Venise, butt I have receyved heare a very unjust affront, being stayed and commanded by this podesta to have gone into the lazaretto, without any cause or suspition alledged. I tooke my first *fede* under the seale of Ratisbone, a place free, and now destined, as your Eccellency knoweth, for the meeting of the Emperor and all the rest of the princes, which yf it had not beene soe, they would not have com thither, it being infected or suspected. Since, in every place as I came, I caused my *fede* to be underwritten, soe that there is no ground for them to lay any suspition upon me. And att this sentence on me by the podesta (that I should goe to the Lazarett) I absolutely refused, and sayd and offered to shewe that I had the pass and recommendation of his Majesty the King of Greate Brittane and of the Emperors Majesty and of my lord Embassador his Excellency, and that I had to goe to princes and men of quality, and that my busines required expedition, and desier'd they would not hinder me, butt, as my passes required, further me and that I mought not bring that suspition and infamy on me, besides my own security, to goe to such a place as lazaretto, whear they use to putt infected persons, and that I had shewed them sufficient *fede*. Notwithstanding all this, heare I am to lye for ought I see in the open base [*sic*] feilds, God knows how long. The podesta refuseth to see or reade my passes, and I cannot cum att him to speake and use my reasons. I am afrayd this lying in the feild will doe me hurt in my health. I beseech your Eccellency to lament hearof. It is unjust to proceed with any man thus without cause and otherwise then Venetians are used in Ingland or soe merrit to be used heare, and otherwise then is fitting for the respects there shold be used to the passes forenamed.

'I pray pardon this scribling on the grass in the feild, and procure with all expedition my freedom from this barbarous usadg. Your distressed frend and humble servant of your Eccellency.' $1\frac{1}{2}$ *p.*

THE SAME *to* THE SAME

1636, Aug. 6/16. Saturday.—'I perceyve heare by there behavier to me how much your Eccellency is pleased ther to stirr and laber for me, for yesterday after I had sent my letters to your Eccelency, they sent sum in a coatch to me, as from the podesta, that I should goe to the other place, wheare I was before (yf I would) or that I should have heare a bed or that he would doe for me what he could, to which I answeared, that since it had pleased him with soe much rigour and cruelty to inflict upon me the greatest misery he could and had brought soe much infamye upon me as to putt me into this lazaretto without any just cause, without any respect of the recommendations I had from my lord Embassador his Excellency or from the Emperors Majesty or from his Majesty my master, not soe much as to reade them or give notice of them in his first dispatch to Venis, nor to make any difference of a servant of his Majestye the King of Greate Brittan, butt by force and threatning of muskets to compell me into the very nasty roome wheare the vitturin and his two servants and saddels lay and not att my request granting me a bed or any commody scarce straw; his offers now weare unseasonable and like phisick when a man was ded and that I had now hardened my self and accomodated as I did content myself and resolved, since it had pleased God by his hands to humble me soe low, I would undergoe it as a pennance and that I had written to your Eccellency and hoped by your intercession within sum few days to have release, and therfore determined to receyve and acknowledg all my comfort from you and to troble the podesta with noe other request but that he would with all expedition free me and shew a respect to my master and my bysines; and debating the bysines and urging them for a reason of all this and that it was unjust to detayn any man and not shew him the cause, or to receyve a man into ther territoryes and then imprison him, they should have denied me entrance att the first and then I had gone sum other way for they should have putt those townes they suspect into ther bands and then I had shunned them or make known att his entrance to every man what he was to doe, otherwise this was to surprize and catch men; and they knowing not well what to answear sumtime alledged that Villach was suspected, sumtime I had not gotten my *fede* subscribed att Conian or Sacile, sumtime that the vitturin had brought a boy with him, his son to gett a master, whose name was not in the vitturins *fede*, soe sumtime I was stayed for him, sum time (they sayd) he and his horses stayed for me.

'Touching ther suspition I answeared Villach took as great care and examined my *fede* as strictly as they could and had given me *fede* of ther safety which they ought in civility to trust, and that the Duke of Alkalay [Alcala] viceroy of Naples with 100 persons choosed to stay there. And that upon bare suspitions of ther owne without any just ground, ought not to be thougt cause enough, to use me in all respects as if I had the plauge for certentye on me, and that if I had had it would they not have granted me in charity a house, bed and succour for my money though all had beene burned after, and I have payd for it. It was agaynst all manhood and charity. And for not having my *fede* subscribed in ther own towns as we passed, they knew well I could com noe other way from Pontevi and that they weare all without suspition and that I was towld, and it was and is in every man's mouth ther was noe neede, and that it was upon accident for our vitturin whoe should have directed us being strangers gott his own *fede* subscribed att Connian, and for the horses we rood on, and did not tell us untill it was to late, thinking his was sufficient. Butt for all these cavills, I sayd the word of an honest man or his oth in this case ought to suffice. I write the larger to your Eccelency of those passages because I know not what they may make of my conference in ther letters that ye may know the truth, and indeed my lord I am a little jealous of them, and to take anny beds now of ther sending, for since ther manners and cruelty hath been soe shamefull to me, and they have soe little reason for what they have done, it would be like the rest of ther proceedings yf they sent me an infected bed to make ther conjectures and suspitions prove true; therfor I choose to ley still to be redeemed by your Eccelency oute of this inocent straw. Yesterday likewise the patron that owed the howse wheare I first took my straw bed (a little poore garden howse full of lumber, durt and knatts, without window or dore, open to the high way att midnight) was to offer me that agayne, because I had chosen that to shun the infamy of this lazaret and the suspition I had that sum infected person had lately bene heare, and from which they forced me with terror of muskets, I write this to shew your Eccelency that all they doe heare upon your stirring is butt formal to salve ther own errors. I tell them I desier nothing of them, or expect or will expect, but only beseech the podesta that I may be att liberty with all expedition, and that att last he will have respect to princes recommendations and to my bysines: and now as I am writing I humbly thanke your Eccelency, your servant is arrived and hath beene with me and is gone to the podesta according to your order. He will tell you of a trick to burn my pass and the injury they have offered me therein.

'When your lordship shale marke how tedious I am in writing I pray give it this interpretation, I have noe other thinge to doe and infinite greedy to be gone, and that I scrible thus, in hast and the want of good pens and inke, etc.

'Yf your Eccellency goe to the Colledg ye may justly lament the little respect this podesta hath given the recommendations I have from my lord Embass. and his Majesty, or the bysines I am sent on, whoe would not soe much as receyve it and read it being offered nor send information thereof to Venis, nor make difference thereupon betweene me and the vitturines servants, would give me noe releife or assistance, not soe much as a barne or stule free to myself butt force that infamy, danger, suspition and base usadg of ther lazarett upon me, not to suffer me to write to your Eccellency untill 5 or 6 howers past, that in the meane time he mought procure an order from Venis to countenance his act and injure me upon unequal relation; and your Eccellency may justly resent that the dispatches to you and bysines of yours should be thus used and not upon your letters released and that ye may have that respect therein which is due, and that I may have reparation and testimony for the burning my pass and for the clearing me of the suspition and infamy of having beene in the lazarett, and my unjust stay, and that I may have agayne my *fede* to make appeare to the world wheare soever I goe that I am cleere, or els that I may have a full *fede* from this state. Yf they make difficulty of my comming to Venis, I pray that I may have sufficient *fede* from hence and I will goe by Padua to Florence and see your Eccellency as I retorne. I pray pardon me for propounding this to your Eccellency whoe know better hearin what is to be done which I doute not but you will performe, that I may be free and we rejoyse together hereafter; and in good sober truth I feare least this ill usadg and base place and the unquiett of my mind may not bring sum sicknes on me this extream hott wether therefor I beseech etc. Your Eccelencys humble servant.' *3 pp.*

DR. HARVEY *to* LORD FEILDING

[1636, Aug. 9/19.] Tuesday afternoon.—'My sweete Lord, this place is soe incommodious to me, and affordeth me soe little comfort, as I beseech your Eccelency to pardon me yf I take the bowldnes herein to make my complaynts unto you. The great longing

I have to be gon and free maketh me thinke these 4 days past (since I had the comfort to see your servant here) to appear so maney yeares, whearin I hoped ether they would have relented of ther cruelty or your Eccelency effected somethinge for my releife. I had thought with joy to have presented my service unto you, and now am sory instead therof to putt your Eccelency to the troble I knowe ye take for me.

'The ill diett I have heare, and the wors usadg hath produced this ill effect that now these two nights I have had a sciatique in my right thigh and legg that much discorageth me, and maketh me lame. I would fayne Signor Francesco [Vercellini] would come unto me. I will pay for his coatch and expence, to direct and advise me, and to deliver him the busynes I have to him from my lord Embassador and the letters I have els to Venis; and yf he bring my freedom with him, I shale have the more joy; yf not, he may gett me heare some garden house, with fier, bed and other necessaryes, least I fale wors. Yf his being there effect better for me, then that som man be hired theare to com and go between, by whom I may heare often what is or can be done, and may certefy me of the receyte of my letters att the least, that I may heare what I may hope or looke for. They tell me heare, yf there be any truth in them, that they have sent to the Duke for my liberty, and that they desier I would write this to your Eccelency, that by your joynt helpe it may be procured. I pray that Signor Francesco would come. Thus in hast, I pray pardon and releve. Your Eccelencys humble servant.' 1 p.

DR. HARVEY *to* LORD FEILDING

[1636, Aug. 12/22.] Friday. Treviso.—'Although I know your care and dilligence for my liberty, and make noe dowte butt your Eccelency doth what is possible and omitteth noe occasion, yett the longing I have to be out of this thraldom and the dayly hope from you maketh me soe often look oute as having not heard from you sinse your man was with me (on Satterday last). I desier much to know how the case standeth, what is the cause, what I may expect. Ther is nothing can beare any color of just objection butt that my *fede* was not underwritten att Conian [? Conegliano] and Sacile, which towns they know well enough are cleare, and by the computation of my journey from Pontevi [Pontebba] it is not possible I could take any other way, butt that I passed those townes wheare it was tould me that it was not necessary for my *fede* to be underwritten since I had the seale of St. Mark att Pontevi, and yett the vitturin had his *fede* underwritte att Connian for him and the horses we rode on and owers had been underwritten too but that he which was to guide us tould us when it was too late, and sayd his underwritten was sufficient, and wheras it was sayd we had one in our company more then we had *fede* for, that was not soe, for that party had a *fede* for himself att Pontevi though after not underwritten.

'I feare lest there may be some other matter in it then I imagin and they meant to stay me, had I the best *fede* could be (as I thinke I have) and that they seeke butt cavills to colour ther intent, otherwise the word of an honest man or his othe would easily give satisfaction for such slight douts; they have since and before letten pass others upon as little testimony. I hoped much on your Eccellencys complaynt to the Colledg butt now because I heare not I dowte much least they neglect you too. I have now bene heare 10 dayes and my *fede* giveth me testimony of health for 40 days almost before that, soe that I cannot guess other then sum malis in this, considering with what cruelty and severity they have proceeded with me. My sciatiq which I gott heare by injurious lodging, I thanke God mendeth well. I beseech you my sweete lord lett me hear from you att least that I may know these letters com to your hands which I write, and what I may hope for, and what reason ther can be of the greate neglect they have used to the recommendation and the passe I brought from my lord Embassador, the King his Majesty and the Emperour. I would be glad since my stay is soe long to have a trusty messenger to send all my letters I have to Venis, and to that end I have sent to Signor Francesco [Vercillini] to whom the greatest parts are, that he would com hither, my lord Embassador in my last letter from Ausburg commendeth him unto your Eccelency, and sayth ther is nothing yett fallen out worthy of your knowledg, otherwise he would have written to your Eccelency er this. Even as this morning I had finished thes lines, came one from this podesta to vew us how we weare in health and sayth within these 2 days we shale have liberty, butt what trust may be given to there words I cannot tell. I feare it is butt a shuffel to deteyne me heare yett a weeke longer, which is the extremity they doe to the worst *fede* and meanest man; likewise it is tould me that Signor Francesco should write soe much to a frend of his heare who is restreyned to his howse, who sent, I thinke, him to me to excuse him. I wonder Signor Francesco, I having written so earnestly to him he did not write a word to me, I know not the passages of your Eccelency being in the Colledg, but suer I am they have used a neclect and contempt of his Majesty's recommendation in his pass and of the Emperor worthy to be hotely complayned of, and to me have done barbarous injustise and incivility. Ther is a post commeth every day from Venis. I beseech your Eccellency to be a comfort to me that I may have butt one word. Of your Eccellency an humble servant and faythfull frend.'

Postscript.—'I humble desier to know when the soonest post goeth for Ratisbone, that I may provide letters.' *3 pp.*

DR. HARVEY *to* LORD FEILDING

[1636,] Aug. 13/23.—'My sweete Lord, becaus I see heare nothing, nothing butt injury, deceyte and jugling every day this eleven days, that to-morrow and att night and to-morrow and shortly I shall be released, and doe not heare from Venis any certenty by any hand; and I ley heare in a miserable case; I pray pardon me yf to your Eccelency I seme in this often sending importune; eccept by your Eccelency his means (in whom is my only hope to gett release from these barbarous oppressions) they delight hear soe to exercise there tirenny as I am like lye for every day they promise a weeke. I feare none of my letters com to your Eccelencys hand or to Signor Francesco; I make noe dout butt your Eccelency hath don for me what is fitting and have procured my releas long befor this time butt that your letters and your help is kept from me. Therefore I pray earnestly I may have but one word in answeare, that I may knowe my letters come to you and what is done, which was my chefest requeste to the gentleman your Eccelency pleased to send to me seven days agoe. The post commeth every day, and even to him that night this podesta sayd he expected from Venise, and soe will doe by his good will I feare this month, to your Eccelencys humble servant.'

DR. HARVEY *to* LORD FEILDING

1636, [Aug.] 16/26. Treviso.—'I wrote to your Eccellency yesterday what a heavy messadg these of the Sanita hear delivered to me from the Senate att Venis, which was that I must stay heare yett untill farther order; and asking how long, they sayd seven or ten or twenty dayes, soe I perceyve they doe butt abuse your Eccellency, to beare you in hand that every day I shale have my liberty, and therin they betray me and make me loose my time, with whom yf they had delt playnly and rowndly, I mought have gone back att the first to Villach and from thence to Gorilia, and there gotten shipping and beene by this time at Rome or Florence, and sene your Eccelency and dispatched my bysines att Venis comming back. Now yf I stay a weeke or ten dayes more heare, I shall loose soe much time as the intent of my jorney wilbe broken, and I must retorne without going farther. Good my lord, I beseech you, putt them spedily and rowndly to it, ether that I presently goe (having now beene 15 days) or that I may retorne, which is a thinge is usuall heare, and a little while agoe they did it, sending ther officer with them untill they weare oute of ther territorye, and in justice they cannot deney your Eccelency one of these and indeed nether, yf ether they did respect any thinge your intercession or would doe justice. I perceyve I am fallen into the handes heare of most base and evel people, and now they begin to accuse one an other, and when I aske them the cause of my stay, they forge lyes, as that I was att Saltburg, and that Villach hath the plauge, and I know not what, and in this place they have talked soe much that to-morrow and to-morrow I should be free, and when they heard your Eccelency stirred in it, expected noe less than present delivery, that now they begin to disesteeme what your Eccelencys favour can doe for me. My lord, I pray therfore urge further the disesteeme and neglect of his Majestys pass, and your intercession, that they stay me for comming from Villach and yett itt is nether a towne in ther bande, and they lett all others pass from thence but me, two having passed by *fede* from thence since I ley here.

'I beseech your Eccelency to pardon me and not thinke this often writing importune, for having soe often written and receyving noe answeare from you, which in all my letters I did soe ernestly requier, and it did so much concerne me to know the particulars as fearing my letters come not to your hands, I send this messenger of purpose to bringe me or write me, whether your Eccelency have any hope, or have or intend anything, and what answeare they give and wheather ye have or intend to complayne of the unjust and bar-barous dealing with me att the first, soe much to neglect the King his Majesty's pass and recommendation as not to reade it, not ther-upon to have made some difference betwene the usadg of me and the vitturin and his servants, butt cheefly in staying me and putting me into ther lazarett, having brought sufficient *fede* and such as they lett others pass with all, butt yf of these they will not be sensible of, to give present reparation, then to demand my *fede* back agayne oute of the Sanita and a testimony of my being heare in lazarett, and my passe burned, and that I may goe back (which I now (yf I cannot goe presently forward) would be glad to doe with Signor Francesco). Ether to goe forward or backward presently they cannot in any justise denye, and I never longed for any thinge in all my life soe much as any way and on any condition to be gone from this base place and barbarous poeple and fearing lest I should be sick and then they would crye me into the plaug, and keep me and cheate and tyrunise over me, God knoweth how long. Signor Francesco was with me on Sunday last and tould me (I humbly thanke you) with what desier and ernestnes your Eccelency dealt for me, and that ye hoped every day, butt other perticulars I could not learne by him, nor since. I send by this bearer the letters I had to deliver att Venis both to your Eccelency and others and a packet for my lord Herbert which was caryed to Ratisbon by James Querk and my lord being not in those cuntryes, is retorned back. Your Eccelency please to pardon this troble which my unfortunat change hath inforced me to put you to. Your Eccelencys humble servant.' 2 pp.

No more is heard of Dr. Harvey after this letter until he writes again and in good spirits from Florence:

DR. HARVEY to LORD FEILDING

[1636,] Sept. 7/17. Florence.—'My sweete lord, with many thanks I humbly present your Eccelency for all the favour I have receyved att my being att Venise. Since I came safe to Florence, I have seene this fayer citty and enjoyed much contentment therin, with health and mirth. The Grand Duke his highness receyved my letters and me with greate curtesy, favour and respect; talked often long and familiarly with me, presented me with frute, fowle, wine &c., gave order for one of his coatches to attend me whearsoever and whensoever I went abroade, shewed me himself many of his rarityes, would have given order for a gally to have carryed me from Leghorn to Naples, and when I thanked his highnes for his affection and love to his Majesty and his affayres, sayd there was nothing in his court or power that was not at the King of Ingland his service, seemed to love and honor him very much, much enquisitive of him, his health and welfare, customs and vertues. I tould him, as your Eccelency commanded me, of your devotion and promptenes and order ye had to doe him all service, which he accepted very kindly, and commended him unto you, and certeynly

yf ye came hither, would doe you all possible honor. It may be his marriadg is shortly to be consummated; it wilbe a fitt occasion to have order to congratulate. I perceyve heare myself to have much acceptance, access and familiarity, whereby it may be (att least I desier) to performe his Majestys service, or for your Eccelency or any your affayres.

'Here is a greate coort. The Duke of Loreyn and his Dutchess, to whom the Grand Duke giveth the hand; the Duke of Guise, his lady and his sonnes, Prince Janviel [Joinville], the Duke of Joyeux and too little ones, knights of Malta, and a daughter marriedgable, besides the Dukes sister, his too brothers, and the Cardinall and one of his uncles. Your Eccelencys humble servant.' 1 *p.*

After this letter there is again a gap in our knowledge of Harvey's movements until 5 October, when he was at Rome. The Pilgrim's book at the English College shows that he dined in the refectory and that Dr. Ent dined there the same night. The two travellers probably met by arrangement, for Ent was born at Sandwich near Harvey's birthplace—Folkestone—and had taken his degree at Padua on 28 April 1636. We owe the publication of the treatise *De Generatione Animalium* to Ent's care.

From this date there is again a gap until 5 November. The King recalled Arundel on 27 September, and Harvey probably received orders to return at once to Regensburg. He visited Lord Feilding at Venice on his way back, and wrote the following letter on his arrival at Regensburg:

DR. HARVEY *to* LORD FEILDING

[1636,] Nov. 5/15. Ratisbone.—'Right honorable and eccelent my sweete lord, I have within the time prefixed at my departure from Venis, now safely atteyned my Lord Embassador att Ratisbone, where I find him ready within too days to depart for Ingland, having his letters of revocation, and yett visited and visiting as yf all weare on better tearmes then as yett it seemeth to me to be, but more certeyne perticulars your Eccelency, I presume, shall understand by himself. I only write thus much to be an introduction to present my humble and harty thankes to your Eccelency for my kinde enterteynement and the rest of your many favors to me, which as I can never forgett, soe will I never omitt any occasion whearin I may

(by performing to your Eccelency any service) testifie my gratuity or
get any opportunity to wish and pray for your Eccelency all happy
success and prosperity. Your Eccelencys humble servant Will
Harvey.' 1 *p*.

The actual journey homewards was begun on Tuesday,
8 November, when the party left Regensburg early, arriving on the third day at Nuremburg, where 'the Lords of
the City came and presented their service to his Excellence
in a long Dutch complement, and after dined with him.
And the next day in the afternoone they came againe with
a present of 40 Flaggons of wine, and three killots of Fish,
which was brought in by thirty men all in red Coats,
guarded [embroidered] on the armes, with white and red
caps . . . and two pictures of Albert Durer and his Father,
done by him . . . and then presented his Excellence with
a Banquet. And from hence to the Castle where the Father
of one of the Lords lived . . . and he presented us with
another Banquet. The next day, which was Sunday, they
all dined with his Excellence. And in the morning being
the 14th day [of November] wee departed, having stayed
heere three dayes, and tooke a convoy of 100 musketiers
along with us to Neustadt—five Dutch miles. The first
night travelling part by torchlight through the woods and
there lay on the straw that night. The fifteenth day earely
to Ketzen, and there lay on the planchers likewise; and
the next day to Wirtzburg . . . staying that night there.
After dinner the Lords of the Towne sent his Excellence
a present of two and thirty Flaggons of wine, Fish and
provision for his Horse'.

It may be noticed that when the Embassy was received
with lavish hospitality the Earl of Arundel had been
making purchases. Thus at Nuremburg he bought the
Pirkheymer library which had belonged to the King of
Hungary. This library was afterwards presented to the
Royal Society by Lord Arundel's son through the good
offices of John Evelyn. At Cologne, on the outward journey, the Bishop of Meyence 'sent one of his Privie Counsell
to invite his Excellency the next day to dinner. He then

sent three of his Coaches for us and gave his Excellency very noble entertainment. The first night his Excellency came, were presented unto him twenty-foure flaggons of severall kindes of Wine, the next day twenty-eight and at every present there was a long speech made to his Excellency in Latine by one that came with the Wine, which came all from the Magistrates of the City in Flaggons with the City Armes on them'.

'The next morning before his Excellence departed from Wirtzburg he was visited by the Bishop of Wesburg, whom wee found in the habit of a Countrey Gentleman, setting aside his Order, which is an enamelled Crosse hanging on a blacke ribbon about his necke; who made very much of his Excellence and presented him with the picture of Our Ladie, done by Albertus Durerus, being one of his best peeces.' The picture must indeed have been a masterpiece, for the Earl says, writing from Frankfort on 5 December: 'I wish you sawe the picture of a Madonna of Dürer which the Bishoppe of Wirtzburg gave me last weeke as I passed by that way and though it were painted at first upon an uneven board and is varnished, yet it is more worth than all the toyes I have gotten in Germanye and for such I esteeme it, having ever carried it in my owne coach since I had it; and howe then doe you think I should valewe thinges of Leonardo, Raphaell, Coregio and such like?'

The seventeenth day of November taking a fresh convoy the party slept at Bishopsheim and started early next morning passing through a hilly wooded country in much danger of the Croats to the number of 6,000 or more who were pillaging and robbing. The 19th day in the morning taking a fresh convoy they came to Selgenstadt still travelling in danger of the Croats, 'where as soon as his Excellence lighted the Grave Vandosme, Governor of the Country for the Bishop of Mentz sent his Excellence a present of half a wild Boar and likewise provision for his Horse, knowing that the town could not afford anything. The twentieth day being Sunday, early in the morning we went thence to Frankfort. And the next morning after his Excellence went to Hannaw to visit Sir James Ramsey, a Scotch Gentleman and Governour of the town. The foure and twentieth day foure of the Burgers of the Citie came and presented their service to his Excellence with twenty flaggons of wine and then dined with him'. A stay of three days was made at Frankfort. The journey by river was begun on Saturday, 26 November. Mentz was reached on the 27th where 'divers poore people were found lying on dunghils almost starved, being scarce able to crawl for to receive his Excellencies almes, and presently returning to our boate to dinner wee afterwards releeved many poor hungry soules with the fragments. Thence to Rudeshem . . . and there cast anchor and lay on the boards likewise.

'Very earely the next morning we weyed anchor . . . and came to Bacharach where some of our Company did but goe ashore (and presently hastened after in a little boat) were pursued by five Musketiers almost to his Excellencies boat, who discharged very often at them, yet by good fortune mist them . . . then going on to a large island an English mile from Coblentz we there cast anchor and lay all that night . . . which night we lay in much danger . . . for as some of our company did but goe a little way from our boat, they were layd hold on, and one that fled had a Musket shot at him and hee that was taken they carried before their Commander. The next morning his Excellence sent againe to the Governor for passage, who like a base fellow made us stay that night also and the next day until three of the clock in the afternoon and would not let us passe for all that his Excellence had sent him the Emperor's Passe and Letter wherein hee was commanded not onely to give passage but to assist him in anything hee required; yet for all this he kept us still and would not give way that our Trumpeter might go to the French in the Castle; but they perceiving how unworthily he did deale with his Excellence discharged four or five cannons at his house and shot quite through it.' Bonn was reached on 30 November and the boats anchored there for the night, but the party durst not land, the plague 'being very sore in it'. Cologne was reached the next day. Coryat [1] says: 'There is a very strange custome observed amongst the Germanes as they pass in the boates betwixt Mentz and Colen, and so likewise betwixt Colen and the lower parts of the Netherlands. Everyman whatsoever he be poore or rich, shall labour harde when it commeth to his turne, except he doth either by friendship or some small summe of money redeeme his labour. For their custome is that the passèngers must exercise themselves with oares and rowing *alternis vicibus*, a couple together. So that the master of the boate (who methinks in honestie ought either to doe it himselfe or to procure some others to do it for him) never roweth but when his turne commeth. This exercise both for recreation and health sake I confesse is very convenient for man. But to be tied unto it by way of a strict necessity when one payeth well for his passage was a thing that did not a little distaste my humour.'

The party stayed three days at Cologne 'until we had exchanged our boats for bigger and every day his Excellence had presented unto him 24 Flaggons of wine sent from the Magistrates who once dined with him.

'And on Sunday the 4th day of December about foure of the clock at night tooke shipping and the next morning at three a clock set sayle.' Toll was paid at Zonz and so to Düsseldorf 'where as soone as we came but neere the shore out came the Noble Duke of Neuburgh and clambered over other ships to come into ours to visite his Excellence being much joyed at his safe returne and had made provision at his house to entertaine his Excellence, but perceiving he would not stay sent for a wilde Bore, wine, and five pictures and presented them to his Excellence and then tooke his leave . . . he staying by the shore and walking along as farre as the water would give him leave and stayed untill we were out of sight. . . . This night wee lay in much danger for there did lye on each side of

[1] *Crudities*, ii. 299.

us parties which robbeth and pillageth all Passengers; for wee saw above fifty in a company going all along by the shore, but a little before wee cast anchor and at 10 of the clocke in the night, being very darke, was a false alarum given by the watch of a partie cumming, which made us all flye to our weapons, at last perceiving it was but one boate and they that were in it crying out "Friends from the Duke of Neuburg" else wee had shot them, who came for to have passage into England'.

Utrecht was reached on 13 December, the previous day being spent in very bad travelling on account of the weather. At Leyden the next day His Excellency viewed the chief things of note in the town, as the Universities and the Anatomy school. From thence after dinner to The Hague. 'Here we stayed until December 21st and then left for Rotterdam. On Saturday being the 24th December (and Christmas Eve by our style) at 11 of the clocke in the night tooke boates and went to our ship called the Garland and about 3 in the afternoone set sayle and sayled over the barre, having a Pilot sayling before us with a lanthorne on the top of his mast sounding for the depth all the way. And the next day at twelue of the clocke cast anchor in the Downs and there rode and could not land for the roughnesse of the sea until Tuesday morning the 27th December and then landed at Deale and from thence by poast to Canterbury and so to Sittingbourne to bed.

'The next day in the morning earely to Gravesend and there tooke water to London, where on the way my Right Honourable Lady met his Excellence, who exchanged barges and there she entertained him with a banquet and so earely the next morning, went to Hampton Court to His Majesty.'

An allowance of £19,262 was made for the expenses of the Mission and of this amount £7,262 remained unspent.

Two or three additional facts about Harvey's accomplishments may, I think, be gathered from this account of his travels. In the first place he must have possessed some technical knowledge of art. It is clear that he had much in common with Thomas Howard, the second Earl of Arundel, and with Basil, Lord Feilding, who were both great collectors. The Arundel marbles given to the University of Oxford in 1667 are still famous. Feilding brought over many pictures from Italy which found their way into the Royal collection. Harvey's interest in art must have been known to and appreciated by King Charles I, himself no mean judge, or he would not have been commissioned to leave the Embassy and proceed to Italy to collect pictures. It is possible, too, that Harvey shared some of the business capacity which had made his brothers successful merchants in London, and if this were the case there is no doubt that the King hoped to have found not only a good judge of art but a shrewd bargainer as well.

The fact that Harvey at the age of 58 undertook so arduous a journey through a country desolated by war shows that he was of an enterprising spirit and loved travel, whilst the little side light in his letter from Linz that 'we drank hard' tends to show that perhaps his gout was acquired and not inherited, for it must have needed some previous training to have enabled him to hold his own at a seventeenth-century Kneipe.

IX

JOHN WARD AND HIS DIARY [1]

GENTLEMEN,—I cannot begin this address without expressing my sense of the great honour you have conferred upon me by placing me in the President's Chair. My unworthiness to fill it is borne in upon me with especial force when I look round and see on the walls of this room the names of my ninety-six predecessors, all eminent in their profession, many illustrious also for their civic and moral virtues. The tradition of the Society is a great one, and will prove hard to maintain in the third year of a war which has dislocated every relationship in life. I can count, however, upon the loyal support of my secretaries and the other officers of the Society, and with their help I hope to hand it on unbroken to my successor.

It is usual for the President to give an address at the beginning of his year of office upon a subject which is of interest to the Society. To some the selection of a topic must have been difficult. I am fortunate in having one ready to hand, because three or four years ago the Council gave me permission to transcribe the manuscript volumes known to us as *John Ward's Diaries*. They have long been amongst the most treasured possessions in our library, and, as the event proved, they have never been adequately examined. It is not known how they came into our possession, but in all probability they formed part of the collection of books belonging to Dr. James Sims, who was President from 1786 to 1809. This long tenure of office caused the schism which led to the foundation of the Royal Medical and Chirurgical Society, which now flourishes as the Royal Society of Medicine.

The note-books are sixteen in number, roughly uniform in size, measuring $5\frac{3}{4}$ by $3\frac{3}{4}$ inches, and have been whole-bound in calf. One volume has 'J. W.' stamped in gold, back and front—the precursor of a book-plate. The

[1] Presidential Address delivered before the Medical Society of London, 9 October 1916.

volumes vary in thickness. The writing is on both sides of the page, sometimes only a word or two, sometimes with blank pages, but for the most part so much crowded that a reading-glass is necessary to decipher it. The volumes follow a sequence of years from 1647–8 until 1673, but the order of date is not followed strictly year by year, though it looks as if a new volume was not usually begun before the previous one was filled. The books are in no sense diaries or records of events from day to day like the diaries of John Evelyn or Samuel Pepys. They are rather of the nature of 'table books', or 'common-place books', in which Ward recorded from time to time notes of what he had read or heard, or ideas and suggestions which might prove serviceable. Although there is nothing of great historical interest, yet the general view gained from reading them affords an insight into the character of Ward which is valuable as giving the opinions and occupations of a scholar and a gentleman during the Commonwealth and Restoration periods.

Dr. Severn's Book on the Diaries

An investigation of the minutes of this Society shows that on 5 October 1838 'a letter was read from Dr. Severn announcing that the MSS. of Dr. John Ward, of Stratford, in the Society's library, contained curious matter relating to Shakespeare, etc. It was resolved that a committee should be appointed to investigate the subject and report thereupon to the Council at their earliest convenience. The following gentlemen were nominated on the committee: Messrs. Clifton, Dendy, Headland, Kingdon, and Roberts'. On 23 November 1838 the committee appointed to examine Dr. John Ward's MSS. reported that, 'although they had found much that was amusing, interesting, and instructive among them, yet they were of too desultory a nature: the historical, medical, and clinical notices too much mingled together for the Society to offer them in their present state to the public, but that, Dr. Severn having made extracts from them, the Society might give him permission to publish them, he acknowledging that it was done with the Society's sanction'. The committee also recommended that the other manuscripts in the Society's possession be catalogued. It was further resolved that permission be given to Dr. Severn to publish extracts from the MSS. of the Rev. John Ward.

Dr. Severn lost no time in availing himself of the permission, and early in the year 1839 there appeared an octavo volume of 315 pages with the title-page,

'Diary of the Rev. John Ward, A.M., Vicar of Stratford-upon-Avon, extending from 1648 to 1679. From the original MSS. preserved in the Library of the Medical Society of London. Arranged by Charles Severn, M.D., Member of the Royal College of Physicians in London, Registrar to the Medical Society of London. Published by permission of the Council. London: Henry Colburn, Publisher, Great Marlborough Street, 1839.'

This volume consists of a dedication to the President and other officers of the Medical Society; of a preface; of some account of the life of the Rev. J. Ward, A.M., and of a series of short articles upon Shakespeare, which together occupy the first 87 pages. The remaining 228 pages deal with the diary itself. It is clear that Dr. Severn had only made a superficial examination, but we owe him a debt of gratitude, not only for calling attention to the volumes, but also for the assiduity with which he gathered such biographical details of Ward as were then available.

Of Severn himself I have only been able to collect the following facts: He was admitted a Licentiate of the Society of Apothecaries on 16 May 1816, and was found qualified to practise in any part of England and Wales, including the City of London and ten miles round. He lived for a time in Jewin Street, E.C., and from there published 'First Lines of the Practice of Midwifery: to which are added Remarks on the Forensic Evidence requisite in cases of Foeticide and Infanticide. 8vo. Lond.: S. Highley, 1831'. He was admitted an Extra Licentiate of the Royal College of Physicians of London on 1 October 1832, and he had then obtained the degree of M.D., but from what university is now unknown. It was not from Oxford, Cambridge, or Glasgow. In 1839 he edited *The Lectures on the Principles and Practice of Midwifery*, by James Blundell, 12mo, published by J. Masters. This little book he dates from the Society's house in Bolt Court, Fleet Street. He died in the summer of 1840, apparently leaving a wife and daughter.

The Society's minute records on 4 September 1840, that 'Mr. Dendy reported to the Committee the decease of Dr. Charles Severn, the late Registrar'. A vote of condolence was passed, and, in accordance with the appreciation of his services, and, moreover, regarding the advanced age and debility of Mrs. Severn, the Council requests the family to remain in the Society's house in order that they may take charge of its property and fulfil the directions of its librarians and secretaries until arrangements may be made regarding the office. Miss Severn performed the duties of Registrar until 5 September 1850, when Mr. Ley was appointed Sub-Librarian. On 9 November 1850 Mr. Dendy called attention to the claims of Miss Severn, and proposed that 'on her leaving the premises in Bolt Court she be paid a year's salary to March next'. This was seconded by Dr. Greenhalgh and agreed to. Miss Severn received £21 in March 1851, the year in which the Society migrated from Bolt Court to George Street, Hanover Square.

Ascertainable Facts about John Ward

Before I give any extracts from the manuscript volumes which lie before you, it may be interesting to gather such facts about the writer as are still available. He was born at Spratton in Northamptonshire in the year 1629, the elder of the two sons of John Ward, M.A., of Pembroke College, Oxford, by Dorothy, a daughter of Richard Pargeter. John Ward the father was a gentleman of property,[1]

[1] His father, Daniel Ward (*d.* 1627), bought the estate and manor of Houghton Parva from Lord Zouche at the beginning of the reign of King Charles I, and also held lands at Stoke Albany and Wilbarston, which he had purchased from Lord Danvers.

who became a lieutenant in Colonel Appleyard's Regiment
of Foot at the outbreak of the Civil War, was taken
prisoner by the Parliamentary forces at Naseby in 1645,
and probably died soon afterwards, for John Ward the
younger makes no mention of his father, though his
mother was living some years later. The younger son,
Thomas, became rector of Stow-on-the-Wold.

John Ward, the writer of the note-books, went to
Oxford in the middle of 'the broken times', as they were
called by Anthony Wood, when the University and College lists were badly kept. It is not surprising, therefore,
that his name does not appear in the registers. He states,
however, that 'I was presented Mr. of Arts about the year
1652 in Easter terme. Anthony Ratcliffe and Philip
Gerard and Mr. Temple with us'.

Ward also speaks of 'our table at Christ Church'—i. e.
the Master of Arts table in Hall, where the resident
Masters dined together. It is fair to assume that Ward
matriculated at Christ Church at the end of 1646 or the
beginning of 1647, graduated B.A. in July 1649, and took
his degree of M.A. on 6 May 1652. It is an interesting
sign of the times that two of his friends had been incorporated from Cambridge, because such migrations at this
time were usually due to political causes. It appears from
various notes scattered through the books that he remained
in residence at Oxford until the Restoration, when the
whole social atmosphere of the University underwent such
a change as to make it uncongenial to those who had lived
in it through the period of the Commonwealth. During
this time his interests lay in history and in science—chiefly
chemistry, botany, medicine—and in general literature.
He never took the degree of Bachelor of Physic, but it is
probable that he held the status of student of medicine, a
status then recognized in the University and only abolished within my own recollection. At any rate, he treated
many sick persons by medicine, though it does not appear
that he performed any operations.

He left Oxford in 1660, perhaps as a direct result of

the Restoration, for, although his father suffered in the Royalist cause, his personal friends must have been of the modified Republican type, who were in residence during the Commonwealth. Casting about for a profession, it is clear that he was sorely tried to decide between the Church and Physic. He took orders in 1660, and his note-books for this year contain numerous divinity notes and sermons. In 1661 he was in London attending lectures on anatomy at the Barber Surgeons' Hall in Monkwell Street, and debating in his own mind whether he should obtain a bishop's licence to practise medicine or an M.D. from a foreign university. He also interviewed 'Mr. Giles, of Lincoln's Inn, who deals in spiritual livings'. He thought first of Brentford, then of Kingston-on-Thames, where his friend, Dr. Bate, the Puritan doctor, is buried, and finally got himself instituted in 1662 to the vicarage of Stratford-on-Avon in succession to Alexander Beane, who had held the living since 1648. Beane was ejected at the Restoration, but his congregation built him a church in the town, and the Congregational Church in Rother Street is still known as the 'Church of the Ejectment'. The presentation to the living was in the hands of the King, but before 1681, when Josiah Simcox, A.M., became vicar, it had passed into the hands of Charles, Earl of Dorset and Middlesex.

Ward held the living until his death on 12 September 1681. He was buried in the chancel near the north wall, and the following inscription was placed on a flat stone: 'Hic jacet Joh. Ward, A.M., Sprattoniae, Northampt., natus, hujus Ecclesiae Vicarius per annos XIX., denatus fuit XII. die Septembris, Anno Domini MDCLXXXI., aetatis suae LII.' The stone disappeared when the church was repaved in 1840, but the inscription was copied and the place of burial was recorded by the Rev. James Davenport, who was vicar from 1787 to 1842. I have little doubt that he was ruptured and that he died of phthisis. Of his domestic relations nothing is known, but as his will makes no mention of wife or child, it is probable that he never married.

The Revival of Science in Ward's Time

A valuable feature of Ward's note-books is the insight which they give into the mental pursuits of the Oxford graduates during one of the most stimulating periods of the University's long career, an insight which is the more valuable because little is known of it except through the crabbed *Life and Times of Anthony Wood*. The note-books give an unvarnished and wholly personal account of the things which were uppermost in the minds of those who 'sate at our table in Christ Church', by one who entered heart and soul not only into the new-born scientific spirit of the time, but into the literary and social life. The books he read, the stories he heard, and the practice he saw, are all faithfully recorded. He shows himself throughout as a well-read gentleman, as insatiably curious as 'the elephant's child', quite clear and decided in his opinions, which are founded on observed facts and not on theories, and yet curiously credulous to our eyes, for as yet science was in its infancy, there was no chemistry, no pathology, and medicine was still medieval in character.

The stern realities of the Civil War, the military occupation of the city, the dispossession of the Royalist Fellows, and the introduction of Independents had finally displaced the authority of the schoolmen and put aside theological controversy. The undergraduates and the younger Bachelors and Masters were more interested in facts gained by observation and experiment than in the disputations and rhetorical displays which had pleased their fathers. Oxford was at the beginning of one of the great periods of awakened interest in natural science such as had occurred in the thirteenth century during the lifetime of Roger Bacon, and during the last quarter of the nineteenth century within our own memory. With the authors of this revival Ward was contemporary, and with many of them he was on terms of friendship.

The seventeenth-century revival of science led to the foundation in 1645 of the Philosophical College, which held its meetings at the lodgings of Dr. Jonathan Goddard in Wood Street, Cheapside. This was followed by the 'Invisible College', or 'learned Junto', which met at Wadham College when Dr. Wilkins was Warden and Dr. Goddard had succeeded William Harvey as Warden of Merton. The Invisible College contained the germ of the Royal Society, of whose foundation Ward says:

'I have heard this guesst abt as ye ground of founding ye Royal Societie. The King well knew yt Harrington who wrote Oceana and such strange fellows as have had their discourses and meetings and have talked of a Commonwealth; whereuppon he instituted another societie, whereof his Royal Self vouchsafed to bee one, in opposition to itt, not thinking fitt to put down ye other by open contradiction.'

The leaders of the scientific revival were nearly all Oxford graduates, though some of the most illustrious, like Wallis and Scarburgh, were only sons by adoption, for they had been incorporated from Cambridge. Most of the founders of the Royal Society were in residence with John Ward, who was born, as you will remember, in 1629, entered Christ Church in 1646 or 1647, and took his M.A. degree in 1652. Dr. Bathurst, of Trinity College, with whom Harvey spent many hours observing the changes in incubated hens' eggs, was nine years older than Ward. Dr. Willis, born in 1621, was eight years older. He entered Christ Church in 1636–7, and practised in a house just opposite Merton. Robert Boyle, the greatest *dilettante* of the set, was born in 1626, and was living in Oxford at the house of Mr. Crosse, the apothecary in the High Street, adjoining University College, in 1654. Richard Lower, born in 1631, entered Christ Church with a scholarship from Westminster in 1649. Christopher Wren, born in 1632, matriculated from Wadham in 1649–50, after he had acted for a time as prosector to Dr. Charles Scarburgh. Dr. Wallis, Glisson's first pupil and the friend of Samuel Pepys, came into residence at Exeter College as Savilian Professor of Mathematics in 1649.

This list of names, incomplete as it is, shows how inspiring must have been the atmosphere to a youth like John Ward, who had a strong inclination towards medicine and science, though he eventually entered the Church. While he was at Oxford Wilkins was considering the problem of perpetual motion; Harvey and Bathurst the development of the chick; Wallis the circulation of the blood; Willis and Lower anatomy in relation to the brain and heart; Barlow of the Bodleian, oriental languages; Bobart, botany, and especially the movements of the sensitive plant. Ward notes of him: 'Bobart ye physick gardiner has had a feavour in 1660 and after itt his hands and his feet peeled, his very flesh came off.' All were interested in chemistry, which was as yet little more than alchemy, whilst physiology had hardly made any headway, for Mayow (1640–79), the gifted Cornishman whose early death was so great a loss, had not yet come to Oxford; Boyle was advancing physics; Goddard was doing something to make medicine scientific, but pathology was non-existent, and physic was little more than folk-medicine.

Extracts from the Note-Books

There is an interesting list of the sermons attended by Ward, with the names of the preachers. Anthony Wood sums up these preachers in a very few words.[1] 'In anno 1646 a little after the citie of Oxon was surrendered to the Parliament forces were sent 6 presbyterian preachers from the Parliament to settle their doctrine there. Their names —Cornish and Langley two fooles; Reynolds & Harrys two knaves; Cheynell & Rabbi Wilkinson two madmen.' Ward therefore attended the sermons of a fool and a madman. He had to make notes of their sermons, which were, no doubt, afterwards read to his tutor, as was done until recently, partly to show that the sermon had been attended and partly that the auditor had listened. Wood further says of the Presbyterian party to which these preachers belonged that 'with their disciples they seemed to be very

[1] *Wood's Life and Times*, vol. i, p. 130, Oxf. Hist. Soc. ed.

severe in their course of life, manners or conversation and habit or apparell: of a Scotch habit, but especially those that were preachers. The other party (The Independents) more free, gay & (with a reserve) frollicksome: of a gay habit whether preachers or not: But both void of public & generous spirits. The former for the most part, preached nothing but damnation: the other not, but rather for libertie. Yet both joyne togeather to pluck doune & silence the prelaticall preachers or at least expose their name to scorne'.

The first volume of the common-place books begins, 'John Ward his booke, 1648 An. Dom. Aug. 26', about a year and a half after he had entered the University, and when he was 19 years of age. It contains an extract of Sir Philip Sidney's *Arcadia*, interspersed with extracts from Sir Thomas Browne's *Religio Medici*, the first edition of which was published in 1642. Perhaps some indication of his politics at this time is given in the statement that 'Parliaments are good physic but ill meat'. He next read *Tite Andronico*, a novel full of sentiment if it may be judged by the sentences he selects that 'shee was grown sick of a surfeit of health', and 'poured soe full and fast compliments uppon him that stifled therewith he could make no answer in return but stood in a swound of amazement'. And in another place: 'The teares trickled down his reverend cheeks as if they had run a race which of them should be foremost,' whilst 'he went out as a Lamp for lack of oil, no warning groan was sighed forth to take his last farewell, but hee smiled himself into a Corps'.

Having finished this novel he started on Sir Walter Raleigh's *History of the World*, but the extracts are not numerous, and he very soon gave it up for *The Unfortunate Politick*, a story of Herod and Mariamne, which was of the same sickly sentimental type as the other romances. He quotes as a part of it, 'Seeing him now at the brink of the grave he flings himself in, expelling by brutish violence that soul which he was ready to surrender up to nature.'

Lectures in Medicine: The Pulse; Purgatives

The book being finished, he returns to history, more especially the History of the Persian Wars, and a few pages later on there are notes of a lecture in Latin on medicine, the subjects being pleurisy, the urine, and menstruation. Other lecture notes deal with the pulse and with the uses and actions of purgatives. Harvey had not yet come to Oxford, and the Regius Professor of Physic does not appear to have accepted his views. He stated baldly that: 'A pulsibus diagnoscuntur statûs vitales. In pulsibus, prout in corde, duo sunt motûs contrarii scilicet systole et diastole.' [The vital conditions are diagnosed from the pulses. There are two contrary movements in the pulses as in the heart, namely, systole and diastole.]

The teaching in regard to purgatives took the following form in Ward's notes: 'The causes of purging medicines: (1) Extreme bitter as in Aloes and Colloquinta [Colocynth]; (2) Loathsome and horrible taste as Agarick and black hellebore; (3) by secret malignity many times not appearing in the taste as Scammony and Antimony: and if anything purge which hath not one of these 2 former virtues in it, it is to be suspected for poison.'

The lecturer then proceeded to say that quantity was an element in the purging capacity, for

'if we drink a great quantity of new milk it purgeth; that a mordication or vellitation of the orifice of the veins especially of the Mesentery veins: that almost all purges cause a kind of twitching and if it be in a high degree it is little better than poison which works by corrosion. The seventh cause of purging is attraction, for purging medicines have in them a direct force of attraction as drawing plaisters have in surgery. So Betony bruised and put into the nose draweth phlegm and water from the head. Those medicines that draw quick draw the fluid humors, those that draw slow work upon the viscous humours. Flatuosity is another cause of purging for wind stirred moveth to expell. Most purges lose their virtue by decoction upon the fire and for that cause they are chiefly infusion, juice or powder.'

I have given the headings of this lecture as they stand,

because it is evidence of the state of medicine in the University before the revival of science at Oxford. It should be remembered, however, that they are the notes of a first year's student.

Ward becomes M.A.: Nature of his Studies

The second volume begins on 27 May 1652, and opens with the exercise for the M.A. degree. The thesis was 'An aestate an hieme plura sunt oblectamenta. Affirmatur quod aestate'. [Whether the delights of summer or winter are the more numerous. It is decided in favour of summer.] The exercise would have taken about ten minutes to read. It ends sententiously with 'Dixi', I have spoken. It is interesting as an example of the Austin disputation which preceded admission to the degree of M.A. Such a disputation or exercise was performed by every Bachelor of Arts once a year unless he had obtained a dispensation. It was held on any Saturday in term time between the hours of 1 and 3 o'clock in the choir of St. Mary's (the University church) and was presided over by the masters of the school, who received either a drachma (4d.?) or a pair of gloves as a fee. Three days' notice was given by affixing the subject of the disputation and the names of the disputants to the doors of St. Mary's Church.

The note-books give no further indication that Ward continued to read romances. They are filled with notes on more serious subjects as soon as he had taken his M.A. degree. After several pages devoted to divinity, to civil and to ecclesiastical law, he returns to natural science as it represented itself to him in alchemical speculations on antimony and mercury. There was still considerable belief in astrology. The philosopher's stone and aurum potabile were still the subjects of serious experimental work and led to the foundation of modern chemistry. The extracts on the chemistry of antimony are 'Ex Angelo Salâ'.[1] His botany he learnt from Bobart, the keeper of the Physic

---

[1] *Angeli Salâ Vincentini Opera Medico-Chymica.* Francofurti, 1647. Salâ was recognized as 'Primus chemicorum qui desiit ineptire'.

Garden in Oxford, by the delightful practice of 'simpling', which meant pleasant summer days spent in walking to Shotover and Forest Hill, or afternoons in the Physic Garden itself. Anatomy he studied in 'Briggs, his Anatomia'; physic in Ramondaeus translated by Tomlinson; surgery in Paraeus rendered into English by Johnson. Incidentally he mentions a case of hysterectomy. 'Dr. Witherburne in London took out ye womb of a woman.' Measles was raging at the time, for he records that the physicians say 'the disease is autogenous like the plague; that the fever is less when the rash is coming out than afterwards, and that the backache before the appearance of the rash in measles is due to an excess of blood in the vena cava'.

Botany

Of Bobart, or Jacob as he always calls him, Ward has many reminiscences, chiefly during the year 1661. There were two Jacob Bobarts, father and son, both Horti Botanici Custodes. Ward must have known both intimately, but it is Jacob Bobart the elder (1599–1680) who taught him botany. He was born at Brunswick, and was appointed superintendent of the Oxford Physic Garden on its foundation by the Earl of Danby in 1632. In 1648 he published a catalogue of 1,600 plants under his care, and this was revised in 1658 in conjunction with his son. The revision, no doubt, was itself being revised when Ward knew him, and it explains his references to Gerard and Tomlinson. Ward's references enlarge our knowledge of the man who must have been one of those characters for which each generation at Oxford has been celebrated. We are told that 'on rejoicing days he used to have his beard tagged with silver', and that a goat followed him instead of a dog. One of the earliest entries is:

'Five sorts of fritillaries Jacob saies they have in ye Garden. Wee saw ym in flour March ye 23 1661 in ye Garden.' 'The 28 March 1661 wee went to Shotover to find Lunaria by Jacob's directions but found none.' 'I was uppon New College wall on ye 17 April

1661 to find Ruta muraria but could find none; but much diastrum nigrum was there.' 'A great piece of horse chestnut. Remember yt I get a cup made of itt.' 'Jacob found a chestnut tree wild near Newburie and many hee hath seen growing in Sion College garden wch brought chestnuts to perfection.' 'Rochet seed scarce to be got. Jacob saies hee had itt not, nor scarce ever saw itt.' 'Jacob hath a very proper orchis wch resembles a Bee wch I saw May ye 4 1661.' 'That Sedum in Bobart's house hath grown up these 8 years only by taking of ye cloth now and then and anointing itt with oil once a quarter and soe putting itt on againe.' 'May ye 9 An° Domini 1661 att ye Physic Garden Jacob told mee there is a gentle-man in Worcestershire who hath made very considerable progress in altering flowers artificially, hee knows not his name.' 'Rhubarb now may bee bought for about 16s. or 18s. ye pound.' 'Bobart had a bunch of grapes once ripe on ye 5 August wch hee presented to ye Swedish Embassador, then att Oxford. Hee brags much of itt still, they usually not soe still ye latter end of August or ye beginning of September.' 'Jacob says hee thinks Parkinson hath 500 plants more than Gerard; only Gerard's paper is better and his cutts better, they being dulled ere they came into his hands.' 'Jacob Bobart spake with Dr. Modesay and says of him, ye whole world yields not ye like man: hee never heard any man talk att yt gallant rate in his life: hee showed ym all his designs in ye new Garden. There are to bee walks in itt of thirtie feet wide as hee saies.'

Anatomy and Physiology

There is an interesting note written in the year 1652 which is valuable, as it affords a test of Ward's accuracy in reporting what he heard. It is interesting because I imagine it formed a part of the talk at the M.A. table in Christ Church Hall, 'our table', as Ward calls it. You will remember that Glisson was one of the original members of the Royal Society, that he was Regius Professor of Physic at Cambridge and a graduate of the University of Oxford; that he first wrote on Rickets and afterwards on the Liver, the capsule of which is still called by his name. A disciple of Harvey, he was 'omnium anatomicorum exactissimus'. of him Ward wrote:

'Asserit Glissonius fuisse Jolivium quendam sibi amicum qui affirmavit dari 4tum genus vasorum distinctorum ab arteriis venis et nervis ut in toto corpore communicationem cujus munus esse aquosam humorem continuo in toto corpore distribuere.

'Glisson says that Jolivius, one of his friends, stated that there was a fourth kind of vessel distinct from the arteries, veins, and nerves, so connected throughout the whole body that their function was to distribute a watery humour through the whole body.'

In 1654, two years after Ward had recorded the story, Glisson published his book *Anatomia Hepatis*, in which the following passage occurs. He is writing of the lymphatics of the liver:

'Incidi primum in eorum notitiam indicio D. Jolivii idque anno 1652 sub initium Junii: quo tempore ille Doctoratus gradus adapturus, me Cantabrigiae in eum finem convenerat. Asseruit nempe dari vasorum 4tum genus, a venis, arteriis nervisque plane diversam idemque ad omnes aut plurimas saltem corporis partes distribui et humorem aquosam in se complecti.

'My attention was first drawn to them by Mr. Joyliffe about the end of June in the year 1652, at which time he was incorporated to the degree of Doctor when I was at Cambridge, and he came to me for that purpose. He stated, forsooth, that there was a fourth kind of vessel clearly distinct from the veins, arteries, and nerves, and that these vessels were distributed to all, or at any rate to most of the parts of the body, and contained a watery humour.'

Jolivius is clearly the Latin name of George Joyliffe, who entered Wadham College in 1637, and migrated two years later to Pembroke College, Oxford. He took his M.A. degree in 1643, being about that time a lieutenant, under Lord Hopton, in the Royalist army. He afterwards studied physic, and with the help of Dr. Clayton, Regius Professor of Physic and Master of Pembroke, discovered the vessels which are now known as the lymphatics. It would seem, says Dr. Munk, that the lymphatic vessels were observed by three different observers in the years 1651 and 1652, and, so far as can be ascertained, independently of one another. Rudbeck, a Swede, saw them first in a dog in January 1651, and published an account of his observations in 1653. Bartholine saw them in December 1651, also in a dog, and published his discovery in 1653. Dr. Joyliffe accidentally noticed them whilst he was examining the spermatic vessel of a dog. He published nothing on the subject, and died at the age of 40 on 11 November 1658. Dr. Timothy Clark wrote about Dr. Joyliffe's discovery in the *Philosophical Transactions* for 1668. Amongst his patients was Mr. Samuel Pepys, for whom he wrote a prescription the day before his lithotomy, on 28 March 1658.

This observation seems to have borne good fruit in Ward's case, for he made some original observations and bought himself a microscope. In 1658 he records that: 'Dr. Willis and Dick Lower opened a Dogg and they first let him blood in the jugulars to discover whether arterial and venal blood did differ in colour and constitution. Mr. Ffrancis told me that he and Dick Lower found much chyle extravasated.'

Dick Lower was Richard Lower, whose name is still familiar in 'the tubercle of Lower'. He was one of the most gifted of the younger generation in Oxford to which Ward himself belonged. Born in 1631, he entered Christ Church in 1649, and he took his degree two years later than Ward. He studied medicine under Willis—the circle of Willis—and assisted his master in the dissections of the brain and nerves which have rendered his name immortal. Lower was especially interested in the movement and colour of the blood and of the chyle. Later in life he lost a good deal of practice owing to his Whig tendencies, but as he left £1,000 to St. Bartholomew's Hospital he must have done well.

Original Scientific Investigations

Lower exercised a singular fascination upon Ward, and it is clear that he assisted in some at least of his investigations in a truly scientific spirit. Here are some illustrations taken at random.

'Dick Lower is answering ye fellow that writes against Willis.' 'Remember to buy Dr. Willis *De Cerebro* for one book and ye fellow's that wrote against Dr. Willis for another.' [This no doubt

was Edmund O'Meara's work against Dr. Willis' work on fevers.]
'Remember in all my dissections to aim at ye discoverie of a passage
betwixt ye stomach and bladder.' 'I look upon ye blood as all other
bodies to consist of three parts, ye thickest part which is first strained
away in ye spleen, by ye arteries, ye thicker next that is strained off
in ye liver, and ye thinest of all after that in ye bodie or ye kidneys.
These certainly are the use of these 3 parts, though Highmore
makes ye spleen to be a kind of a focus [furnace?] to ye stomach to
impart heat to it, and ye very consistence or hardness and porosities
of whose part does argue as much.'

There are several other references to the spleen and its
uses, so that Ward had this organ under consideration for
a long time. Thus, at one time he was asking himself—
'Whether when there is a redundance of ferment in ye
stomach and spleen this ferment may not passe along with
ye aliment and in several parts, especially ye joints, may
not be laid aside again and so cause ye gout.'

And again—'Whether ye spleen borrows its ferment
from the stomach or the stomach from it: Qy. whether
a too much ferment in ye stomach is not ye true cause of
ye cardialgia together with wind and some other things.'

Such theories were probably inspired by Dr. Willis, but
the practical influence of Lower can be seen in—'Things
to be inquired into in dissecting Mr. Toone's dogg: at
first whether his spleen is any whit grown again since it
was taken out; 2ndly, whether its dulishness does not proceed from ye ill crasis of his blood not being duly fer-
mented and heightened by ye fermentation of ye spleen.'

In another instance he notes that—'A dog's spleen
taken out by Mr. Day, afterwards ye same spleen and ye
dog was stole by Mr. Hartford and brought up to London
and there dissected.'

Other evidence of experimental work in a scientific
spirit is seen in the statements that—

'The recurrent nerves in a dog's neck being cut ye dog afterwards
could not bark.' 'Mr. Lower cut a dogges windpipe and let him run
about. Hee had a week so hee could not smell, but would eat anything as I am told.' 'When one would discover ye ductus chyliferus

of Pecquet presse ye Mesenterie somewhat hard and a thinne pel-lucid liquor will come out at ye top.' 'The nerves have their original rather from ye cerebellum or medulla oblongata cerebri than from any other part.' 'Inquire whether there is any such thing as a woman having a suture down her forehead as people commonly report. I searched 34 skulls or thereabouts, and of these all I found but 4 wch had a suture downe ye forehead to ye very nose: another wch seemed to have a squamiferous suture upon ye vertex and which I admired much att. I suppose nature does vary in such things and I wish I could discover something of her operations, especially whether epileptick persons have any sutures.'

An equally good piece of original work, putting theory to the test of experiment, also due to Lower's influence—for he afterwards published a work on the subject—is the following:

'View ye blood of all animals as to its thickness or thinness; yt of Turkies seems to me to be very thick.' 'Turkey's blood again a 2nd time observed and found to be thick immediately after its being out, wch well might bee in regard of its fulness of spirits wch soon flies away and so leaves ye masse very thick, or whether ye blood naturally is thicker yn that of other animals. Remember to kill a turkey and another fowl together and observe wch blood soonest coagulates.'

Medicine and Physicians

The extracts relating to medicine and physicians are numerous, and show that practice had not advanced, and was not being investigated in the same way as anatomy and physiology. Symptoms, of course, were alone treated, and often by a nostrum.

'Dr. Wagstaff hath a water made of Roman vitriol and plantain water. He calls it aq. coerulea.' 'Dr. Wagstaff uses Mastick pills very much and amongst them oil of aniseed for the stone.' 'Mrs. Woolmer having a great weakness one time when she lay in, Dr. Wagstaffe applied cantharides to blister the inside of her foot and so draw, and drew three days untill letting out ye blister. At last she had a sore in ye place and a Lameness which she could never recover afterwards. She hath since had a numbness or palsie on one side of her head and bodie, but it hath passed away presently without any considerable matter of damage.' 'Inquire of Mrs. Woolmer whether ye numbness she complains of is on ye side where ye blisters were used and again advise her to keep open her issue in the other leg and stop it up in that which hath ye sore running in it.' A good many years later 'Mrs. Woolmer had a tympanie. Att last it inclined to breaking and rose to a head about her navel and one day she runne a pinne into itt and itt streamed out extremely. Her advice with Mr. Hall, who wished her to lie on her back and let it out by degrees, after they got a tapp. A quarter of a year, with much stench and filth, after yt closed up and well.' 'Dr. Wagstaffe calls Laudanum extractum hypnoticum and extractum cordiale.'

Ward died a bachelor, but he seems from the following extract to have learnt something of the wiles of women: 'Dr. Wagstaffe's daughters have a cosmeticke wch would make ye skinne peel off a little and after they lookt very fair: only they kept in every time they used it about 2 or 3 dayes: and once in 6 months they used it.'

As an illustration of the methods of contemporary practice he states:

'Dr. Willis imparts his receipts chiefly to 2 Apothecaries in Oxford so farre as I can perceive, Mr. Hazlewood and Mr. Crosse. Hee hath a syrup of sulphur wch hee makes much use of. Itt is his owne composition and no Apothecarie hath itt or knowes itt but ye two forementioned. Itt may be taken and is so usually with a Liquorish stick. It is a compound not above 4*d*. an ounce, but it is most used in Colds and distempers of the Lungs.

'Two ounces and a half of quicksilver given by Dr. Conyers to a patient yt was troubled with ye Iliack passion. Itt is very good for yt distemper. Dr. Willis uses to give more: ye more you give ye less is ye danger. Itt does by its own weight passe quickly. Doe but mix itt with a plaister and heat itt a little and presently itt flies away, but boyling hurts itt not at all.'

Dr. Conyers, born 1622, was educated at Merchant Taylors' School, was a Fellow of St. John's College, and took the degree of M.D. at Oxford in 1653. He was one of the few physicians who remained in London during the Great Plague, says Munk, and fell a sacrifice to it. Of Dr. Conyers, Ward also says: 'Hee uses nothing else almost but his emetick powders,' and that 'he knows some families yt for many years, they say some hundreds, have not had ye pocks: and soe it is not in ye blood of ye mother'.

References to Sydenham, Willis, and Ent

There is a short reference to Sydenham in the passage—

'There was a great phlogosis in ye Duke of Cambridge his bowels. Dr. Sydenham kept ye Duke of Cambridge alive 3 weeks and the Dutchess thought hee would really have cured him. Hee did itt by some cooling water or other wch hath got him some credit. Hee was allso with Sir Richard Bishop for his gout but did little except pultisse him with milk and crumb of bread. He advised Mr. Bishop to fast one day in a week for his rheumatismus so as yt humour would spend ittself.'

Of Dr. Willis he says: 'My Lady Windsor is dead: her brain was good as Dr. Willis said, but her liver was rotten and corrupt much. Dr. Willis lays much store uppon ye brain nowadays.'

The relationship of Willis to Lower is well shown in the fact that—'Dr. Lower found out ye famous well near King's Sutton though hee was willing itt should goe under Dr. Willis his name.' 'Dr. Willis hath got a new way of opening ye Brains, as to cut them on all parts from what holds them and so to turn them upside down.'

Of Willis, too, he tells the following story of a strangulated hernia: 'Stephen Toon's rupture was laid open, as ye phrase is, and caused a peristaltic motion of ye guts. At last eased by a plaister and a grain of laudanum wch Dr. Willis said hee was too weak to take, the Dr. left him with these words: "Stephen, God comfort thee".'

Stephen Toone did not die of his rupture. He was the apothecary with whom Ward lodged in Oxford. He was the son of Thurstan Toone of Collingborough, Northants, and was 'Privilegiatus' 14 September 1666, aged 30. His will was proved at Oxford on 1 October 1681. The teaching of Willis and Lower is again exemplified in the passage:

'Some Drs. especially in Oxford now are of opinion yt hysterical fitts are caused by ye indisposition of ye Brain. Most in Oxford, as

Mr. Ffrancis said, are of yt opinion and that men have ye same thing which some women have, and that Mr. Elyot had a patient that hadde itt and was cured by anti-hystericall things though hee was a man. That there is no passage for fumes into ye Brain by way of valves.'

Sir George Ent, the friend of Harvey, to whom we owe the publication of the *De Generatione*, is mentioned more than once.

'I heard that Dr. Ent going to Warwick Castle, my Lord Brook having a man very sick of ye griping of ye gutts, My Lord asked ye Dr. what was good for itt. He answered white wine plentifully drank if itt was not too sharp would doe itt, hee would lay his life of itt.' 'Dr. Ent said to Mrs. Lucy one time when she was sick yt hee had intended to have let her blood, but afterwards perceiving shee had ye jaundice hee said hee would not for a hundred pound yt he had done itt.'

Dr. Bate and Scurvy-Grass

There are many references to Dr. Bate, whom Ward always calls Bates, of New College. He practised in and around Oxford, especially 'among precise and puritanical people, he being then taken to be one of their number'. He moved to London, was physician to the Charterhouse, and attended Cromwell in his last illness. At the Restoration he became physician to Charles II, and dying in 1669 was buried at Kingston-on-Thames. Ward says: 'I have heard that Dr. Bates writt few bills wherein hee did not prescribe scurvy grass, hence some have styled him in my hearing, as relating itt for others, ye Scurvigras Dr., imagining, I suppose there might be a tang of itt in most diseases.'

Anthony Wood [1] says that scurvie grass drink began to be frequently drunk in the mornings as a physic drink in March 1659. Ward says, 'Put a quart of scurvy grass all fresh to 3 gallons of ale, if strong put in more.'

There is an account of Bate in *Longman's Magazine* for August 1894, pp. 364-75. 'Dr. Bates told Dr. Barke that

[1] *Life*, i. 273.

he had used ragwort with scabby people in ye hospital for 40 years with good success.' He might therefore have said, as did Dr. Ballard to Lady Peniston, 'Madam, I could advise you to a chymical medicine wch should cost you 10 shillings, but I am a friend of what grows under a hedge.' Of his end Wood relates in 1663: 'June 1 or 2 Dr. [George] Bates died at London of French pox and confessed on his death-bed that he poysoned Oliver Cromwell with the provocation of two that are now bishops, viz. . . . and his majestie was privi to it.' The date is as incorrect as the accusation. 'Mr. Hodges of Gloucester was sick of a kind of phthisis and hee consulted Dr. Bates, who prescribed him some kind of Almond milk, then a wash of oil of Almonds and after ye chewing of tobacco to make him vomit and this cured him· cleverly. After ye eating of oil and hony much gravel came away from Mr. Hodges as appeared by his urine.'

Dr. Dickenson and the Use of Antimony

He records the following case, which was under the care of Dr. Dickenson, Linacre Lecturer at Oxford and of Eton and Merton Colleges. 'Mr. Gwinne of our house vomited up long pieces of blood wch had heads like fishes. They carried them to the Apothecaries and cut them but knew not what to make of them.'

A few pages later comes the end of the case—

'I saw Mr. Gwinne of our house dissected but could perceive nothing in him that might cause his death, his spleen was somewhat flaccid, so was his heart and one of his kidnies, but his lungs had some kind of scyrrhus in them and in these scirrhuses a sabulous kind of matter, but that could not kill him. They pretended hee had a contusion of the liver in regard ye concavity of it was a little stained or possibly itt was nothing else but a settling of ye blood when death came. There was a membrane coming from his side to his lungs on each side wch some ignorant people would have interpreted a growing of ye lungs to ye side, but Mr. Boghill said he had seen it severall times in sound men yt hee had opened. His heart was large, about as large as ye heart of an ox but not perisht at all.'

Edmund Gwynne, 'serviens', matriculated from Christ Church on 25 July 1655. The post-mortem examination shows that he had suffered from a tuberculous pleurisy with a dilated right heart, and the long pieces of blood may have been formed in a dilated bronchus. 'Mr. Gwinne of our house' was under the care of Dr. Dickenson, the physician who tried to prove that the Greeks borrowed the story of the Pythian Apollo and all that rendered the Oracle of Delphi famous from Scripture and especially from the Book of Joshua. Dr. Sheldon thought so highly of his work that he recommended its author to devote himself to divinity and take orders. Dickenson preferred, however, to study chemistry, a subject in which he soon became *facile princeps*. After practising in the High Street, Oxford, he moved to London and became physician in ordinary to Charles II, and afterwards to James II. Troubled by old age and stone in the bladder, he died in 1707, and is buried in St. Martin's-in-the-Fields.

He was the kindly senior who helped Anthony Wood when he was an undergraduate. For 'after he had concluded his speech, he was taken doune by Edmund Dickenson, one of the bachelaur-commoners of the house: who with other bachelaurs and the senior undergraduates made him drink a good dish of cawdle, put on his gowne and band, placed him among the seniors and gave him sack. This was the way and custom that had been used time out of mind to initiate the freshmen'.

Ward records in another passage that—

'Antimonie:—Mr. Boghill made a balsam of itt wch hee gave to one whose lunges were distempered with excellent success. Hee spake with a great chymist who said if one could take away ye vomiting part of itt and make itt a medicine purely purging downward itt would be a great thing; now Crosse said Dr. Dickenson gave a Lady a pill wch worked 20 times without making her sick and hee told mee confidently yt there was nothing but Antimonie in itt. Hee highly commends Dr. Dickenson for his strong pains taken in prosecuting of itt, and says that certainly hee hath admirable remedies.' Mr. Boghill hath his elaboratories about Chelsey.'

Boyle, it will be remembered, lodged with Crosse, the apothecary, in the High Street, Oxford. Of Turner Ward tells 'a merrie storie': 'Dr. Turner being to bee examined by ye College for his admission thereto ye young Dr yt examined him askt him how many chapters there were in such a book of Galen? Hee made answer yt he had read Galen before he was divided into chapters'. This Dr. Turner was probably John, a Doctor of Medicine of Leyden, who was admitted a Licentiate of the Royal College of Physicians on 4 June 1630.

'Mr. Topham of Christ Church if hee sat at disputations with his hat off hee used to pisse blood.' This was, I suppose, a case of paroxysmal haemoglobinuria, the attack being precipitated by a chill. Mr. Topham was Richard Topham, B.A., incorporated from Trinity Hall, Cambridge, on 6 December 1652. He took the degree of M.A. from Christ Church on 11 December 1652.

Surgery

Ward kept himself abreast of the surgery of his day, for he says: 'Remember to bring Woodal's Chirurgerie, he was a rare fellow in his time doubtless.' This was John Woodall, surgeon to the East India Company, and author of the *Viaticum, being the Path-way to the Surgeons Chest* as well as *The Surgeon's Mate*—the two text-books of naval surgery for many years. 'Remember to purchase, as soon as possible, Pareus his chirurgerie and Mr. Woodall, and in the meantime to borrow Woodal of some of my parish.' Paré, translated by Johnson, was published as a second edition in 1649. Ward also supplied himself with surgical instruments, as is seen in the note: 'Remember to get a speculum oris and other instruments fit for chirurgerie when I goe to London and a great case to hold them.' He did not aspire to a great armamentarium, for—

'I saw one day all Gill's instruments and hee told mee ye names of ym all and their use and what ye whole case cost him: hee wanted a small spoon and some other things in ye case: yt and his Launcets and his syringe and his salvatorie were all ye necessarie tools of a chirurgion.' 'Gill said yt Mr. Day hath amputated 5 armes, 3 legges and somewhat else since hee came to him and but 1 of all these died and hee was a person of 60 years at leaste.' 'There are two of ye Molines in London. Ye one Edward ye eldest is excellent at stone-cutting and curing of fistula in ano or Lachrymale; ye other Gill told mee is ye better chirurgion. Hee told mee very many pretty stories of his exquisiteness in dissecting bodies wch hee saw admirably performed, taking out ye muscles and letting ym only hang by ye tendons by wch they were inserted. Mr. Moline hath a great many excellent cutts and pictures of ye liver and other inward parts.'

Some Surgical Cases

He gives a graphic account of the surgical treatment of the time:

'A man coming out of a bed by chance jabbing his bare breech down on ye side of ye bed a needle ran up his breech just by his anus. Hee sent for a surgeon of Abbington to pull itt out and hee catching hold of itt with his forceps but not being able to hold itt but itt slipped and afterwards attempting itt hee thrust itt in further within ye cuticula. After wch Mr. Smith, an Oxford Chirurgian, was sent for; but ye fellow had made an incision and cut ye haemor-rhoidal veins wch bled abundantly att wch ye fellow, being dis-couraged, threw down his instruments and ranne away leaving him bleeding. They got a woman in ye town to dress him. Smith could see no signe but went and made a great incision 2 inches deep in ye Menbrana adiposa and thrust in his finger and turned itt about and felt it; then getting an instrument under hee drew itt out cleverly and gave itt him. Ye fellow when he sawe itt, took him in his arms and kisst him and made exceeding much of itt. Hee made not his incision betuixt ye needle and ye anus as did ye other fellow but on ye outside and so no danger of ye sphincter.'

Abingdon is a good seven miles from Oxford, so that, by the time the double journey had been accomplished, to get Surgeon Smith to the patient, some hours must have elapsed. Mr. Smith, the Oxford surgeon, also appears in the following passage: 'A way to stop a flux of blood. Take long needles and take up ye flesh first on one side ye vessel, yn beyond on ye other side and soe drawe ye flesh over itt and itt stopps. But itt seems an odd kind of way, tried by Smith ye Oxford Chirurgion in one, but hee died.'

A Case of Tumour of the Breast

Here is the treatment of tumour of the breast:

'A cancer in Mrs. Townsend's Breast of Alverston taken off by 2 surgeons the one's name was Clark of Bridgnorth, another's was Leach of Sturbridg. First they cutt ye skinne cross and laid itt back; yn they workt their hands in ytt one above and the other below and so till their hands mett and so brought it out. They had their needles and waxt threads ready but never used them, and allso their cauterising irons, but they used them not. Shee lost not above ℨvi of blood in all. Dr. Needham coming too late staied ye next day to see it opened. Hee said itt was a Meliceris and not a perfect cancer, but it would have been one quickly. There came out a flow of a great quantity of waterish substance as much as would fill a flaggon. When they had done they cutt off one one bitt and another another. Put a glass of wine in and some lint and so let it alone till next day. Yn they opened itt again and injected Myrrhe, Aloes, and such things as resiste putrefaction and so bound itt up again. Every time they dressed itt they cutt off something of ye cancer yt was left behind. Ye chirurgions were for applying caustick, but Dr. Needham said "No, not till ye last, since she could endure ye knife ". They prepared her body somewhat, yn let her blood ye day before. She endured it with infinite patience all along, not offering to lay her hand uppon itt to ease itt, but a warme cloth to ye other breast all ye time.

'One of the chyrurgeans told her afterwards that shee had indured soe much yt hee would have lost his life ere he would have suffered ye like; and ye Dr. said hee had read yt woman would indure more yn man, but did not beleeve itt till yn. The way how and where itt should be cutt away was markt out with Ink by one Dr. Edwards, who lives at Bridgnorth. Mrs. Townsend likt him very well. Hee said iff they could prevent a Gangraena there was little fear, but itt might be a cure iff she fell not into a feavour.

The extract is interesting as showing how completely the surgeon was subordinate to the physician. The case was clearly one of Brodie's tumours of the breast, so that Dr. Needham was correct in saying it was not a true cancer. Caspar Needham, of Peterhouse, Cambridge, took his M.A. in 1648, and then went to Oxford for the sake of the public library, and was incorporated 1655. He was one of the early Fellows of the Royal Society, and died at the age of 57 in 1679. He is buried in St. Bride's, Fleet Street, but nothing more is known of him. Dr. Edwards was Richard Edwards, of Bridgnorth, who was admitted an extra Licentiate of the Royal College of Physicians on 19 December 1662.

There is a good instance of a long-standing pathological error in the next note about a patient who clearly had tetanus: 'A worme in ye Gutts caused such a convulsive motion in one yt hee carried his heels and his head violently backwards, and so carrying his bodie into a roundness tumbled up and down with groaning.'

Ward's Medical Observations and Sacerdotal Duties

Ward must have had a singularly bad memory, for sandwiched between these details are such entries as, 'Remember to excommunicate ye 2 persons yt committed Adulterie: ye woman yt turned Catholick: and to [warn] drunkards and ye like.' The warning seems to have taken the form of a sermon, for a few lines farther on he says, 'Remember to preach on 35 Jeremiah, 14, 15, and to prove yt man is readie to obey man rather yn to obey God.' The text is:

'The words of Jonadab the son of Rechab, that he commanded his sons not to drink wine, are performed; for unto this day they drink none, but obey their father's commandment: notwithstanding I have spoken to you, rising early and speaking; but ye hearkened not unto me.

'I have sent also unto you all my servants the prophets, rising up early and sending them, saying, Return ye now every man from his evil way, and amend your doings, and go not after other gods to serve them, and ye shall dwell in the land which I have given to you and your fathers: but ye have not inclined your ear, nor hearkened unto me.'

Sometimes it would seem that his medical observations

must have interfered with his sacerdotal functions, or, at any rate, that his attention was divided, for—

'A woman yt died in childbed. I saw her just before shee departed. Shee was much troubled with convulsive motions wch are twitchings of the heart just before her expiring.' 'Full-chested people are long a dying as was observed in Mrs. Williamson . . . and such people as they are long in dying so are they long likewise ere they come to die.' 'Remember to write to Mr. ffrancis for a reason why a blow under the ear kills so suddenly rather yn in another part.' 'One used to say of his patients that when they were ill they are saints and when they are well they are devils.'

Humorous Stories: Folk-medicine

He was fond of good stories, thus: 'One seeing Dr. Bailey goe by a shop in Oxford said instantly, "Why, there goes ye Dean of Swarum instead of ye Dean of Sarum".' Dr. Richard Baylie matriculated as a plebeian from St. John's College 3 July 1601, aged 15; D.D. 16 July 1633; President 1632; expelled 1648; restored 1660. Chaplain to King Charles I and Laud; Archdeacon of Nottingham 1628; Dean of Salisbury 1635; died 1667. The extract throws a light on the Dean's language.

'One having to say something in the close of a funeral sermon in commendation of ye person deceased he began itt thus: "It is an old saying De mortuis nil nisi verum. It was Mr. Doolie's brother of Alverston at ye death of our Mr. Lane who lived in Mr. Bishop's house."

'Dr. Prideaux said of ye man in ye Gospel yt made excuse because hee had married a wife: says hee, What a fool was hee not to bring his wife with him for yn he had been the more welcome.

'Remember when I goe to London to buy Gusman and Jacobus de Voragine and some other such merrie authors to peruse in winter nights and keep up cheerful innocent mirth.

'My Lord Paget seeing a little bit of mutton in a great platter of pottage put off his doublet. Itt being askt what he intended to doe hee told them hee intended to swimme for ye bit of mutton. This I have heard.'

Here and there pieces of folk-medicine are given, as: Children get ye Nephriticke disease by pissing in ye fireplace say nurses; and some say to pisse in a pot where some man hath pissed before is doing wrong, ye spirits without communicating with those within.'

This appears to belong to the same class of superstition as the preservation of nail-parings and hair-clippings.

'Advise Mr. Benjamin Trapp to touch his swelling in his wrist with a dead man's hand wch may gett itt away.' 'For a person yt hath lost his stomach injoyn him every morning to eat a piece of Cheshire cheese strong of ye Rennet.' 'I have seen Cobwebs prescribed inwardly to be taken in conserves of red roses in a Bill [prescription] at Mch Potters, Nov. 28, 1658'

Conclusion

I have entitled this Part I, as it only deals with the first six volumes of the MSS., and, owing to pressure of work, it has been impossible to make myself acquainted with the remaining ten. These six volumes I have transcribed myself; the rest have been abstracted by Mr. Bethell, your indefatigable Registrar. I hope in the future [1] to deal with his work, for he tells me that it is full of interest; indeed, did time allow, there is much that could have been added from the note-books I have read. They show us Ward as an epitome of his age, well read, quite clear in his opinions, with knowledge based on experiment, and yet with a naïve credulity which is surprising until we recall how little was known for certain and how much that is now certain had still to be learnt. His religion, so far as can be ascertained, dealt more with the broad aspect of truth and morality than with any speculative theology. His object was clearly to help his parishioners in their daily trials rather than to teach them the mysteries of the faith.

[1] On 10 May 1920 Sir D'Arcy Power delivered the Annual Oration before the Medical Society of London on 'The Rev. John Ward and Medicine' (*Tr. Med. Soc. Lond.*, 1920, xliii. 253; vide Bibliography, p. 342).

X

WHY SAMUEL PEPYS DISCONTINUED
HIS DIARY [1]

MR. President and Gentlemen,—It is the pleasant duty of the officers of the club to fill a gap when there is a temporary dearth of papers. I have been called on to perform that duty, and I have naturally chosen the medical aspect as being the one with which I am most competent to deal. I have selected for to-night's paper a short account of the conditions which led Mr. Pepys to end his Diary prematurely, and to the loss of history, at the early age of thirty-six.

I may premise for your information a few facts about the eyesight which are obviously commonplace to the members of my own profession, though they may not be quite so well known to the majority of my audience this evening.

Some Preliminary Remarks on Eyestrain

The eyes are in a normal condition when they see both near and distant objects with equal facility. The power of seeing near objects—i.e. objects not more remote than 20 feet, a distance that has been arbitrarily fixed—depends upon an alteration in the thickness of the crystalline lens which is situated within the eyeball. This alteration in the thickness of the lens is accomplished by a muscular effort. The lens in early life is transparent and elastic, so that the muscular effort is small, but as age increases the lens gets firmer in consistence and less transparent; a greater muscular effort is then required to produce the same effect; whilst as we become older the retina or receptive surface at the back of the eye is somewhat less sensitive. Near objects, therefore, are seen with increasing difficulty as people get older, though vision for distance remains un-

---

[1] An address delivered at a meeting of the Samuel Pepys Club held on 5 April 1911.

D d

altered. The difficulty is usually noticeable between the ages of forty and fifty. It is called presbyopia, for it is a perfectly natural result of increasing years. It is easily remedied by the use of suitable convex spectacles, which act by relieving the muscular effort of accommodation, whilst at the same time they magnify, and so render the impressions on the retina more definite.

The most common divergence from normal vision is long-sightedness or hypermetropia, a condition which results from too great a flatness of the eyeball. All images, whether from near or distant objects, are then focused behind the retina, so that nothing is seen distinctly when the eye is at rest. The lens is focused by a delicate muscular mechanism, and in the slighter cases of hypermetropia objects can be focused by an effort of this—the ciliary—muscle. The power of focusing is called accommodation. It is performed quite involuntarily, but is nevertheless a muscular effort. The muscle thus employed continuously either becomes over-fatigued, when the sight is blurred, or it passes into a state of spasm, which sets up a train of reflex symptoms known collectively as eyestrain. If there is a great amount of hypermetropia the ciliary muscle is unequal to the task of focusing images—especially of near objects—and vision is then so imperfect that there is no eyestrain. The amount of hypermetropia is often unequal in the two eyes, and it may then happen that the patient only uses one eye, the other eye being turned adrift, so to speak, for it is never used. It becomes practically blind, and its loss of function is proclaimed by a squint which follows in course of time.

Another defect of vision is often associated with hypermetropia and is called astigmatism. It is due to the fact that the transparent media of the eye are not equally curved in every direction, and this defect, like hypermetropia, throws an undue strain upon the accommodation, which has to be constantly altered in order to obtain a fairly accurate adjustment both for far and near objects. The accommodation, therefore, is never at rest whilst the patient is awake if he suffers from hypermetropia or from astigmatism. A combination of hypermetropia and astigmatism is necessarily more trying than either defect separately, and it is more likely to be troublesome when it is present in a low degree and in both eyes than when it is high, and higher in one eye than in the other. When the defect is of low degree the patient sees fairly well by a constant effort of the accommodation, but suffers from eyestrain; when it is of high degree he gets no eyestrain, because he cannot see sufficiently well to do much work with his eyes. He does not use them, therefore, to any great extent, or he obtains spectacles which enable him to see better. A comparatively low degree of hypermetropia with some astigmatism gives rise to the train of symptoms which are now known to depend upon eyestrain or an overuse of the mechanism of accommodation. These symptoms are often reflex in character, and, as at first sight they do not appear to bear any relation to the cause, they long passed unrecognized.

Chief amongst the symptoms of eyestrain are watering of the eye; a glueing together of the eyelids on awakening in the morning; headache, the position and character of which vary with each individual. It may be neuralgic or it may be deeply seated, as was the case with Wagner the musician, who was complaining constantly of 'the nerves of his eyes'. The headache is often replaced by an inflammation of the eyelids, especially in young and healthy persons who also have a little conjunctivitis with a feeling of tension or fullness in the eyes which may become real pain of a dull aching character, the eyeballs being very tender on pressure. Sometimes there are vertigo and sickness, with dyspepsia, palpitation, and even difficulty in breathing. Sleeplessness is a very frequent symptom, due in part to the excessive flow of blood to the brain and in part to the low tone of the whole nervous system.

The symptoms of eyestrain appear sooner in those who lead a confined and sedentary life, who follow occupations which need a constant use of the eyes in bad or unsuitable light, and in those who are debilitated from any cause. The symptoms appear later in those of coarser fibre, who pass much of their time in the open air or who follow occupations which do not need a prolonged use of the eyes for close work. Clerks, therefore, often wear spectacles, whilst it is rare to see them amongst an agricultural population. With increasing years presbyopia is added to the hypermetropia, and the patient is then reduced to the same condition as he would have been if he had originally suffered from a high degree of hypermetropia. He must either give up using his eyes or he must obtain suitable spectacles. The spectacles in such a case would be convex glasses to correct the hypermetropia, ground in such a manner as only to permit the rays to be focused in that meridian through which the patient sees best if he also suffers from astigmatism. The glasses, therefore, are convex and cylindrical.

Let us see how these facts fit in with the record which Mr. Pepys has left us in his Diary. I quote from our President's edition in ten volumes.[1]

Mr. Pepys's Account of his Visual Troubles

The first record of any complaint about his eyes is made by Mr. Pepys on 19 January 1663/4, when he was nearly thirty years old, and had been rather worried by an unreasonable jealousy of his wife. He writes: 'I to my office till very late, and my eyes began to fail me, and be in pain which I never felt to nowadays, which I impute to sitting up late writing and reading by candle-light.' Again, on 1 April 1664 he complains: 'This day Mrs. Turner did lend me, as a rarity, a manuscript of one Mr. Wells, writ long ago, teaching the method of building a ship, which pleases me mightily. I was at it to-night, but durst not stay long at it, I being come to have a great pain and water in my eyes after candle-light.' On 4 May: 'So home to dinner, and after dinner to my office, where very late, till my eyes (which begin to fail me nowadays by candle-light) begin to trouble me.' And on the following day: '. . . to

[1] *The Diary of Samuel Pepys*, edited by H. B. Wheatley, London, 1893–9.

the office ... and thence betimes home, my eyes beginning
every day to grow less and less able to bear with long
reading or writing, though it be by daylight: which I never
observed till now.' On 5 October 1664 he set about getting some assistance for his sight, for 'then comes Mr.
Cocker to see me, and I discoursed with him about his
writing and ability of sight and how I shall do to get some
glasse or other to helpe my eyes by candle-light: and he
tells me he will bringe the helps he hath within a day or
two, and shew me what he do'.

On 11 October 1666 there is a memorandum to the
effect that 'I had taken my Journall during the fire and
the disorders following in loose papers until this very day,
and could not get time to enter them in my book till
January 18th, in the morning, having made my eyes sore
by frequent attempts this winter to do it'. On 13 December 1666: '. . . for these three or four days I perceive my
over-working of my eyes by candle-light do hurt them as
it did the last winter, that by day I am well and do get
them right, but then after candle-light they begin to be
sore and run, so that I intend to get some green spectacles.'
Three days later: '. . . home by water and so to supper and
to read and so to bed, my eyes being better to-day, and I
cannot impute it to anything but by my being much in the
dark to-night, for I plainly find it is only excess of light
that makes my eyes sore.' A few days later, on Christmas
Eve, he writes: 'I do truly find that I have overwrought
my eyes, so that now they are become weak and apt to be
tired, and all excess of light makes them sore, so that now
to the candle-light I am forced to sit by,' adding, 'the snow
upon the ground all day, my eyes are very bad, and will
be worse if not helped, so my Lord Bruncker do advise as
a certain cure to use greene spectacles, which I will do'.
However, it did not depress him much, for he continues:
'So to dinner, where Mercer with us and very merry.'
And later on the same day: 'I this evening did buy me
a pair of green spectacles, to see whether they will help my
eyes or no. . . . Then home to the office, and did business

till my eyes began to be bad and so home to supper.' On New Year's Eve he was busy with his accounts 'till my eyes became very sore and ill, and then did give over, and supper, and to bed'.

Pepys does not again complain of his eyes until 12 April 1667, when: 'I close at my office all the afternoon getting off of hand my papers, which, by the late holidays and my laziness, were grown too many upon my hands, to my great trouble, and therefore at it as late as my eyes would give me leave.' And on the following day: '... then to the office, where sat all the afternoon till late at night, and then home to supper and to bed, my eyes troubling me still after candle-light, which troubles me.' A few days later, 22 April: 'Did business till my eyes were sore again, and so home to sing, and then to bed, my eyes failing me mightily.'

Mr. Pepys makes no further complaint, after this, until 3 August 1667, when, after he had been very busy with the Admiralty accounts to show that the total debt was £950,000, 'my eyes began to fail me, which now upon very little overworking them they do, which grieves me much'. On Sunday, 4 August, he writes again: 'Busy at my office from morning till night in writing with my own hand fair our large general account of the expence and debt of the Navy, which lasted me till night to do, that I was almost blind.' Two days later: 'I to the office, busy as long as my poor eyes would endure, which troubles me mightily.' On 19 August he writes: 'I home to supper and to read a little, (which I cannot refrain, though I have all the reason in the world to favour my eyes, which every day grow worse and worse, by over-using them).' On 24 September: 'At business till twelve at night, writing in short hand the draught of a report to make to the King and Council to-morrow. . . . This I did finish to-night to the spoiling of my eyes, I fear.' The next day: 'My eyes so bad since last night's straining of them that I am hardly able to see, besides the pain which I have in them.' This pain lasted at least over the next day, because on 26 September 1667 he concludes the report of the day's proceedings with, 'and for the ease of my eyes to bed, having first ended all my letters at the office'.

At the beginning of this winter Pepys took some trouble to get his defective sight improved, for on 4 November: 'I took a coach and went to Turlington, the great spectacle maker, for advice, who dissuades me from using old spectacles, but rather young ones, and do tell me that nothing can wrong my eyes more than for me to use reading glasses which do magnify much'. Mr. Turlington's advice was superlatively bad, for he was clearly recommending Pepys to use concave glasses when in reality he needed convex ones. It is probable that the spectacles were tried and found unsuitable, for he never bought them, and on the 14th—a fortnight later—he writes: 'So home to supper and to bed, my eyes being bad again; and by this means the nights nowadays do become very long to me, longer than I can sleep out.' In his survey of April 1668 he says that he is in 'some trouble for my friends . . . and more for my eyes, which are daily worse and worse that I dare not write or read almost anything'.

We read no more about the state of Mr. Pepys's eyes for the next six months, until 20 June 1668, when there is an entry: 'So we home and there able to do nothing by candle-light, my eyes being now constantly so bad that I must take present advice or be blind. So to supper, grieved for my eyes, and to bed.' His eyes must have been more than usually painful at this time, for on 29 June— nine days later—he writes: '. . . toward St. James', and I stop at Dr. Turberville's and there did receive a direction for some physic, and also a glass of something to drop into my eyes: who gives me hopes that I may do well.' On the following day: 'Supper about eleven at night: and so, after supper, parted, and to bed, my eyes bad, but not worse, only weary with working. But, however, I very melancholy under the fear of my eyes being spoiled and not to be recovered: for I am come that I am not able to read out a small letter, and yet my sight good for the little while I can read, as ever they were I think.' On 13 July: 'This morning I was let blood, and did bleed about fourteen ounces, towards curing my eyes.' Two days later, on 15 July: 'Up, and all the morning busy at the office to my great content, attending to the settling of my papers there that I may have the more rest in winter for my eyes by how much I do the more in the settling of all things in the summer by daylight.' On the 29th again he notes: 'My eyes for these four days being my trouble and my heart thereby mighty sad.' Again on 31 July he concludes his diary for the month with the reflection: 'The month ends mighty sadly with me, my eyes being now past all use almost; and I am mighty hot upon trying the late printed experiment of paper tubes.' The next day, 1 August, he again says: '. . . at night to bed, my eyes making me sad.' Indeed, they were so bad at this time that he made his boy (2 August) 'read to me several things, being nowadays unable to read myself anything for above two lines together, but my eyes grow weary'. But on 4 August he was obliged to sit up until 'two in the morning drawing up my answers (for the Committee of Tangier) and writing them fair which did trouble me mightily to sit up so long because of my eyes'. A few days later, on 11 August, he was 'at the office all the afternoon till night, being mightily pleased with a little trial I have made of the use of a tube-spectacall of paper, tried with my right eye'. The result of the trial seems to have been satisfactory, for on the 12th he went to the play and saw *Macbeth* and 'then home, where the women went to the making of my tubes'. But the improvement was not long maintained, as on the 15th: 'So home and to my business at the office my eyes bad again, and so to bed.' And on the 17th again: '. . . late, reading over all the principal officers' instructions in order to my great work upon my hand, and so to bed, my eyes very ill.' On 21 August he went to 'Reeves's and bought a reading glass'. His eyes became rather less troublesome, for on 23 August: 'After dinner to the Office, Mr. Gibson and I, to examine my letter to the Duke of York, which to my great joy I did very well by my paper tube without pain to my eyes.' His wife and others often read to him, and thus relieved the strain upon his eyes, for it is not until the end of November in his review of the month that he again complains about them, saying: 'But my eyes are come to that condition that I am not able to work'; and again on 16 February 1668/9:

'. . . my eyes mighty bad with the light of the candles last night, which was so great as to make my eyes sore all this day, and do teach me by a manifest experiment that it is only too much light that do make my eyes sore. Nevertheless, with the help of my tube and being desirous of easing my mind of five or six days journall, I did venture to write it down from ever since this day se'nnight, and I think without hurting my eyes any more than they were before, which was very much, and so home to supper and to bed.'

A few days later he complains again: '. . . myself out of order because of my eyes which have never been well since last Sunday's reading at Sir William Coventry's chamber.' Even at the playhouse in a good place among the Ladies of Honour he 'was in mighty pain to defend myself from the light of the candles'.

From his thirty-sixth birthday onwards the complaints about his eyes become even more frequent and always in the same strain, 'pretty merry only my eyes which continue very bad', and they were so painful on many occasions that he was obliged to curtail even his play-going. At the end of March 1668/9 he was

'to my great grief put to do Sir G. Downing's work of dividing the customs for this year between the Navy, the Ordnance, and Tangier; but it did so trouble my eyes that I had rather have given £20 than have had it to do.'

This extra work led him to make another attempt to get relief, for on 25 April:

'Up and to the office awhile and thither comes Lead with my vizard, with a tube fastened within both eyes; which with the help which he prompts me to, of a glass in the tube, do content me mightily, and then . . . he being gone, to write down my Journal for the last twelve days; and did it with the help of my vizard, the tube being fixed to it, and do find it mighty manageable, but how helpful to my eyes this trial will show me.'

Pepys had the tubes altered with his usual ingenuity, for on 8 May 1669:

'Up and to the office and there comes Lead to me and at last my vizards are done and the glasses got to put in and out as I will; and I think I have brought it to the utmost, both for easiness of using and benefit, that I can; and so I paid him 15s. for what he hath done now last in finishing them, and they I hope will do me a great deal of ease. At the office all this morning and this day the first time did alter my side of the table after eight years sitting on that next the fire. But now I am not able to bear the light of the windows in my eyes, I do begin there, and I did sit with much more content than I had done on the other side for a great while, and in winter the fire will not trouble my back.'

The vizard and the change of position proved of small use, however, for on 16 May 1669:

'Dined at home . . . and I all the afternoon drawing up a foul draught of my petition to the Duke of York about my eyes for leave to spend three or four months out of the Office, drawing it so as to give occasion to a voyage abroad, which I did to my pretty good liking.'

The next few days were spent in trying to find an opportunity of presenting the petition to the Duke, and it was not until 19 May

'dinner done, I out, and to walk in the Gallery [at White Hall] for the Duke of York's coming out. . . . By and by the Duke of York comes and readily took me to his closet and received my petition and discoursed about my eyes and pitied me and with much kindness did give me his consent to be absent and approved of my proposition to go into Holland to observe things there of the Navy, but would first ask the King's leave, which he anon did, and did tell me that the King would be a good master to me, these were his words, about my eyes.'

Leave being thus obtained, the remaining days of the

month were spent in making preparations for the holiday, and the Diary ends on 31 May 1669.

'And thus ends all that I doubt I shall ever be able to do with my own eyes in the keeping of my Journal, I being not able to do it any longer, having done it now so long as to undo my eyes almost every time that I take a pen in my hand; and therefore whatever comes of it I must forbear; and therefore resolve, from this time forward, to have it kept by my people in long-hand, and must therefore be contented to set down no more than is fit for them and all the world to know; or, if there be anything, which cannot be much now my amours to Deb. are past and my eyes hindering me in almost all other pleasures, I must endeavour to keep a margin in my book open, to add here and there a note in shorthand with my own hand. And so I betake myself to that course which is almost as much as to see myself go into my grave; for which and all the discomforts that will accompany my being blind, the good God prepare me!'

Cause of the Condition and the Remedy

Any one who reads critically the account which Mr. Pepys has given of the state of his eyes must feel sure that he suffered from hypermetropia with some degree of astigmatism, and that his fear of becoming blind was wholly unfounded. These errors of refraction were not very great, though they were sufficient to cause eyestrain and undue sensitiveness of his retinae. He did not suffer from headache, or he would have said so; he did not squint, or his portraits would have shown it. The eyestrain came on when he was about thirty. He had been accustomed to lead an outdoor life, but he now settled down at his office, began to use his eyes for long spells of work, and was concerned with masses of figures which often required the closest attention. The paper at this time was coarse, the writing was crabbed, and the candle-light by which he worked was insufficient. Considerable strain, therefore, was put upon his accommodation, and the latent defect soon became manifest.

I asked my friend, Mr. Ernest Clarke, what spectacles he would recommend for a young man who came to him complaining of similar symptoms, and he replied at once: +2D. or +2·5 D. convex glasses. I have very little doubt that Mr. Cocker and Mr. Lead supplied this strength of glass, but the eyestrain continued. There was some cause, therefore, additional to the hypermetropia, and this was the slight degree of astigmatism. Mr. Pepys complained that his eyes were especially troublesome when he had been reading music, or working long at figures, and these are exactly the conditions which are most trying to the astigmatic. I have therefore added to Mr. Clarke's prescription: +0·50 D. cylinders axis 90°. The prescription reads, therefore:

For Samuel Pepys Esq.

Spectacles—

+2 D. c. +0·50 D. cyl. axis 90°.

This prescription Mr. Edward C. Bull, who is the manager of the Birmingham branch of Messrs. C. W. Dixey's business, has put up in the silver frames which it is most likely that Mr. Pepys would have had, for they are similar to a pair which went to America in the *Mayflower* in 1620. With these glasses the Diary might have been continued at any rate for several subsequent years.

Such a prescription, however, would have been impossible. Convex and concave spherical glasses for spectacles seem to have been the outcome of the marvellous twelfth and thirteenth centuries. Roger Bacon is generally credited with their invention, and Hirschberg says: 'From the middle of the fourteenth century convex spectacles were commonly known.' From that time the older people of the Old and New Testaments, as depicted in pictures, stained-glass windows, and statues, are provided with spectacles. Spectacles are referred to in public transactions, valuations of property, and wills. They were still somewhat costly. Towards the end of the fifteenth century their use became general as the result of the invention of printing. Spectacle-makers are mentioned as early as 1482 at Nürnberg. But lenses were only known in their stronger forms; and as late as 1841, Mr. Bull tells me, +0·75 was the weakest lens made by Chevalier, the great optician, and it was left to Sichel to employ a $+0.50$ D.

Concave glasses for short sight were introduced later than convex glasses, for they seem to have been first used in Paris some time before the middle of the sixteenth century, although Roger Bacon is said to have suggested them. But it was not until well on in the nineteenth century that the proper question of treatment by glasses received the serious attention of ophthalmic surgeons, and it was after the middle of the century before this matter had been put on the scientific basis which determines the practice to-day.[1]

Astigmatism was known to Young at the beginning of the nineteenth century; it was named by Whewell and popularized by Donders (1818–89). Chamblant first made the tools for working cylindrical glasses in 1820, and Mr. Bull tells me that the first cylinders made in England were by Fuller, of Ipswich, for the use of Sir George B. Airey, the great astronomer. Chevalier said, however, in 1841, that the cylindrical glasses invented by Gowland had long been abandoned.

It is clear, therefore, that the hypermetropic astigmatism from which Mr. Pepys suffered could not have been cured by glasses during his lifetime, for science was not sufficiently advanced to recognize the condition. But astigmatism can be relieved by allowing the rays of light to pass through only a single meridian of the irregularly curved cornea or lens. It is tantalizing to think that Pepys might have stumbled accidentally upon this method if anything had caused him to read through a slit whilst he was wearing his glasses. This might easily have happened had he sat upon his tubes and crushed them, or if in the agitation of speaking he had squeezed them flat in his hands. He would then have found his eyestrain removed; his acute mind would have set itself to determine the

---

[1] G. A. Berry: The Presidential address delivered before the Ophthalmological Society of the United Kingdom. *Transactions of the Ophthalmological Society*, 1910, xxx. 15.

cause; he would have pasted strips of black paper on each side of his glasses, and the Diary might have been continued to the end of his life; whilst the paper he would certainly have read on the subject before the Royal Society would have added still greater lustre to his name and might have revolutionized the laws of dioptrics.

XI

THE CENTENARY OF THE ROYAL COLLEGE OF SURGEONS OF ENGLAND, 1900

THE Royal College of Surgeons of England, like its predecessors, the Barbers' Gild, the Fraternity of Surgeons, the Barbers' Company, the United Company of Barbers and Surgeons, and the Surgeons' Company, has always performed two great duties. It has taught all and sundry interested in surgery, by means of lectures in anatomy, physiology, and surgery, the lectures being delivered by the most able men of the time. It has examined its apprentices at the end of their servitude, and only after an examination of greater or less severity has it been possible to become a member of the body corporate. To these duties the Royal College of Surgeons has added the care of the great museum founded by John Hunter, and has enriched it with the additions of a hundred years, and it has founded and maintained a noble library of anatomical, surgical, and scientific books.

The College as a Corporation

The Royal College of Surgeons was established on 22 March 1800 by letters patent under the Great Seal of Great Britain from George III, granted at the humble petition of James Earle, a late Master of the Surgeons' Company. Earle was born in 1755, was appointed assistant surgeon at St. Bartholomew's Hospital in 1770, and surgeon to that institution in 1784. He married a daughter of Percivall Pott, whose works he edited with a memoir. His position as surgeon extraordinary to George III enabled him to exercise his influence in obtaining the charter for the College of Surgeons, and in 1802 he received the honour of knighthood. He was Master of the College in 1807, and died in 1817.

The charter founded the Royal College of Surgeons in London for the promotion and encouragement of the study

and practice of the art and science of surgery in direct
succession to the Surgeons' Company, which had been
dissolved in the year 1796. The college was granted a
common seal, and was allowed to hold land, &c., to the
yearly value of one thousand pounds. It was to be independent of the City of London, to which members of the
previous companies had always been attached as full citizens with the franchise, but it enjoyed all the other privi-
leges and possessions of the older corporations. It was
particularly enacted that the company should continue to
provide a proper place within four hundred yards from the
place of execution for the purpose of conveniently dissecting and anatomizing the bodies of such murderers as
should be delivered to them by virtue of an Act of Parliament passed in the twenty-fifth year of the reign of King
George II, intituled 'An Act for the better preventing the
horrid crime of murder'.

The governing body of the college was to consist of a
Court of Assistants of twenty-one persons, of whom ten
were to be constituted examiners of surgeons, and of these
ten one was to be the principal Master of the Company
and two others were to be Governors. The entire management was given to the Master, Governors, and Court of
Assistants, and the members had no voice at all in the
college affairs. The charter named the first members of
the governing body and was granted to Charles Hawkins,
one of the principal serjeant surgeons, who was designated
the first Master; William Long and George Chandler
being the first Governors; Joseph Warner, William Lucas,
Samuel Howard, William Cooper, James Earle, Thomas
Keate (Surgeon-General of the Forces), and Charles Blicke
being the first examiners. Charles Hawkins had been the
last master of the Surgeons' Company. Joseph Warner
was remarkable from the fact that he was a member of
the three Corporations of Surgeons. He was the favourite
apprentice of Samuel Sharp, the great surgeon of Guy's
Hospital, and was admitted a member of the Barber-
Surgeons' Company on 1 December 1741, was chosen a

member of the Court of Assistants of the Corporation of Surgeons on 5 April 1764, and was nominated to the Court of Examiners of the Royal College of Surgeons when it was founded. He was of such strict integrity, and so punctually attentive to truth, even in small matters, that to the end of his life when he met his colleagues at the Court of Assistants he invariably accosted them thus: 'How d'ye do, gentlemen? I am glad to see you all, except Mr. Cowell', for Cowell, by an underhand proceeding, had supplanted Warner by getting himself elected surgeon to Guy's Hospital whilst his opponent was out with Cumberland, suppressing the Scottish rebellion, in 1745. Warner shared with Bromfield, Sir Caesar Hawkins, and Sharp the civil surgical practice of London, and it was the success of these surgeons which prevented John Hunter sooner coming to the front. He died on 24 July 1801, leaving behind him the reputation of being the first surgeon to tie the common carotid, an operation he performed in 1775. Charles Blicke was born in 1745, was educated at St. Bartholomew's Hospital, where he succeeded to the office of surgeon, on 17 July 1787, in the place of Percivall Pott, who then resigned. In 1779 he was living in Mildred Court, and received John Abernethy as apprentice in surgery. He made a considerable fortune, was knighted in 1803, during his year as Master of the College, and died in 1815, being, according to Abernethy, fonder of money-making than of science. He turned his fortune to good account, however, in the service of the college, for he bequeathed it a sum of money to be spent on the library.

The charter allowed the members of the governing body of the college to nominate new colleagues as occasion required. They were appointed for life, but the Masters and Governors changed annually, the day of their election being fixed for the first Thursday in July, no Master or Governor to be elected unless he was already a member of the Court of Examiners. The Court of Examiners from time to time, upon request of the Commander-in-Chief and the Lords of the Admiralty, were required to examine all army and navy surgeons, their assistants, and mates.

It is clear from the provisions of the charter here enumerated that no advance was made by the new college, but that it was intended to occupy exactly the same position as that held by the Surgeons' Company. This company, though it had only been constituted in 1745, when the surgeons of London had separated themselves from the barbers, had long been a byword amongst the better class of surgeons. In 1790 Mr. Gunning had delivered himself of a most scathing speech at the end of his year of office as Master. He had pointed out that the books of the company had been kept in a very irregular manner. No entries had been made of what passed at the Court of Examiners, and as to the Minutes of the Court of Assistants they had never been signed by the Master. The bills were brought in late, paid late, and audited late, until at last they scarcely made their appearance at all. The clerk himself had absconded with eight or nine hundred pounds belonging to the company, and with the very security for his fidelity in his own possession. Before each examination the Court of Examiners met at a quarter to four at a tavern and dined almost immediately afterwards. He then went on to say, 'You have a theatre for your lectures, a room for a library, a committee-room for your court, a large room for the reception of your communities, together with the necessary accommodations for your clerk. But how great soever your intentions were, I am sorry to observe they have been very ill-executed. Your theatre is without lectures, your library room without books is converted into an office for your clerk, and your committee-room has become his eating parlour, and is not always used even in your common business, and when it is thus made use of it is seldom in a fit and proper state. If your committee-room is to be converted into an eating parlour, why should we not eat in it ourselves? Your dinners at the tavern are exceedingly inconvenient and expensive, and attended with great loss of time. You meet at the hall, you adjourn to the tavern, you return to the hall again, and all this when you have a house of your own inhabited at a great expense to you, and where if you have not already all the conveniences you want, you may at any time be furnished with them.' Surgeon-General Gunning was actuated by no spirit of pique in these observations, but the mischief had extended too deeply for any reforms, and the company had so far lost the confidence of its members that its downfall was assured.

The establishment of the new college on the old lines, therefore, did not receive the approval of the younger members of the profession, and for many years the college was quite out of harmony with its environment. In 1815 it lost the opportunity of taking a representative place, and allowed the Society of Apothecaries to act as sponsor to the modern system of medical education formulated in the Apothecaries' Act of that year. It was not until 1843 that it threw off its lethargy, and by abolishing the system of co-option and life appointments paved the way for a more liberal policy. The order of Fellows was then founded, and the college has gradually assumed a position equal to its importance.

The College as a Qualifying Body

It is not very easy to ascertain the cost of becoming a member of the College of Surgeons in the early years of the century. But the curriculum, with its necessary expenses, was somewhat as follows: Every one who wished to obtain the membership had to serve as an apprentice for a term of seven years. Before his indentures were signed, if he was to serve in London, or within seven miles, he was brought before the Court of Examiners to be examined as to his knowledge of Latin. If his answers proved satisfactory he was duly bound to the surgeon, his master, for seven years, and paid a fee of 10 guineas to the college, this sum being allowed off his diploma at the end of his servitude. For the apprenticeship the usual charge was £100, the master undertaking to feed and house his apprentice, to find him suitable clothing and pocket-money, according to his station in life, and medical attendance when he was ill. The fee for apprenticeship varied greatly, and the surgeons to the large London hospitals charged from £500 to £1,000. It was tacitly agreed, however, in these cases, that the apprenticeship carried with it a chance—if not the right— to succeed by seniority to the master's place. This 'hospital system', as it was called, became an abuse in process of time, though it only ended when apprenticeship fell into desuetude after the passing of the Medical Act in 1858. Although the term of apprenticeship was seven years, yet the last portion was always spent in London 'walking the hospitals' and attending systematic lectures, and a pupil rarely spent more than five and a half or six years with his master. He appeared in London, usually for the first time, on 29 September, and entered himself at one of the hospitals. At St. Bartholomew's Hospital in 1797 the fee for a surgeon's pupil was 25 guineas a year, and if allowed to dress the patients 50 guineas. A like sum of 25 guineas, paid by a physician's pupil, gave him the privilege of an unlimited attendance. At St. Thomas's Hospital the fee for the surgeon's pupil was £25 and £50 for a dresser, and it is expressly stated that if the surgeon's pupils go round with the physicians while prescribing, a further fee of $5\frac{1}{2}$ guineas is taken of each. At Guy's Hospital the pupils for a year paid as at St. Thomas's. The surgeon's pupils entering for a year at either hospital were allowed to see the practice of both and might attend for two seasons. At the Westminster Hospital the physician's or surgeon's pupils paid 20 guineas each. At St. George's Hospital a physician's pupil paid for a year 20 guineas, and was perpetual for 24 guineas. A surgeon's pupils paid 20 guineas for a year, but none were admitted as perpetual students. At the London Hospital the fee for the surgeon's pupils for a year was 30 guineas and a physician's 20 guineas, whilst at the Middlesex the physician's and surgeon's pupils each paid 20 guineas a year. A little later—about 1830—the time-table laid down for the hospital student was as follows: Midwifery from eight till nine a.m. Chemistry from half-past nine to eleven, three days a week. The practice of medicine at the same hour the three alternate days. Walking the hospitals every day from one till two. Anatomy from two to four. Demonstrations of anatomy in the morning at eleven. Physiology from six to half-past seven twice a week. Surgery from half-past seven to nine the same evening. Materia medica twice a week in the evening. Lectures on natural philosophy (optional); and, finally, a meeting of the Hospital Medical Society every Saturday evening, also, fortunately, optional. A student who carried out this programme conscientiously found that he had three or four hours a day for food, exercise, and recreation, with Thursday evening free for the play. The fee for the diploma of the college was £21, and a stamp duty of £1, paid to the Government. For a certificate of qualification as surgeon in the Army, Navy, East India Company's or merchant service, 5 guineas. For a certificate of qualification as assistant surgeon or mate in the Army, Navy, or East India Company's service, 2 guineas.

The College and its Examinations

From the earliest times of which there is any record surgeons who desired to practise in London, or within seven miles of the City, were obliged to become members of the Gild or Company of Surgeons or of Barber Surgeons. Before they were admitted to this privilege it was usual to serve an apprenticeship and afterwards to be examined, though persons of special attainment, or with peculiar influence, were sometimes exempted. The character of the examination varied from time to time and, at any rate from the year 1497, there were two grades, i.e. the ordinary examination for apprentices held *in camerâ*, and the much more formidable examination for 'the Grand Diploma', which was conducted in public after the candidate had called upon his examiners to invite their attendance. The grand diploma was taken by men like Pott,

Cheselden, and Sharp, who wished to attain the rank now held by a Fellow of the College.

The Surgeons' Company seems to have conducted its examinations with as much laxity as the other business. The Court of Examiners met on the first and third Thursdays of every month to admit members and examine surgeons and surgeons-mates for the Army and Navy. Members who meant to practise in the country paid only half the admission fees, but signed a bond to pay the remainder in case they came to reside and practise in London, or within seven miles. The admission fee for the full membership was £27 11s.

Smollett gives an account of the ordeal which had to be undergone in his time by candidates for an assistant surgeoncy in the Navy or the Army. His picture is probably true in substance, though there may be a little spice of malice to flavour it, as we read that Smollett had received a qualification from the United Company of Barbers and Surgeons after he had failed on the first attempt. Roderick Random says:

'I preserved my half guinea entire until the day of examination, when I went with a quaking heart to Surgeons' Hall in order to undergo that ceremony. At that instant a young fellow came out from the place of examination, with a pale countenance, his lip quivering, and his looks as wild as if he had seen a ghost. He no sooner appeared than we all flocked about him with the utmost eagerness, to know what reception he had met with, which (after some pause) he described, recounting all the questions they had asked and the answers he had made. In this manner we obliged no less than twelve to capitulate, which, now the danger was past, they did with pleasure, before it fell to my lot; at length the beadle called my name, with a voice that made me tremble as if it had been the sound of the last trumpet. However, there was no remedy; I was conducted into a large hall where I saw about a dozen of grim faces sitting at a long table, one of whom bade me come forward in such an imperious tone that I was actually for a minute or two bereft of my senses. The first question he put to me was, "Where was you born?" to which I answered, "In Scotland." "In Scotland," said he, "I know that very well; we have scarce any other countrymen to examine here; you Scotchmen have overspread us of late as the locusts did Egypt; I ask you in what part of Scotland was you born?' I named the place of my nativity, which he had never before heard of. He then proceeded to interrogate me about my age, the town where I served my time, with the term of my apprenticeship, and when I informed him that I served three years only, he fell into a violent passion, swore it was a shame and a scandal to send such raw boys into the world as surgeons, that it was a great presumption in me and an affront upon the English to pretend to sufficient skill in my business having served so short a time, when every apprentice in England was bound seven years at least; that my friends would have done better if they had made me a weaver or a shoemaker; but their pride would have me a gentleman (he supposed) at any rate, and their poverty could not afford the necessary education. This exordium did not at all contribute to the recovery of my spirits, but on the contrary reduced me to such a situation that I was scarce able to stand; which being perceived by a plump gentleman who sat opposite to me, with a skull before him, he said Mr. Snarler was too severe upon the young man, and turning towards me, told me that I need not to be afraid, for nobody would do me any harm; then bidding me take time to recollect myself, he examined me touching the operation of the trepan, and was very well satisfied with my answers. The next person who questioned me was a wag, who began by asking me if I had ever seen amputation performed; and I replying in the affirmative, he shook his head and said, "What! upon a dead subject, I suppose? If," continued he, "during an engagement at sea, a man should be brought to you with his head shot off, how would you behave?" After some hesitation, I owned such a case had never come under my observation, neither did I remember to have seen any method of cure proposed for such an accident in any of the systems of surgery I had perused. Whether it was owing to the simplicity of my answer, or the archness of the question, I know not, but every member of the Board deigned to smile, except Mr. Snarler, who seemed to have very little of the *animal risibile* in his constitution. The facetious member encouraged by the success of his last joke, went on thus:—"Suppose you were called to a patient of a plethoric habit, who had been bruised by a fall, what would you do?" I answered, I would bleed him immediately. "What," said he, "before you had tied up his arm?" But this stroke of wit not answering his expectation, he desired me to advance to the gentleman who sat next him; and who, with a pert air, asked what method of cure I would follow in wounds of the intestines. I repeated the method of cure as it is prescribed by the best chirurgical writers, which he heard to an end, and then said, with a supercilious smile, "So you think by such treatment the patient might recover?" I told him I saw nothing to make me think otherwise. "That may be," resumed he, "I won't answer for your foresight, but did you ever know a case of this kind succeed?" I answered I did not, and was about to tell him I had never seen a wounded intestine, but he stopped me by saying, with some precipitation, "nor ever will. I affirm that all wounds of the intestines, whether great or small, are mortal." "Pardon me, brother," says the fat gentleman, "there is very good authority." Here he was interrupted by the other with, "Sir, excuse me, I despise all authority, *Nullius in verba*, I stand upon my own bottom." "But, sir, sir," replied his antagonist, "the reason of the thing shows." "A fig for reason," cried this sufficient member, "I laugh at reason, give me ocular demonstration." The corpulent gentleman began to wax warm, and observed that no man acquainted with the anatomy of the parts would advance such an extravagant assertion. This innuendo enraged the other so much, that he started up, and, in a furious tone, exclaimed, "What, sir! do you question my knowledge in anatomy?" By this time all the examiners had espoused the opinion of one or the other of the disputants, and raised their voices all together, when the chairman commanded silence, and ordered me to withdraw. In less than a quarter of an hour I was called in again, received my qualification sealed up, and was ordered to pay five shillings. I laid down my half guinea on the table and stood some time until one of them bade me begone: to this I replied, "I will, when I have got my change": upon which another threw me five shillings and sixpence, saying, I should not be a true Scotsman if I went away without my change. I was afterwards obliged to give three and sixpence to the beadles, and a shilling to an old woman who swept the hall. This disbursement sunk my finances to thirteenpence halfpenny, with which I was sneaking off.'

One might suppose that the previous meeting of the examiners at the tavern had something to do with the argumentative display here satirized, but whether the facts were true or false the popular ideal of the examination remained unchanged. The accompanying caricature (Plate XII), bearing the date 1811, shows that very little improvement

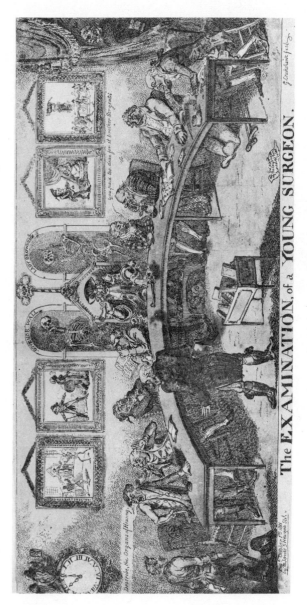

The **EXAMINATION, of a YOUNG SURGEON.**

XII. An examination at the College in 1811

had taken place in the chief surgical examination in England in the space of sixty years.

The sketch was executed by George Cruikshank in the early part of the year 1811 at the age of nineteen. The master is Sir Charles Blicke. The two serjeant-surgeons sitting, in virtue of their office, immediately to the left of the master, are Sir David Dundas, appointed in 1793, and Sir Everard Home, the pupil and brother-in-law of John Hunter, appointed in 1808 upon the death of Charles Hawkins, the first master of the college. Okey Belfour, the secretary, sits on the extreme left of the table with the fees and a money-bag in front of him, whilst William Taylor, the beadle, is visible behind the curtain in the background.

Some of the other examiners in 1810 were James Earle, Thompson Forster, William Blizard, Henry Cline, and Thomas Keate, and as Keate was the immediate past master of the college he sat next the chair, and is probably depicted as the surgeon reading a book on the right of the master.

The skeletons are in allusion to the statutory duty of the college to anatomize the bodies of murderers. Governor Wall was hung at Newgate in 1802 for the murder of Benjamin Armstrong, whom he caused to be whipped to death at Goree in Africa, in 1782. Mr. J. T. Smith gives an account of the execution in his *Book for a Rainy Day* (p. 165). 'Lady Brownrigg' was hung at Tyburn in 1767, for whipping to death Mary Mitchell, her apprentice. She was midwife to the St. Dunstan's workhouse, and her crime excited such reprobation that the crowd nearly tore her to pieces on the way to the gallows. The picture next the skeleton of Governor Wall is a representation of the Hottentot Venus, whose model is still a familiar object to visitors at the college. The pugilistic display with Death seems to be a sly allusion to the fate which nearly befell 'black Sambo', whose physical configuration was so perfect that the college obtained a plaster cast of him. When the plaster set, his thorax was fixed, and he nearly died of asphyxia, for his natural colour prevented the operators noticing that he was more 'black in the face' than usual. The worship of the golden calf explains itself, but I do not know the significance of the fourth picture.

Many of the more liberal-minded members of the college used to insist that the examination was no fair test of knowledge, but ·their protests remained unheeded. The obstacles to reform lay in the facts that the examiners, ten in number, were appointed for life, receiving a salary of £300 a year apiece, a sum by no means excessive when the responsibility, the tedium, and the interruption to other work is taken into account: that the examinations were absolutely private, as neither teachers nor members had any access to them, whilst the whole examination was conducted at one sitting in such widely divergent subjects as anatomy, physiology, pathology, surgery, and the practice of physic connected therewith, and animal chemistry. Even as lately as 1860 these various subjects were discussed at a continuous sitting of an hour divided into four separate quarters, and a candidate who had been subjected to no examination since his indentures were signed emerged from the college in Lincoln's Inn Fields an admitted member and a duly qualified practitioner. From the college he usually passed straight to the dingy little pothouse in Clare Market, where successive generations of successful examinees had signed the book and wetted their diplomas in the style then approved by the somewhat Bohemian community of medical students. Recent improvements in Portugal Street, next to Sheffield Street, have swept away the 'Black Jack' with its memories, and with it has disappeared the celebrated book containing the autographs of many who afterwards became famous, of a few who became infamous, and of the majority who, though obscure, did useful, if humble, service in many a village and country town at home and abroad.

Plate XIII is another caricature of the examination at the Royal College of Surgeons of England, as it was conducted in 1844. The diploma existed, in the opinion of the

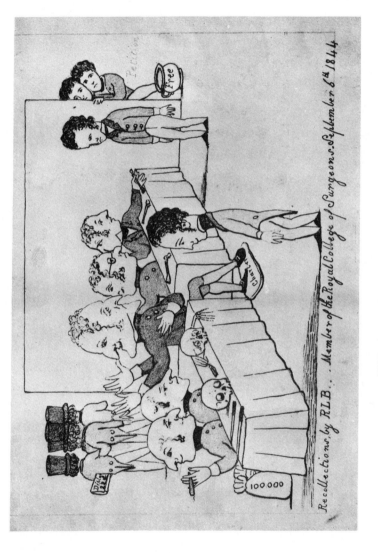

XIII. An examination at the College in 1844

caricaturist, for the pecuniary benefit of the examiners, as representatives of the college, for what was free, though useful, was of small value. The Janus-headed President is Sir Benjamin Collins Brodie, who is trampling under foot the new charter of 1843. Amongst his colleagues on the Court of Examiners were John Painter Vincent, George James Guthrie, Anthony White, Samuel Cooper, William Lawrence, Benjamin Travers, and Edward Stanley.

The modern system of examination began in 1875, when the Court of Examiners delegated some of their authority to certain Fellows of the College who were authorized to examine candidates in anatomy and physiology, the principle having been already approved in 1868, when Dr. Peacock and (Sir) Samuel Wilks were appointed examiners in medicine. In 1886 this system was further improved, and a conjoint examination was held by the Royal College of Physicians of London, and the Royal College of Surgeons of England, in the subjects of medicine, surgery, and midwifery, the successful candidates receiving a licence from the physicians, and the diploma of membership from the surgeons.

The College and its Lectures

The records of the Barber-Surgeons and of the Surgeons' Company show that the older Corporations were always intent on teaching their apprentices and members by a system of lectures. Many worthy men filled the office of lecturer, and determined efforts were made from time to time to keep the teaching in the hands of the surgeons. But the demand for lecturers exceeded the supply, and it was impossible to obtain a succession of capable surgeons to fill the post, even though it was dignified and lucrative. Time after time, therefore, it was necessary for the Companies to turn for help to the Royal College of Physicians, who were always willing and able to lend some of their younger fellows to instruct the surgeons. The great advance which took place in surgical teaching in the last quarter of the eighteenth century has enabled the College of Surgeons to dispense with this help, and the List of Lecturers and Lectures at the Royal College of Surgeons of England, 1810–1900, compiled by Mr. Victor G. Plarr in 1900, shows that, with very few exceptions, all the college lectures have been delivered by Members or Fellows. The object of the lectures, too, has changed very greatly; at first simply instructive, the Treasury agreement which gave to the college the custody of John Hunter's Museum made them explanatory of his collection, whilst of late years the tendency has become more marked to render them vehicles of original research on subjects of pathological and surgical importance.

Blizard and Home delivered the first course of lectures in 1810 and they were followed by Astley Cooper, Abernethy, Lawrence, Brodie, Wilson, J. H. Green, and others of equal reputation. The lectures were delivered twice a week, on Tuesdays and Fridays, at three o'clock in the afternoon, and consisted of a course of fifteen lectures on comparative anatomy or of nine lectures on surgery. Mr. South gives a most graphic account of those which he himself attended when he was an apprentice of Mr. Cline. The year was 1814; (Sir) Astley Cooper was Professor of Comparative Anatomy and Abernethy was lecturing on John Hunter's theory of life.

'The lectures', says South, 'were given in an amphitheatre which was, I think, the most incommodious of any I have ever seen: it was semi-elliptical, with a small semi-elliptical alcove thrown back from the long diameter of the audience part of the building, and the long floor space on which the professor and his table stood was elliptical. A bust of King George III was placed high up on a bracket in the centre of the alcove, and on the floor at each end was a door, the eastern communicating with the court room and front entrance of the college, and the western door led through a little lobby into the museum. Immediately in front of the elliptical floor rose up very sharply tiers of seats to within about 4 feet of the wall, against a tall partition, behind which was a standing gallery, the floor of which was about 8 feet below the semi-elliptical dome and lantern by which the room was lighted. The tiers of seats were very carefully arranged in reference to the dignity of those by whom they should be occupied. The first four rows were appropriated to distinguished visitors and the Court of Assistants, and the Master's chair occupied the middle of the first row, raised to a level with the second; they were admitted by the eastern door on the floor. This more favoured part of the audience was separated by a partition from the members, who occupied several tiers of seats, all, indeed, except two or three rows immediately below the gallery. They were admitted by a little narrow inconvenient door on each side just behind the court, and they were in turn separated by another partition from the upper seats and the gallery occupied by the pupils, who scrambled in by a narrow door at its eastern end. The entrance to the members' and pupils' seats was from Portugal Street, at that time a filthy street, with butchers' and costermongers' carts belonging to Clare Market close by. The doorway was not more than 3 feet 6 inches wide, and opened on a winding, steep, stone staircase, scarcely so wide, which ascended to a landing, at which there was a wicket giving entrance to the members through a passage to their doors in the theatre; but the pupils had to ascend another flight till they reached the wicket by which they got admission to their gallery and seats. Nothing could be more inconvenient and disagreeable than this Portugal Street approach, as for many years the celebrity of the professors was very great, and thus the number of the audience and the desire to get good seats was such that they often stood in a crowd in the dirty street till the appointed hour for opening the door arrived, when the pushing and rushing upstairs could only be compared to the driving up the gallery stairs of a playhouse. Withal, however, though the scuffling often caused rows, and now and then a blow or two, and always a scrimmage with the doorkeepers—who were not of the most pleasant behaviour if the ticket was not ready, or the pupil's arms were so pinioned by the pressure that he could not get his hand into his pocket—yet still, there was plenty of fun, and the youngsters did not feel their dignity offended.

'After much crushing and pushing we, the pupils, got into the theatre; the more fortunate soon filled the seats, the rest had to stand or lean on the gallery rail, and be squeezed by those behind for about twenty minutes, as the students' allotment was soon filled. The more easy-going members avoided the crush, but they, too, gradually filled their seats. The lower tiers, however, remained untenanted for a time.

'As we still wait and admire, from the eastern door stalks in, in a most lordly fashion, a very tall, hard-featured man, who throws a hasty glance upwards, and orders any chance hat which is remaining on the owner's head to be taken off, sees his orders obeyed, and retires; but comes in again, it may be once or twice, and the same scene is repeated.

'At last the clock strikes four, and immediately the College Secretary, Mr. Belfour, appears through the eastern doorway, and heralds a long train of visitors of all degrees and professions to the upper of the reserved seats, and disappears. Immediately appears the beadle in his black robes, and carrying his staff of office, with the silver scutcheon of the college arms, and fixes himself like a statue by the doorway. Now again enters the tall, ungainly man we had already seen popping in and out, and exorcising the hats, but he is now clad in the Master's heavy silk robe, and bears an enormous three-cornered hat. He walks in a most dignified manner to the chair, steps up, remains standing whilst the other members of the Court range round him, then bows very formally to the audience, takes his seat, puts on the formidable hat, and the whole dignity of the college is sustained in the person of Sir William Blizard. He is directly followed by our favourite teacher, Professor Astley Cooper, who comes in with his bright, joyous smile, and evidently as much excited as a boy to make his holiday speech, to be received with long-continued applause, which sadly disturbs the dignified notions of the Master, who rises from his chair, and having in vain tried to put it down, is fain to resume his seat; the cheering gradually subsides, and the lecture begins.'

The lectures were rather a strain upon Cooper, for not being deeply read in the subject of comparative anatomy he resolved to see what industry could do, and restricted himself to three or four hours' sleep that he might gain additional time for the dissection of animals. He also employed several assistants to dissect for him, and the result was that his specimens came by coach-loads to each lecture. Mr. Clift remarks of one lecture: 'This was indeed an overpowering discourse and highly perfumed, the preparations being chiefly recent, and half-dried and varnished.' His lectures were very successful, though there is no doubt that he would have preferred lecturing on surgery, which was allotted to Abernethy.

Although these passages were written by a celebrated surgeon, himself President in 1860, and Hunterian Orator as early as 1844, who died in 1882, they have a curious old-world flavour about them, for they tell of matters which would not be tolerated for a moment at the present time. It will be noticed that the head of the college is spoken of as the Master. The old names of the governing body—the Master, Wardens, and Court of Assistants— had been inherited by the college from the Surgeons' Company, who in turn had obtained them from the United Company of Barbers and Surgeons, established in the reign of Henry VIII, who again had carried on the titles from the Barbers' Company, founded in 1462, whilst there had been Masters and Wardens of the Gild of Barbers sworn yearly at the Guildhall from 1416, and Masters only from 1308. These ancient titles were changed by the charter granted on 13 February 1822, when the chief officers became the President and Vice-Presidents, and the Court of Assistants was called the Council. In the same charter George IV expressed his will and pleasure that 'it shall and may be lawful to and for the said college at all times hereafter, and upon all such occasions as they shall think proper and expedient, to exercise and enjoy the right and privilege of having a Mace, and of causing the same to be borne by such an officer as they shall appoint for that purpose'. The heavy three-cornered hat, emblem of Presidential authority, is still laid on the table—though it is too dirty to wear—at each meeting of the Society of Antiquaries of London, and is familiar to those who possess the engraving of Samuel Medley's picture of the Medical Society of London, where James Sims, who occupies the chair, is actually wearing it.

John Abernethy, President of the College of Surgeons in 1826, deserves special recognition, because he brought to bear upon its affairs a sturdy common-sense and a business-like capacity which afterwards bore good fruit and enabled the college to attain its present exalted position. He promoted the cult of John Hunter, and it is largely to his energy and foresight that the college owes its present magnificent library. Born in 1764, the son of a merchant, he was apprenticed to Sir Charles Blicke, and in 1786 he succeeded at St. Bartholomew's Hospital to the vacancy caused by the resignation of Percivall Pott. As a pupil of John Hunter, he was attracted rather to the physiological than to the anatomical side of surgery, and a prolonged experience of the out-patient room of his hospital taught him to consider many local conditions as manifestations of a constitutional taint. This doctrine he developed to the uttermost in a work abounding with acute and original observation and exhibiting comprehensive and philosophical views: *Surgical Observations on the Constitutional Origin and Treatment of Local Diseases.*

'He reserved all his enthusiasm', says P. M. Latham, 'for his peculiar doctrine; he so reasoned it, so acted it, and so dramatized it (those who have heard him will know what I mean); and then in his own droll way he so disparaged the more laborious searchers after truth, calling them contemptuously "the Doctors", and so disported himself with ridicule of every system but his own, that we accepted the doctrine in all its fulness. We should have been ashamed to do otherwise. We accepted it with acclamation, and voted ourselves by acclamation the profoundest of medical philosophers, at the easy rate of one half-hour's instruction. The great Lord Chatham, it is said, had such power of inspiring self-complacency into the minds of other men, that no man was ever a quarter of an hour in his company without believing that Lord Chatham was the first man in the world, and himself the second; and so it was with us poor pupils and Mr. Abernethy. We never left his lecture-room without thinking him the prince of pathologists and ourselves only just one degree below him.'

Of Abernethy as a lecturer Pettigrew says, 'his mode of entering the lecture-room was often irresistibly droll— his hands buried deep in his breeches pockets, his body bent slouchingly forward, blowing or whistling, his eyes twinkling beneath their arches, and his lower jaw thrown considerably beneath the upper. Then he would cast himself into a chair, swing one of his legs over an arm of it, and commence his lecture in the most *outré* manner. The abruptness never failed to command silence and rivet attention'. The fame of Abernethy's teaching spread far and wide, and he must be regarded as the true founder of the great school attached to St. Bartholomew's Hospital.

Sir Robert Christison, who attended his lectures in 1820, describes Abernethy as a very little man, but in figure and countenance uncommonly handsome. He had not strength enough to become a great operator, nor was he fond of the operating theatre. Cullen, who was his anatomical assistant, says that he had seen him in the retiring room, after a severe operation, with big tears in his eyes, lamenting the possible failure of what he had just been compelled to do by dire necessity and surgical rule. The diagnosis and constitutional treatment of surgical diseases was his favourite field of practice, and in this work he acquired a considerable fortune from the dyspeptic free-livers who abounded then as they do now. Endless are the stories told of his rudeness and eccentricity when such patients applied to him for advice. He is reported to have been consulted by the late Duke of York, before whom he stood whistling, and with his hands in his pockets. The Duke, astonished as this conduct, said, 'I suppose you know who I am?' 'Suppose I do,' said he, 'what of that?' And his advice to his Royal Highness was given thus: 'Cut off the supplies, as the Duke of Wellington did in his campaigns, and the enemy will leave the citadel.' Lord Tennyson had a favourite story which he used to tell of Abernethy. A farmer went to the great surgeon complaining of discomfort in the head—weight and pain. The doctor said, 'What quantity of ale do you take?' 'Oh, I taaks my yaale pretty well.' Abernethy (with great patience and gentleness), 'Now, then, to begin the day, breakfast; what time?' 'Oh, at haafe-past seven.' 'Ale then—how much?' 'I taakes my quart.' 'Luncheon?' 'At eleven o'clock I gets another snack.' 'Ale then?' 'Oh, yees; my pint and a haafe.' 'Dinner?' 'Haafe-past one.' 'Any ale then?' 'Yees, yees; another quart then.' 'Tea?' 'My tea is at haafe-past five.' 'Ale then?' 'Noa, noa.' 'Supper?' 'Noine o'clock.' 'Ale then?' 'Yees, yees; I taakes my fill then. I goes to sleep arterwards.' Like a lion aroused, Abernethy was up, opened the street door, shoved the farmer out and shouted after him, 'Go home, sir, and let me never see your face again. Go home, drink your ale, and be damned!' The farmer rushed out aghast, Abernethy pursuing him down the street with shouts of 'Go home, sir, and be damned'. Yet if Abernethy was merciless to patients of this class, he was unsparing in his attentions to those who were deserving objects of pity, and he often sacrificed his private practice to the needs of his hospital patients. He died at Enfield on 18 April 1831, when the college lost an able administrator and the profession a first-rate surgeon.

The College and John Hunter

The college deserves well of all lovers of John Hunter, for even in its darkest days and when it was most ill-advised it struggled to preserve and increase his reputation. The museum was displayed, catalogued, and increased. Lecturers were chosen to formulate the knowledge stored in it, and since 1814 a distinguished surgeon has been selected to deliver an oration at regular intervals and on 14 February, Hunter's reputed birthday, to celebrate John Hunter's name and fame, the oration being followed by a love feast. Hunter, as is well known, spent his life, or, at any rate, every instant which he could spare from his surgical practice, in amassing a collection of specimens illustrative of comparative anatomy, physiology, and pathology. It was his peculiar merit that he compared, so far as his resources would allow, like with like, and he thus formed the beginnings of series of objects which have since been increased with the most happy results. The simplicity of the plan is as great as its originality, whilst its utility is such that if Hunter could again visit the museum in Lincoln's Inn Fields he would at once be able to resume the threads of his work though he died on 16 October 1793, on the same day, and perhaps hour, that the unfortunate Marie Antoinette, Queen of France, was beheaded in Paris. It is easy to imagine what would be his surprise and pleasure, first, at the old and well-remembered preparations in fresh jars and clean spirit, then at the catalogues made by the master hands of Paget, of Owen, and of Flower; afterwards at the additions to each series, for where he left fifty skulls there are now more than 3,000, and the pathological preparations have more than doubled. Lastly, we may feel sure that he would work eagerly at the new methods, both of preparation and research, and that his receptive mind would soon grasp the use of the microscope and the manifold problems of bacteriology.

The present position of the museum was not attained until it had passed through many vicissitudes. Hunter's death left his collection at 13 Castle Street, at the back of his house in Leicester Square. Here it had been slowly and laboriously gathered together, and here it remained till midsummer, 1806, when the lease expired, and the preparations and manuscripts were removed to Lincoln's Inn Fields. Hunter willed that his collection should be offered to the Government in one lot, then to any foreign Government, then sold by auction in one lot. The Government in 1794 was not in the mood for spending money on anatomy. 'What! Buy preparations,' said Mr. Pitt, 'why, I have not money enough to buy gunpowder.' Lord Auckland and, to a lesser extent, Sir Joseph Banks interested themselves in the matter. The House of Commons appointed a committee to take evidence as to the value of the collection and the cost of its maintenance, and on 13 June 1799 the sum of £15,000 was voted for its purchase. There was some idea that it should be transferred to the College of Physicians, or to the British Museum, but the College of Physicians refused to have it because it would require so much money to keep it up. The Surgeons' Company, quite as poor, did not hesitate a moment, and by a unanimous vote on 23 December 1799 agreed to take charge of the collection and do the uttermost not only to preserve it, but to make it serviceable to the public.

The Treasury, in handing over the Hunterian Collection to the Court of Assistants of the Surgeons' Company, stipulated that it should be open four hours in the forenoon every week for inspection and consultation of the Fellows of the College of Physicians, the members of the Company of Surgeons, and persons properly introduced by them; a catalogue of the preparations, and a proper person to explain it, being at those times always present in the room. That a course of lectures, not less than twelve in number, upon comparative anatomy, illustrated by the preparations, should be given twice a year by some member of the Surgeons' Company. This clause was altered in the following year, at the wish of the company, to the much more comprehensive one that one course of lectures, not less than twenty-four in number, on comparative anatomy and other subjects, illustrated by the preparations, should be given every year by some member of the company, instead of two courses of twelve lectures. The Government further stipulated that the preparations were to be kept in a good state of preservation, and the collection in as perfect a condition as possible, at the expense of the college. It was to be under the management of a Board of Trustees, consisting of sixteen members by virtue of their public offices, and of fourteen others to be appointed in the first instance by the Lords of the Treasury and afterwards to be elected, as vacancies should occur, by a majority of the remaining trustees. The museum was to be inspected annually on a given day by the trustees acting collectively as a board.

The catalogue was at first very imperfect and consisted at the time the museum was bought of twenty-four fasciculi relating to the gallery preparations, i.e. the physiological part of the collection: two separate volumes describing the pathological series, and one other volume relating to the fossils. These catalogues had been compiled from old catalogues formed under the superintendence of John Hunter, and they contained an admirable and perfect account of Hunter's views and opinions in the formation of his collection, though they were very deficient in the explanation of the individual preparations. In 1830 a new catalogue was prepared, but it was unsatisfactory in many ways, and in 1842 (Sir) James Paget, working at first with Stanley, began the great work of his life in the preparation of the *Descriptive Catalogue of the Pathological Specimens contained in the Museum of the Royal College of Surgeons of England*, the separate volumes appearing between 1846 and 1849. The catalogue was a model of its kind, and Paget had so put his heart into the work that in 1878, when a new edition was required, he undertook to bring it out with the assistance of Dr. Goodhart and Mr. Alban Doran, though he was then in the height of his great practice.

The Hunterian collection for many years remained quite inaccessible to visitors. After its removal from Castle Street it was deposited in the dwelling-house belonging to the Royal College of Surgeons in Lincoln's Inn Fields. In 1806 the trustees recommended to Parliament that a grant of £15,000 should be made towards the building, and in 1810 a further sum of £12,500 was voted towards the completion of the building. The college found upwards of £21,000, and the first museum was opened in the year 1813. The rapid increase of the museum and library soon made this building inadequate, and in 1835–6 the college was practically rebuilt by Sir Charles Barry. In 1847 the college purchased the premises of Mr. Alderman Copeland in Portugal Street, and in 1852 erected thereon the Eastern Museum (see p. 247). The warehouse belonging to Copeland's premises was originally the Duke's Theatre. The college premises were again materially enlarged in 1888. Two new museums were added, and the house occupied by the conservator on the eastern side was pulled down, and the Erasmus Wilson *annexe* to the library was built upon its site.

No account of the Hunterian Museum would be in any way complete without mention and recognition of the loving care bestowed upon it by William Clift. Clift was

born on 14 February 1775 at Burcombe, near Bodmin.
He was brought up, says Mr. Stephen Paget, in his ad-
mirable life of John Hunter, in poverty, went to school at
Bodmin, had a taste for drawing, and used to adorn the
kitchen floor with sketches in chalk. Mrs. Gilbert, of
The Priory, Bodmin, who had been a schoolfellow of
Mrs. Hunter, took notice of him and sent him to London
to her old friend. Young Clift came to Leicester Square
on 14 February 1792. He was apprenticed without fee to
Hunter. Board and lodging were given to him in Castle
Street, and he was set to write and to make drawings, to
dissect and to take part in the charge of the museum. For
a year and eight months he saw and wondered at the inces-
sant rush of work and fashion through the great house in
Leicester Square; then came the end of it all, and he took
up again with poverty and lived year by year with an old
housekeeper in the dreary Castle Street house on seven
shillings a week; and at one time, from the war with
France, a quartern loaf was two shillings. He kept things
together and watched over the museum when it was often
difficult to obtain spirit to supply the waste from evapora-
tion in badly sealed bottles; yet such was his care and
assiduity that the whole collection was twice removed
without suffering any damage, and when it left his hands
at the end of this trying time of transition, it was actually
in better condition than when his master, the owner, had
left it. Clift says that from the beginning of 1794 to 1806
he had no books to read except the manuscripts of John
Hunter, and having possession of them, 'I frequently
availed myself of the opportunity to read them. They
related entirely to the subjects of the museum, and as I was
not in the least restricted, and thinking that there was a
great deal of useful information in them, I made large
extracts from some of them, and hope that I have been
instrumental in preserving the substance of nearly half of
the papers destroyed by Sir Everard Home. The manuscripts were the histories of cases in the museum.'
Clift was appointed the first conservator of the museum

in 1800, at a salary of £100 a year, an office in which he was succeeded, in 1842, by (Sir) Richard Owen, who had married his daughter, Caroline Amelia, in 1835. His son, William Home Clift, appointed assistant conservator in 1824, had died from a cab accident in 1833.

The museum contains many interesting preparations, but few, perhaps, show evidence of such careful and skilful work as the injected specimens to be seen both at Lincoln's Inn Fields and in the museum of William Hunter at Glasgow. William Hunter and his pupils, Hewson, Sheldon, and Cruikshank—denominated by Dr. Johnson, whom he attended in his last illness, as 'a sweet-blooded man'—were busily engaged, during the years 1768 to 1786, in a series of elaborate dissections to show the anatomy of the lymphatic system, and their researches led them to some interesting experiments in embalming. Sheldon proved himself a master in this gruesome art, and in some respects was superior, I think, to William Hunter, his master, and to Cruikshank, his fellow-worker.

Both Hunter and Sheldon employed the method of embalming originally introduced by Ruysch, the great anatomist of Amsterdam, where he filled the Chair of Anatomy from 1666 to 1717. He brought the art of embalming to such perfection that Peter the Great is said to have kissed the lips of a child, which Ruysch had preserved, thinking it was asleep. Ruysch's method is still employed, and consists in forcing a preservative fluid into the body through the blood-vessels, in opposition to the older plan of mummification. The methods of the two great English embalmers differed a little in detail. Hunter used Venice turpentine, one pint; oil of lavender, two fluid ounces; oil of rosemary, two fluid ounces; oil of turpentine, five pints. Sheldon used as his preservative camphor dissolved in spirit, in the proportion of one ounce of camphor to six ounces of spirit. In most cases, too, Sheldon removed the viscera and coated them with tar, making a similar application of tar to the visceral cavities before he returned their contents. Both Hunter and Sheldon laid their subjects upon a bed of dry plaster of Paris to absorb any moisture.

John Sheldon was in many respects a most interesting personage; born in 1752, the son of John Sheldon, an apothecary in Tottenham Court Road, he was educated at Harrow, where he was flogged for making a boat and floating it. He learnt anatomy at Watson's anatomical school in Tottenham Court Road, which was wrecked by a mob during his pupilage, and in 1777 he opened a private anatomical school in Great Queen Street. He was appointed Professor of Anatomy at the Royal Academy in 1782, in succession to William Hunter, and was elected F.R.S. in 1784. He became surgeon to the Westminster Hospital in 1786, but his health broke down in 1788 when he resigned his post and removed to Exeter, his house in Great Queen Street being taken and his teaching continued by James Wilson. Sheldon was elected surgeon to the Devon and Exeter Hospital, 25 July 1797, and died on 8 October 1808. He was the first Englishman to make an ascent in a balloon, with Blanchard the aeronaut. It is said that when the balloon unexpectedly descended, Blanchard was very urgent with Sheldon to dismount, and by lightening the car allow the balloon to continue its voyage. Sheldon would not comply, and a short dispute took place. 'If you are my friend', says Blanchard, 'you will alight. My fame, my all, depends on my success.' Still Sheldon was positive. On which the little man in a violent passion swore he would starve him—'Point du poulet—you shall have no chicken, by Gar,' says Blanchard, and saying this he threw out every particle of their provision, which lightening the machine, they once more ascended. It was a good French notion, that the best way to get rid of an Englishman was to throw out the eatables.

The college, as might be expected, possesses many interesting personal relics of John Hunter. There is his mahogany escritoire, his consulting-room table, a chair made from part of his bedstead, his clock which still keeps

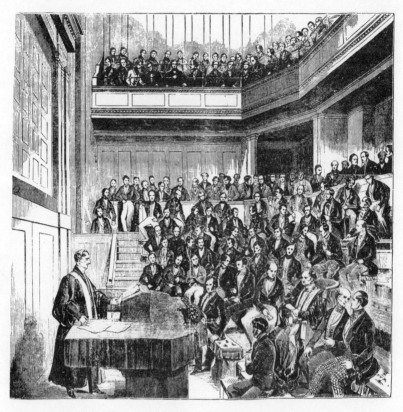

XIV. John Flint South delivering the Hunterian Oration in 1844

good time, his pocket scales in a wooden box, some of his lancets, and many portraits, books, and papers chiefly gathered by the care and assiduity of the late Mr. J. B. Bailey, librarian to the college.

The Hunterian Oration

An annual lecture, called the Hunterian Oration, was instituted in 1814 with a special sum of money vested in the public funds, presented by Dr. Baillie and Sir Everard Home, Hunter's executors. The object of the lecture is to keep green the name of John Hunter and to commemorate dead surgeons worthy to be remembered. At first the oration was given annually, except on a few occasions when it was omitted, but since the year 1853 it has been delivered every other year by the most thoughtful, the most learned, or the most fluent member of the Council of the Royal College of Surgeons of England. In the earlier years of the century the orators were the relatives, friends, and pupils of John Hunter, and we owe them a debt of gratitude, for they have preserved for us many reminiscences which must otherwise have been lost.

The Hunterian Oration depicted in Plate XIV is that delivered by the late Mr. J. Flint South in 1844, J. G. Andrews being President. He commenced by giving an account of the early 'Maisters of Chirurgery', exemplifying the priority of surgery over all the other branches of the healing art, and going on to speak of the incorporation of the Company of Barber Surgeons, and of their ultimate disunion at the foundation of Surgeons' Hall. The orator then traced the rapid upward progress of surgery to its present exalted station, and concluded with a brief memoir of his late colleague at St. Thomas's Hospital, Frederick Tyrrell. The oration, unfortunately, was never published, though from Mr. South's well-known care and accuracy it would have formed a valuable addition to the history of surgery. It is said to have been remarkable because John Hunter was never mentioned. The orator began his theme on so large a scale and at so remote a period, that his allotted time had expired before he reached the middle of the eighteenth century.

The writer has in his possession the following account written by Mr. South of the day's work. It is somewhat in the style of Pepys:

'Wednesday, 14th February, 1844. Up early and hard at work, only finished the principal part of the oration—and an unsatisfactory beginning—obliged to have to trust to only extempore for some part. Went up in glass-coach, took Anny [his wife], with Dolly and Dick, and finished as we went along in a manner. At Fishmongers' Hall discharged the children, took in John, Peter, Annie Towse and Tom Wrench, who had come up from Stouting this morning. Then to college; found myself in good spirits and pluck; went in. Theatre brimming, but plaguey hot before I got to the end. Time would not let me go further than Ranby, where I stopped and finished with speaking of poor Tyrrell. Green congratulated me after. God knows that I am indeed deeply thankful for having acquitted myself, I hope, not discreditably. The number in the theatre, 350. To Freemasons' Hall, where I found Edmund Holroyd and Wyon, who I had asked, and Will. Clowes came in at dinner time. We all sat together with Green, Barlow and Paget opposite and were merry, but the dinner bad and very heavy—left about half-past ten —then to the [Fishmongers'] Hall to pick up Anny and children, and home about twelve.'

The Library

The United Company of Barbers and Surgeons possessed a good library, and one which, if it had been preserved intact, would have been of great value, for it consisted of presentation copies from the great Elizabethan and Stuart writers on surgery, and the following entry shows that the United Company took care of their books.

1638–9. The charge and setting up our books and ancient manuscripts in our new library:

Paid for 36 yards of chain at 4*d*. a yard, and 36 yards at
  3*d*. the yard cometh to . . . . . . xxii*s*. vi*d*.
Paid to the coppersmith for casting 80 brasses to fasten
  the chains to the books . . . . . xiii*s*. iv*d*.
To porters at several times to carry these books . . ii*s*.

Paid to the bookbinders for new binding 15 books   .   xlviii*s*. vi*d*.

Paid for clasping 19 large and small books and fastening
all the brasses to the iron chaines to three score and four
books in the library, new bosses for two great books 8*s*.,
setting on old bosses, i*s*., mending old clasps, ii*s*.   .   xxxi*s*. viii*d*.

Paid for making rings, swivels, and fitting on all the iron
chains   .   .   .   .   xii*s*.

Sum is   .   .   vi*li*. x*s*. viii*d*.

When the separation of the company occurred the clerk
of the Barbers' Company reported on 16 July 1747 that
the library, skeleton, and curiosities had been offered to the
Corporation of Surgeons at a price of twenty-five guineas.
The surgeons, however, replied that they considered themselves entitled to the library under the Act of 1745, but
that, to avoid controversy, they would be willing to refer
the matter to counsel. The opinion was unfavourable to
the surgeons, for on 5 July 1749 it is 'ordered', by the
Barbers' Company, 'that the library of books formerly
belonging to the late lamented company be forthwith sold
for the most money that can be gotten for the same'. All
trace of the books thus dispersed seems to have been lost;
none are to be found, so far as I know, in the British
Museum or in the Bodleian, and the library of the present
College of Surgeons has hitherto failed to yield any example
that can be recognized. Within the last few months, however, I learn that the University Library at Cambridge
contains a copy of John Halle's works—'a gift from the
author to the hall of the Barbers and Surgeons, 15—', as
an inscription on its title-page attests.

The Surgeons' Company remained without a library
until its dissolution, though a room was provided in which
to store the books that were never collected. It was a part
of John Hunter's comprehensive scheme to attach a library
to his collection in the manner successfully accomplished
by William Hunter, his brother. But his energies were so
engrossed in the illustration of life in all its bearings, that
the library never occupied any prominent place in his
thoughts. In 1786, however, he addressed a letter to the

Surgeons' Company, pointing out that the absence of a public surgical library in London is 'a circumstance so extraordinary that foreigners can hardly believe it'. He suggests that all members of the company should send copies of their works to the library, and to give practical effect to the proposal he presented the books he himself had published. But nothing further was done in the matter, and in 1790 Surgeon-General Gunning, the Master, complained that 'Your library room without books is converted into an office for the clerk', and suggested that a sum, not exceeding £80 per annum, might, with advantage, be appropriated to form a library, which should be open, under certain conditions, to students in surgery for their information.

The College of Surgeons at first was as supine in this matter as its predecessor, the Surgeons' Company. A grant of a sum not exceeding £50 towards the purchase of books was made in 1800, and for many years the annual cost was less than the modest £80 suggested by Gunning. Sir Charles Blicke, in 1816, invested the sum of £300, the interest of which was to be spent on the library, and he was, in addition, a liberal donor of books. But the college long laboured under the reproach of having no library, and the members made a constant and special point of this grievance. It was not until the year 1827 that any real effort was made to form a library worthy of the college. In the years 1827–9 the sum of £5,269 was spent on the purchase of books. A reading-room was opened on 1 January 1828, and Robert Willis, a graduate of the University of Edinburgh, was appointed librarian upon the recommendation of Abernethy. The reading-room had risen to the dignity of a library in 1831, but at first it was not greatly used, for during the years 1832–3 it was only visited by 650 persons. When the college was rebuilt in 1835–6 the library department was well provided for, and it has remained practically unchanged since that date, except that in 1888 the Council built an eastern portion, which has added materially to its utility. Willis, the first librarian, proved himself a careful and competent official, who is now known by his scholarly translation of Harvey's works, to which he prefixed an excellent life. He resigned in 1853, and was succeeded by John Chatto, who died in 1887, and was replaced by James Blake Bailey, B.A., Oxon., 'the prince of medical librarians', whose all too early death left the office vacant for the present occupant, Mr. Victor G. Plarr, M.A., Oxon.[1] The library contains a large collection of engraved portraits, and is remarkable for the very large number of serial publications upon surgery and the allied sciences. In 1893 Mr. T. Madden Stone, assistant in the library 1832–53, and clerk 1853–82, enriched the library by presenting it with his extensive and valuable series of portraits and autographs, and Miss Hunter-Baillie has given a very interesting series of letters from Boerhaave, John and William Hunter, Dr. Arbuthnot, Joanna Baillie, and others.

The College Buildings

The surgeons were homeless after their separation from the barbers in 1745, and at first met to transact their business in Stationers' Hall. They soon leased a piece of ground in the Old Bailey, on the site of the present sessions house, erected 1809, and built a hall upon it from the designs, it is said, of William Cheselden, the surgeon to St. Thomas's Hospital. The theatre of this building was used for the first time in August 1751, and the hall was occupied by the Surgeons' Company throughout its corporate existence. On 19 May 1796 'The Master informed the Court that in consequence of a survey and examination made some time since by Mr. Neill, a surveyor called in for that purpose, it appeared that the hall and theatre were very much out of repair, and that the first estimate for these repairs exceeded £1,600. That the tenure by which they are held is only about 55 years, sub-

---

[1] Victor Plarr died on 28 January 1929. After a Council Meeting on 11 April 1929 Sir D'Arcy Power was invited to become Honorary Librarian of the College.

ject to a ground rent and taxes amounting to £240 a year. It had been frequently a subject of consideration among the members of the Court of Examiners whether it would not be for the benefit of the company to dispose of the hall and theatre, and to erect new premises upon freehold ground.' In consequence of this report instructions were given to the clerk to sell the property by public auction if a suitable bid could be obtained. The property was accordingly offered for sale, and in July 1796 it was reported that as no one had bid within £200 of the reserve price, the property had been bought in. It was then let as a drill-hall for the City militia, and it was not until some time afterwards that it was transferred to the City authorities for the sum of £2,100. The company in the meantime had purchased for £5,500 a freehold house in Lincoln's Inn Fields, belonging to Mr. Baldwin, and here a Court of Assistants of the Surgeons' Company was held on 22 November 1797.

When the College of Surgeons was founded in 1800 the house was taken over from the Surgeons' Company, and in 1806 it was modified by G. Dance, R.A. (1741–1825), the designer of Newgate and of St. Luke's Hospital, to enable the Hunterian Collection to be displayed more effectively. Dance encased the original front of the house with stone, and added a portico with round pillars.

The rapid increase of the museum, and the provision of a library, soon made this accommodation insufficient, and in 1835–6 the college was practically rebuilt by Sir Charles Barry, as is seen in the annexed sketch (Plate XV) by George Scharf (1788–1860). The sketch shows, amongst other points of interest, that the pillars of Dance's portico were not taken down but were fluted as they stood. The stone front was also extended from 84 feet to 104 feet, and the front then consisted of a noble portico with fluted columns with a bold entablature, and an enriched cornice bearing the inscription, which may still be read: ÆDES . COLLEGII . CHIRVRGORVM . LONDINENSIS . DIPLOMATE . REGIO . CORPORATI . A.D. MDCCC.

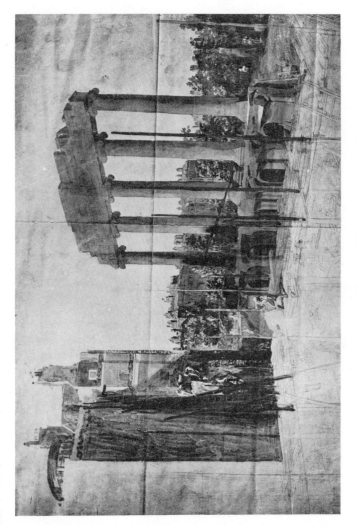

XV. Rebuilding the College in 1835

Water-colour sketch by George Scharf

More space was again needed in 1848 and the college bought the china warehouse of Messrs. Copeland and Spode, upon which the Eastern Museum was built in 1854. The warehouse faced Portugal Street, where is now the long blank wall marking the back of the college buildings. It had a long and interesting history and I, for one, rarely pass down the Comparative Anatomy Museum without thinking of the classic ground upon which it stands. The warehouse had been an auction room, and the auction room was once a barrack, but before it became a barrack it was the Duke's Theatre, where Macklin killed Mr. Hannam in 1735, where Quin played his best parts; the home of the *Beggar's Opera*, 1727–8, 'making Gay rich and Rich gay', as the wits of the time said, alluding to the author and the manager. Here Pepys first saw Nell Gwyn, and here it is said that female characters were first played by women. Tradition still tells that the theatre was closed after a representation of the pantomime Harlequin and Dr. Faustus, because, when a tribe of demons necessary for the piece were assembled, a supernumerary devil was observed, who showed a devil's trick by flying up to the ceiling and making his way through the tiles. He tore away a fourth of the house in his progress and so affrighted the manager that the proprietor never afterwards had courage to open the house. When the college bought the building the only parts of the theatre that remained were the outer walls built on an arched cellar, a large Queen Anne staircase, a saloon on the first floor, and an attic, lighted by windows in the roof, which had been probably the scene-painting loft.

The college premises were again materially enlarged in 1888 with funds derived from the Erasmus Wilson bequest. The frontage was increased upon either side and an additional story was added. Two new museums were thus obtained, the library was greatly improved, a common room was provided for the Fellows and Members, and greater facilities were given to those who wished to pursue original work in connexion with the Hunterian Museum.

Until 1886 the college was self-contained, for even the examinations and all the clerical work in connexion with them were carried on in the building at Lincoln's Inn Fields. But after the union with the Royal College of Physicians more adequate accommodation was obtained by building the Examination Hall on the Victoria Embankment at the foot of Waterloo Bridge. The foundation stone of the building was graciously laid by H.M. the Queen, in March 1886, in the presence of a large assemblage of medical men, clothed for the most part in academic costume. Behind the Examination Hall is a series of laboratories munificently maintained by the two colleges, where excellent and most useful scientific work is carried out under the able supervision of Dr. T. G. Brodie.

It is thus clear that the position occupied by the Royal College of Surgeons of England in 1900 differs *toto coelo* from that which it occupied at its birth in 1800. The college, at the beginning of its career, was hardly representative of the discredited oligarchy which governed it. Then it was penniless, and was lodged in an ordinary dwelling-house. Now it is ruled upon broad lines, which can be still further enlarged as may be required by the continued advance of democracy in the medical profession. It is rich, and is housed in palatial buildings. It acts harmoniously with its sister College of Physicians to secure a thorough training for all its students. It has an anatomical, physiological, and pathological collection second to none in the world, and a library which is renowned, whilst the expenditure on the laboratories shows that the surgeon of to-day looks to pathology for the advance of his art just as our old masters looked to anatomy. All this and more, too, was foreseen by John Hunter, and it may justly be said that had there been no John Hunter there could have been no English College of Surgeons in its present position. In honouring Hunter, therefore, the college honours itself, and may it ever continue to do so, for it could have no greater or more worthy example.

XII

SPENCER WELLS' FORCEPS: A SURGICAL EPONYM

WHEN I was house surgeon to Sir William Savory at St. Bartholomew's Hospital in the year 1883, a single pair of spring forceps was alone provided to arrest the bleeding even in so large an operation as amputation through the middle or upper third of the thigh. At that time, and for some years afterwards, it was the duty of the assistant surgeon always to be present to help his chief at every operation. Amputations, the removal of tumours, ligature of arteries in their continuity, and the relief of strangulated herniae were the usual operations, and by long association the assistant surgeon had learnt every movement of his chief, who always operated for speed. The control of the bleeding was not as difficult as might be thought. The main artery was controlled by digital pressure in cases of amputation, and, as the surgeons had all graduated through the dissecting room, each vessel was picked up in turn, ligatured with silk, and when all the normally situated vessels had been thus tied the pressure on the main vessel was relaxed and any smaller bleeding points were tied.

The need for improved mechanical means to stop bleeding was felt in places, where such skilled assistance as in the older institutions was not attainable, and where abdominal surgery was beginning to be practised.

Attempts were made, certainly as early as 1860, to replace the spring forceps by others with scissors handles and a catch on the shanks, but a single pair was still considered sufficient for each operation, and multiple forceps did not come into use until the little bulldog forceps which, as physiologists, we used to call Krönecker's forceps spread from the physiological laboratory to the operating theatre.[1]

[1] Mr. Alban Doran, in the typed copy of a *Descriptive Catalogue of*

Mr. Spencer Wells published his 'Remarks on Forci-
pressure and the use of Pressure-Forceps in Surgery' in the
British Medical Journal [1879, i. 926]. He there says:

'Mr. Spencer Wells (Samaritan Hospital) has introduced a kind
of artery and torsion forceps, which very conveniently replace the
old spring artery-forceps of Liston and the bull-dogs used for *the
temporary stoppage of bleeding vessels during operations*, while they
are the most readily applied of any of the varieties of torsion-forceps
met with in the shops. They... were first made for Mr. Wells by
Krohne and Sesemann. The grasping and holding extremity is
roughened by rather deeply cut transverse teeth, so that *the bleeding
vessel is forcibly compressed, and its coats squeezed or almost crushed
together*. This is alone often sufficient to stop the bleeding without any
torsion, especially if the instrument be left on the vessel for a minute
or more. But if the vessel be large, then two or more rotations may
be added. Instead of the spring-catch, the fastening is effected by
a Mathieu's catch in the handles. This is quite as easily fixed and
opened as the spring, and is much less likely to get out of order.
The instrument is made of steel, but is coated with nickel, which
prevents any rusting after use.'

This passage, quoted from an article which appeared in
the *British Medical Journal* of 10 January 1874 [1874, i.
47], proves, says Mr. Spencer Wells,

'that before 1874 I had employed forcipressure, not only for the
temporary arrest of bleeding during surgical operations, but had de-

---

*Gynaecological Instruments in the Museum of the Royal College of Surgeons
of England*, gives the following note on the 'Development of the Pressure
forceps. In 1853 Webber invented his anti-ligature forceps. Spencer
Wells used bulldog forceps in all his earlier ovariotomies. In 1858, Charrière introduced his dressing forceps with handles, bows or rings as in
scissors, and a catch on the shanks just above the handles. In 1862 Koeberlé
applied a Charrière's forceps to a bleeding ovarian artery: it came away
spontaneously on the sixth day. In 1865, Verneuil secured the bleeding
stump of a uterine polypus by leaving a polypus forceps attached to it for
two days. In December 1865 Elser constructed Koeberlé's *pince hémo-
statique*: after October 1867 that surgeon removed the forceps at the end
of the operation instead of leaving it on the vessel for a day or longer. In
1868 Gueride constructed for Péan an instrument for forcipressure—a modi-
fication, like Koeberlé's, of Charrière's, with Charrière's lock. In 1872,
Spencer Wells first employed this pressure forceps after testing several
designs, and in 1878 he adopted the later form with superimposed blades.'

signed forceps for the express purpose of so squeezing or crushing the coats of the bleeding vessel together, as *permanently* to stop bleeding from vessels of moderate size.... I do not wish to enter into the discussion between MM. Koeberlé and Péan, nor to prove that I had preceded both of them by many years in the use of forci-pressure. My chief object is to bring more prominently before the profession the many and great uses of this simple and rapid mode of stopping bleeding, and describing what I believe to be the best form of pressure-forceps hitherto constructed.

'I can hardly recollect when I first began to use forceps instead of the fingers of an assistant for temporarily stopping bleeding during operations; but I believe I learned it from Mr. Bowman before he left King's College. I had often admired in the private and hospital practice of Sir William Fergusson the ready way in which Mr. Henry Smith and the late Mr. Price would instantly stop a spouting vessel by the finger, and tie it at a glance from the great operator. But I well remember seeing Mr. Bowman extirpate a very large tumour from the neck, and quietly put a "bull-dog" upon every considerable vessel as he divided it. This must have been in 1854; because when I went to the Crimea in 1855, I took a number of "bull-dogs" with me; and after my return in 1856, I never went to any serious operation without several of different sizes. I used them in all my earlier cases of ovariotomy (beginning in 1858) for stopping any vessel which bled in the abdominal wall divided in the first incision.... I cannot remember precisely when I began to find that the "bull-dogs", used at first only as a means of temporary com-pression, were sufficient to close permanently vessels of moderate size; but, in 1863, I began to increase the size of the "bull-dogs", and to attach long pieces of silver or iron wire to them, so that when used on omental vessels, or on bleeding vessels from torn adhesions on the inner surface of the abdominal wall, they should not be for-gotten or lost. Then, as torsion came into more general use, and various forms of torsion-forceps were contrived, I arrived at the form of instruments described above.... Mr. Krohne tells me that he made the first of these forceps for me early in 1872.... Koeberlé's [and Péan's instruments] have the great disadvantage of an open space between the blades, which admits of entanglement of one instru-ment with another, or of the passage of omentum or other structures. This was a fault in my own earlier instruments. It has been com-pletely corrected in the later instruments made for me by Mr. Hawksley, without at all lessening the compressing power exerted

on the vessel. In October 1878, Mr. Hawksley carefully tested
the compressing power of different forceps when opened by a piece
of leather one *millimètre* thick between the jaws of the forceps, and
covering about four teeth from the points. The following table
gives the result, as well as the force required to be exerted by the
hand in closing the handles or fastening the catch or catches under
each condition.

*Pounds avoirdupois exerted by four teeth of the end of
the forceps when one millimètre apart.*

Forceps.	First Catch.	Second Catch.
Koeberlé . . .	—	$3\frac{1}{4}$
Péan . . .	8	12
S. Wells (old) . .	$22\frac{1}{2}$	—
Ditto (new) . .	12	$22\frac{1}{2}$

It may be seen that in my old instrument there is only one catch.
And in my new one, the second catch only exerts the same power
as the first catch of the old instrument. But this is six or seven times
greater than the second catch in Koeberlé's—and nearly double that
of Péan's. When only the first catch in Koeberlé's instrument is
closed, the points are separated about half a *centimètre*, so that they
only compress anything more than that thickness. I have used all
these instruments, but find them much less handy than my own, in
which the handles meet without leaving any opening between them.
The rings do not admit the thumb and finger too far; and the end
which compresses the vessel is so bevelled, that, if it be desirable to
apply a ligature, the silk will easily slip over the forceps, and not tie
them together. Thus my instrument is not only useful in forci-
pressure and in torsion, but enables the surgeon to dispense with any
other kind of artery-forceps, if he wish to apply a ligature.'

The history of the pressure forceps is to be found in
an interesting article by Mr. Alban Doran in the *British
Medical Journal* [1915, i. 555]. It is headed: 'The Develop-
ment of the Pressure Forceps (Webber's—Koeberlé's—
Péan's—Wells's). In Chronological Order from the
Original Reports.'

Thomas Spencer Wells was born at St. Albans in 1818,
the eldest son of William Wells, a builder. He early

showed an interest in natural science, and was apprenticed to Michael Thomas Sadler, a highly respected general practitioner at Barnsley in Yorkshire. He lived for a year with the parish doctor at Leeds, and there attended the lectures of the second Hey and the elder Teale, whilst he followed the practice of the Leeds Infirmary. In 1836 he entered Trinity College, Dublin, and received instruction from William Stokes, Sir Philip Crampton, and Arthur Jacob. Three years later he came to St. Thomas's Hospital in London, where his education was completed under J. H. Green, Benjamin Travers, and Frederick Tyrrell. At the end of his first year he was awarded a prize for the most complete and detailed account of the post-mortem examinations made during the time of his attendance at the hospital. He was admitted a Member of the Royal College of Surgeons of England in 1841, and joined the navy as assistant surgeon. He served in Malta for six years, combining civil practice with his naval duties, and acquired so good a reputation as a surgeon that the honour of a Fellowship of the Royal College of Surgeons was conferred upon him in 1844. He left the navy in 1848, and paid a visit to Paris to see the gunshot wounds from the barricades in the June of that year. He afterwards visited Egypt with the Marquis of Northampton and made some observations on malaria. In 1853 he began to practise in London as an ophthalmic surgeon, and in the following year he was elected surgeon to the Samaritan Free Hospital for Women and Children, which was then little more than a dispensary, and he was appointed editor of the *Medical Times and Gazette*. He resigned his posts on the outbreak of the war in the Crimea and proceeded to Smyrna, where he became surgeon to the Civil Hospital. He returned to London in 1856 and took up his former post of surgeon to the Samaritan Hospital.

In 1848 Wells believed ovariotomy was an unjustifiable operation as surgery then stood; in April 1854 he assisted Baker Brown at his eighth operation for the removal of an ovarian tumour. The patient died, and it was not until 1858 that Wells himself operated for a similar condition. The remainder of his life was practically a history of the operation from its earliest and imperfect stage until it became one of the routine operations of surgery. Ovariotomy was accepted by the medical profession as a legitimate operation about 1864, and its acceptance was largely due to the wise manner in which Wells conducted his earlier operations. He invited men of authority to see him operate; he published series after series of cases giving full descriptions of the successful as well as of the unsuccessful results, and he constantly modified his methods, always in the direction of greater simplicity. His operations were models of surgical procedure. He worked in absolute silence; he took the greatest care in selecting the instruments, and he submitted his assistants to a rigid discipline.

Wells may thus be looked upon as the founder of modern abdominal surgery. He found ovariotomy a discredited operation, but even before the introduction of antiseptic methods his success was sufficient to render its performance justifiable. Coupled with the improved surgical procedure introduced by Lister, the principles governing the operation of ovariotomy have been applied to the uterus, the kidneys, the liver, the spleen, and the intestines, all of which are now subjected to surgical interference and often with the happiest results. Yet Wells had at first no easy battle to wage. The whole weight of surgical opinion was against him. His perseverance, his transparent honesty, his absolute sincerity, and his fighting powers at last overcame all opposition, and he lived to see his operation approved, adopted, and fruitful beyond all expectation.

Wells had many interests outside his profession. He was an ardent advocate for cremation; he was a good judge of horses, rode well, and, in later life, was to be seen daily driving himself in a phaeton with a well-matched pair of horses from his house in Golders Green to his rooms in London.

He was President of the Royal College of Surgeons of England in 1883, and in the same year he was created a baronet. He died near Cannes in 1897, and his body was cremated at Woking. He left five daughters and one son by his wife, Elizabeth Lucas, daughter of James Wright, solicitor, of Sydenham, who practised in New Inn.

XIII

IMAGINARY ANNALS OF THE SECTION OF COMPARATIVE MEDICINE [1]

I AM told that it is the duty of the incoming President to open the proceedings of the session with a short address. Mindful of my own limitations and acting upon the sound advice laid down by Apelles, the Athenian painter, that a shoemaker ought not to criticize outside his trade, I cast about for a subject upon which to speak to you this afternoon. It occurred to me that if I told you something about those who might have been qualified for election as Honorary Members of this Section you would perhaps gain some information as to the manner in which comparative medicine came into being. We shall then see that, like a river, it had a common source in natural history, that it divided into the two streams of human and veterinary medicine—both empirical—and that these two streams have united to form comparative medicine, which it is the business of this Section to place and maintain upon a scientific basis.

There can be no doubt, I think, that Hippocrates would have been chosen as our first President unless, indeed, we had made him our Patron. His keen Greek intellect recognized that the diseases of men and of animals are closely allied, and either he or one of his pupils actually wrote on the diseases of animals. Aristotle would have joined our Section at once: 'The Master of all that know', as he is described by Dante. A great investigator and a great thinker, he would have taught us much that was long forgotten and has now only been re-discovered.

But our first candidate for election as an Honorary Member would have been a man of colour, for he must certainly have been Mago, the Carthaginian, who was known as the 'Father of Agriculture'. He wrote a work in twenty-eight volumes comprising all branches of the

[1] Presidential address delivered before the section of Comparative Medicine of the Royal Society of Medicine, 27 October 1926.

subject. The work was so highly prized that after the destruction of Carthage, when the libraries which had fallen into the hands of the Romans were distributed amongst the princes of Africa, an exception was made in favour of Mago's work and the Senate ordered it to be translated into Latin. A Greek version appeared afterwards and an epitome in six books was made by Diophanes of Bithynia.

Xenophon, too, would certainly have been with us. We are accustomed from our schoolboy recollections of him to think only of his *Retreat of the Ten Thousand* and of his *Cyropaedia*, but he had a very real interest also in horses and seems to have had some practical experience in their management.

Sir Frederick Smith has epitomized Xenophon's rules for 'The Choice, Management and Training of Horses', and says that he tells horse-owners that nothing but close supervision will prevent their horses being robbed of their food, and that standing in dirty stables ruins their feet. The horses, of course, were not shod, and he recommends that the stable flooring should be of stones, each the width of a horse's foot. By increasing the slope of the stable floor —which he specially directs—and placing the horse on cobble-stones, he secures the feet being kept dry and the sole exposed to air-currents. Xenophon sums up his principles of management in the words, 'keep the hoofs hard and the mouth tender'. He deals also with the ordinary stable operations of grooming, removal of litter, and the bridling of horses at a time when there was no saddle. He gives detailed instructions for grooming and condemns the habit of washing the legs, which, he says, should be hand-rubbed in order to remove the dirt. He impresses upon his readers what he calls his first and best precept, which is, never to be angry with a horse.

Vegetius was well qualified to hold office amongst us, for he says, in his *Ars Veterinaria*, that to assist him in the compilation of veterinary matters he had called to his aid existing veterinarians and physicians, though he forgets to add that he owes a great deal to the works of Mago, the Carthaginian, of whom I have already spoken. Vegetius was far in advance of his time, for he ridicules the idea of disease being evidence of Divine wrath and recommends that dead animals should be buried deeply.

Pliny would undoubtedly have been invited to become an Honorary Member of the Section. Like the Master of Balliol he took all knowledge for his province, and his *Natural History* is still one of the most readable and entertaining books in existence. I would strongly advise all of you to dip into it from time to time. If you can get Philemon Holland's translation you will even go to the expense of buying an arm-chair with a reading-desk to support its great weight, and the long winter evenings will pass all too quickly whilst you read how

'Horses', of all other creatures, teeth wax whiter by age, for in the rest they turn to be brown and reddish. The age of Horses, Asses and Mules is known by a mark in the teeth; a horse hath in all forty. At the end of thirty months he loseth his fore teeth of either jaw as well above as beneath: the year following as many, even those that be next, namely at what time as they put out those which be called the cheek-teeth. At the beginning of the fifth year he loseth other two, but there come up new in the place in the sixth year. By the seventh year he hath all, as well as those that should come in others place as those which are firm and never change. A gelding never casts his teeth, no not his sucking teeth, in case he were gelded before; Asses in like manner begin to shed their teeth at the thirtieth month of their age, and so forward from six months to six months; and if they foal not before they have shed their last teeth, they are for certain to be held barren. Kine and Oxen when they be two years old do change their teeth. Hogs or swine never have any teeth to fall. Now whenas these marks are gone out which show the age of horses, asses and such like, ye must (to know their age) go by the overgrowth and standing out of the teeth, the greyness of the hair over their brows and the hollow pits thereabout, for then are they supposed to be sixteen years of age.'

And so Pliny goes babbling on, sometimes of the breed of mice and rats, sometimes of the pestilence which, beginning in the south, goeth to the west and continueth but three months. Everything he writes of is interesting—the old mingled with the new and the book containing half the folk beliefs of the world.

Next to Pliny we must have elected Cornelius Celsus, a writer of whom it is still in dispute whether he was a practising doctor, a veterinary surgeon or merely a literary Roman gentleman with scientific aspirations. I place him after Pliny because his scope is more limited and his style is less interesting. I am to some degree biased against him, perhaps because I was obliged to read him for examination purposes when I took my M.B. degree at the University of Oxford. He would undoubtedly have been welcomed here because he said that: 'No one thing is a sole cause, but that is taken for the cause which seems mainly to have contributed to an effect. That which singly has not the power of exciting disturbance may do so in the highest degree when it acts conjointly with other causes.'

He says, too, that: 'The art of medicine hardly admits any precepts of general application, and even cattle doctors since they cannot learn the idiosyncracies of dumb animals insist on observation rather than on theories in cases of disease.'

Leaving the ancients we should have admitted Conrad Gesner to our ranks with the utmost joy. He was named the German Pliny, but he did more than Pliny, for he awakened natural science from its long medieval sleep, and his *Historia Animalium libri II* deals at large with the habits and diseases of animals. He was certainly one of the best beloved men of his time and he was the most learned. He practised for many years at Zürich, and when he died at the age of forty-nine from the plague Beza wrote of him:

> Natura te omnis denique suorum
> Fidum antistitem plorat sacrorum; muta
> Futura deinceps, ni loqueris mortuus.

I sometimes think that our first President, Sir Clifford Allbutt, was Conrad Gesner reincarnated; both, at any rate, had the same type of encyclopaedic mind.

Gervase Markham is next on the list of candidates for

the Honorary Membership. He might have been elected, but it is very likely that he would have been badly black-balled. He wrote his Masterpiece in 1644 saying that it contained 'all knowledge belonging to the smith, farrier or horse-leech touching the cure of all diseases in horses drawn with great pain from the public practice of all the foreign horse markets in Christendom and from the pri-vate practice of all the best farriers of this kingdom'. The promise seems fair at the outset, but hear what is said of him by Major-General Sir Frederick Smith:

'He was a soldier, a scholar, a gentleman of fortune, a minor poet, a literary hack and a social parasite. He was a most versatile person and wrote with facility and assurance on any subject. For reasons of pelf he chose during long periods of his life to write on veterinary matters and to pose as a practitioner. He knew nothing of his subject and was not only a mean plagiarist but a violently untruthful person.'

On the other hand he was observant and had a trained mind, so that perhaps if he had been elected a Member of the Section we might have made him a real authority in comparative medicine.

Robert Lovell we should have admitted because of his *Compleat History of Animals and Minerals with their Place, Natures, Causes, Properties and Uses.* He was a student of Christ Church, Oxford, and was the exact antithesis of Conrad Gesner, for he stood on the old road and his book is a mere restatement of what was well known to the naturalists of classical times. It reads as if he had compiled it from the Bodleian and Christ Church Libraries. Still he was a gentleman, and had an interest in men and animals, so that we should have been glad to see him amongst us.

Thus far the tradition of Comparative Medicine had been kept alive by physicians who had interested them-selves in natural history. It now passed to the surgeons and to a few veterinarians, like Sainbel, who introduced some knowledge of their art from France, where it had long occupied a higher position than it had done in England.

John Hunter would assuredly have been elected our first President had the times been ripe for inaugurating a Society of Comparative Medicine during his lifetime. He loved to found small and friendly societies—such as ours—where men could meet informally and discuss the problems in which they were mutually interested. Some of these little coteries even met at his own house, for he was an admirable host. If such a Society had been formed he would certainly have enlisted the youth and energy of Astley Cooper to act as Secretary, whilst the elder Cline and Samuel Foart Simmons would as certainly have been put upon the council. Edward Jenner would have been seduced into reading a paper, and perhaps Monro secundus, of Edinburgh, might have demonstrated before us the stomach pump which he had invented for the relief of acute tympanites in cattle.

Charles Vial de Sainbel would have come to the meetings to show his appreciation of John Hunter's help when he founded the Veterinary College in Camden Town. His contributions would have been of great value, for he was the first to introduce into England the science of veterinary practice as it was understood in France as a result of the teaching of Claude Bourgelat.

Coming to our own time we should have elected William Kitchen Parker and his great expositor, Thomas Huxley, Honorary Members of the Section, less for their knowledge of disease than for their great scientific attainments in comparative anatomy, and they would have helped us in many points of anatomical detail.

Parker I knew well, as he was a personal friend of my father, and when I was a boy we often went in to watch him at work on a summer evening. He lived at 18 Bessborough Street, Pimlico, and used to preach on Sundays in the Wesleyan Chapel in Claverton Street. He was the son of a small Lincolnshire farmer, and he told us that one day after a morning's ploughing he came home and said: 'Father, I am fit for something better than this. I'll go to school and plough no more.' He obtained the L.S.A., married, had a large family, and made a scanty livelihood by the practice of his profession. His interests lay wholly in science, and, when we knew him, he was working at the homology of the shoulder girdle and the structure of the vertebrate skull—work which secured his election as a Fellow of the Royal Society and afterwards the award to him of the Gold Medal of the Society. Dining there once in the middle of the day we had a cod's head and shoulders, and we were warned to be very careful not to injure the bones 'because father was going to make a skeleton of them afterwards'. Parker was a morphologist pure and simple. It was a delight to see him working at a frog's skull, his only instruments being a pair of dissecting forceps, a pair of scissors, and two darning needles fixed in small splinters of wood for handles. His demonstrations were easy to follow, for he showed every point as he spoke, but with the enthusiasm of genius he soon wandered off and, speaking in the language of the Bible, Shakespeare, and Milton—works he knew literally by heart—he soon lost us in realms of thought which even Huxley was not always able to make clear to our lower intellects. To us in this Section he would have been of the greatest value, for his knowledge of developmental processes in the vertebrate skeleton would have explained many of the structural variations occurring in men and in animals.

It thus comes to pass that by a gradual process of development and the spread of knowledge, a Society for the study of Comparative Medicine has become possible. We owe much to Sir Clifford Allbutt and also to Sir German Sims Woodhead, who wished to establish a Society of Comparative Pathology at Cambridge many years ago. The advantages of such a Society had been shown us at the Pathological Society, for the medical members learnt much and had their ideas greatly widened whenever we had the good fortune to get a member of the veterinary profession to take part in any discussion that was going forward. The veterinary surgeon, we found, viewed things from an entirely different angle and was often able to add pertinent facts of which most of us were wholly ignorant. The project of forming a Society of Comparative Pathology was talked about, the usual objections to its existence were raised, but on the whole it was agreed very generally that such a society would be of great value. No one, however, came forward as an active spirit to call it into existence, and it was not until the veterinary side of the profession took up the matter that the long-wished-for scheme became an accomplished fact. The original proposal to have a purely scientific society dealing only with comparative pathology was widened, and I think wisely, into one dealing with comparative medicine, and it was decided to make it a Section of the Royal Society of Medicine. The influence of your first President, Sir Clifford Allbutt, and the energy of your second President, Major Hobday, together with the zeal of your secretaries has already made the Section a conspicuous success, and it remains for all of us to maintain and even to enhance its present position by contributing of our knowledge and taking part in the discussions. The work of the Section embraces a vast field extending on the one side to the most difficult problems of human medicine, and on the other to the interrelation of human and veterinary science, showing thereby that the processes of disease are identical whether they occur in men or in animals. It touches, too, the confines of tropical medicine, the most virile, the most progressive, and to us—as Englishmen—the most valuable of all branches of medicine, for we are a great colonizing race, whose interest it is to make the tropics healthy for our countrymen.

There is one final remark I should like to make. As a writer of many papers may I say, without giving offence, that when you have promised a communication and have yielded to the seductive voice of the Secretary 'just to put together your experience in a little paper', you should write it at once. Pressure of work is no excuse for putting off the evil day, for then the matter as well as the style suffers. I know there is high authority for postponement, for Sir

Rickman Godlee tells us that Lord Lister usually wrote his addresses at the last minute and sometimes left them so late that they were never finished, and that he had to trust to his memory for the concluding sentences. I have the highest admiration for that great surgeon, but in this I think he erred.

The Presidential address is ended and I have only to wish the Section God-speed.

XIV

HOW THE TRADITION OF BRITISH
SURGERY CAME TO AMERICA [1]

AS I am credited with knowing something of the development of surgery in Great Britain, I thought it might not be out of place if I tried to show you to-day how the British surgical tradition arrived in this country, a tradition which has enabled you in a very short time to build up a science of surgery which it took us many centuries to obtain. You have, indeed, learned something from us at the beginning, and our tradition was formerly of use to you. But for many years past you have developed surgery along lines laid down by yourselves to our advantage, for we have learned much by watching your progress.

Go back as far as we will in English medicine, we have always had well-defined grades of medical practitioners— the physician, the surgeon, the family doctor, the apothecary, the dentist, and the quack, who usually posed as a specialist and was itinerant. I show you pictures of each of them, and you will see that they are as clearly differentiated by their dress as they were by their education and uses. No grade trenched upon the preserves of another. The *physician* was generally an ecclesiastic, with a greater knowledge of books than of practice; he was essentially a teacher of the theory of medicine. The *surgeon* was a practical man—stout-hearted, for he was willing to run risks; not always of unblemished reputation in early days and rather greedy in the matter of fees. The *family doctor* would be called a herbalist nowadays, for he treated his patients for the most part with infusions of plants growing in his own garden or in the hedges; but he used his common sense and called in a surgeon when in difficulties just as he still does. The *apothecary* was a tradesman, who made and sold the more complicated remedies, like theriac, which contained several hundred ingredients, and the plasters which it was beneath the dignity of the

[1] Address delivered before the American Surgical Association at Baltimore, Spring 1924.

physicians to manufacture and was too long and expensive a job for the surgeon or family doctor to undertake. The *dentist* was itinerant; he travelled from place to place, carrying the teeth he had extracted in a bandolier, that all might see his skill. He announced his advent with the musical cry of 'touch and go, touch and go, says kind heart the dentist', which was heard in London well on into the eighteenth century. The *quacks* were the couchers for cataract, the curers of rupture, the cutters for stone, and the bone-setters; they were a pestilent brood, with some rough skill and with a terrible mortality.

There were advantages and disadvantages in practising medicine in the early days of which I am now speaking. Our predecessors made no bad debts; they were rarely accused of malpractice, and they were, if I may dare to say so, a remarkably close trades union; they had, on the other hand, no social position, and their lot sometimes fell in very evil places.

The physician as an ecclesiastic was protected by the Church, and was usually attached to the court or to the person of some great nobleman. He was, therefore, always sure of protection. The surgeon—at any rate in London—was a member of the fellowship of surgeons, a fraternity whose members co-opted each other, and who usually selected their own apprentices. The barbers, or barber surgeons, who were the family doctors in all the large English towns, could not practise at all until they were free of the gild or company of barbers, to which they must have been apprenticed for five or seven years. The apothecaries were all members of the very important gild of pepperers or grocers, and their wares were officially inspected from time to time, and were cast into the open street if they were not up to a rather high standard of purity.

I said a little while ago that the surgeons were of necessity stout-hearted people, though they were not always of unblemished reputation. They were stout-hearted, because if an operation were not so successful as had been represented beforehand to the patient and his friends the surgeon sometimes came to an untimely end. King John of Bohemia, for instance, from whom Edward the Black Prince is said to have taken his cognizance of three ostrich feathers at the battle of Crecy, was operated upon for cataract. The king said that he could see no better after the operation than before, so the surgeon was tied up in a sack and was thrown into the Oder. We know that similar sequelae sometimes happened in England. It is no matter of surprise, therefore, that the surgeon was always careful to take his fee beforehand, and, as it was the custom for him to live in the patient's house until the cure was completed, it happened from time to time that he rode off some fine morning without saying where he was going, when he had dressed the wound and found that it was not looking as well as he would have wished.

A somewhat lurid light is thrown upon the habits of surgeons when it is said: 'A wise surgeon will do well to refrain from stealing anything while he is actually attending a patient, and he should be careful not to employ notoriously bad characters as his assistants, for these things may spoil a good operation and thus detract from the dignity of medicine. A surgeon, too, should not talk to the women of the house with closed doors, whether she be mistress or servant; he should never speak improperly to her nor make eyes at her, especially in the presence of the patient. Such actions may cause a patient to lose confidence in his surgeon, and thus the operation may prove unsuccessful, because the patient has lost the good opinion he had of the operator.' On the other hand, it is said, 'The rich have a nasty habit of coming to the surgeon in old clothes, or, if they are properly dressed, as befits their station, they invent all kinds of excuses for beating down his fees. They say charity is a flower and think that a surgeon ought to help the unfortunate, but they never consider that a like rule is binding upon themselves. I often say to such folk,' the writer adds, 'well, then, pay me for yourself and for three paupers and I will cure them as well as you. But they never make any answer.'

I have only been able to find one action for malpractice in these early days, and that was in the year 1424, when a citizen of London, called William Forest, sued John Harwe, an 'enfranchised surgeon', John Dalton and Simon Rolf, 'barbers admitted solely to the practise of surgery', for an injury to the muscles of his right thumb. It appeared from the evidence that the plaintiff had cut his thumb and that there had been recurrent haemorrhage on six occasions, which the two barbers, practising surgery, had stopped successfully, but temporarily. It recurred a seventh time with such violence that John Harwe, the surgeon, was called in, who finally applied the actual cautery and arrested it. Harwe had fortunately told the patient in the presence of witnesses that the thumb would never be as useful as it had been, and the man had said that he would rather suffer mutilation of his hand than bleed to death. The arbitrators, therefore, had no hesitation in giving their award in favour of the defendants, which was to 'impose perpetual silence on the said William about this affair; moreover, we find that the surgeon and the barbers are so free from the fault attributed to them, and have been defamed so maliciously and undeservedly that, as far as in us lies, we restore to them their good name unsullied. We further declare that any defect of the aforesaid hand thus wounded, or the mutilation, or its ugly shape, is the result of the injury occurring when the moon was dark and in a bloody sign, namely, under the very malevolent constellation Aquarius, on the last day of last January, or else from some peculiar defect or injury in the said Forest'. It must have been a comfortable time for a surgeon when a bad result could be attributed to the influence of an evil planet! We still recall this state of thought when an event is spoken of as being 'ill-starred'.

The family doctors went their way through the centuries without much change, but it was quite otherwise with the surgeons. They gradually came to be so completely subordinate to the physicians that they could order nothing but the commonest remedies unless the prescription was countersigned by the physician, and they could not perform a major operation except in the presence of a physician. The surgeon, therefore, had no knowledge at all of what would now be called inner medicine or physic, and his calling was looked upon as so much inferior that it was almost impossible for one who had been practising surgery ever to become a physician.

An attempt was made during the reign of King Henry VIII, about 1540, to raise the standard of surgery from a mere trade into a recognized profession, partly by improving the education of the apprentices and obliging them to pass examinations before they were admitted to become masters, and partly by eliminating the quacks, who flourished in great numbers. Surgeons in London, Maidstone, and Nottingham took part in the struggle, but it proved futile, and when these pioneers died no one was found to fill their places, so that for another hundred years surgery remained in a subordinate position.

The régime began when the surgeon became a gentleman—that is to say, when he became educated to the level of the better classes among his contemporaries. Such men at first were few and far between. Richard Wiseman was perhaps the first, a surgeon who had seen much service in the Civil War during the middle of the seventeenth century. He died of haemoptysis, and says that he was often obliged to stop operating on account of a sudden burst of bleeding from his lungs. The illness was bad for him, but good for us, because during the periods of enforced idleness he wrote his *Severall Chirurgicall Treatises*. He tells in these treatises of the cases he had seen and, collating like with like, he draws conclusions as to their nature. His predecessors had contented themselves with the publication of individual cases of rare conditions without any useful commentary. But Wiseman was as one born out of full time, for after his death, in 1676, there was again a barren period in British surgery until the profession as distinct from the trade of surgery came into permanent existence. It began, I think, about 1711, with William Cheselden, surgeon to St. Thomas's Hospital, a skilful lithotomist and oculist, anatomist and architect, a friend of the great literary characters of his day. The poet Pope wrote of him:

> Late as it is I put myself to school
> And feel some comfort not to be a fool.
> Weak though I am of limb and short of sight,
> Far from a lynx and not a giant quite,
> I'll do, what Mead and Cheselden advise,
> To help these limbs and to preserve these eyes.
> Not to go back is somewhat to advance,
> And men must walk at least before they dance.

Cheselden was followed by Sharp and Percivall Pott, surgeons and educated men, to whom John Hunter owed something. They were great operating surgeons and teachers, but they were men of their time. Hunter differed entirely. He was a great thinker, and for the first time he raised surgery in England to the dignity of a science. Where his immediate predecessors had been little more than anthropotomists and clinical surgeons, he was a comparative anatomist, a physiologist, and a pioneer in surgical pathology. He was original in thought and put his ideas to the test of experiment. He was a great teacher, as well by example as by precept, and he founded a school in which you and we are, I hope, apt pupils.

You may perhaps ask why I have told you all this which at first sight has nothing to do with American surgery. It is because I wanted to show you something of our surgical tradition and how we were helped as well as hindered by its existence. Our physicians remained physicians, our surgeons remained surgeons, our family doctors remained family doctors. It has been different with you, for a large and new country, with a scattered population, had to evolve new methods and develop on different lines. Still we speak a similar language, and, although as a nation you are less homogeneous than we are, we appear to think very much along the same lines. But if we are alike in our ideas the course of development has been very different. Self-

reliance has been your most marked characteristic. Every
doctor had to do everything, and for many years there was
no opportunity for specializing even in the larger towns,
except that, as must always happen, one man would show
a bent for inner medicine, another for surgery, and yet
another would be more interested in midwifery. With us
self-reliance was not fostered. For many hundred years
every surgeon and every family doctor was obliged, under
penalty of fine, imprisonment, or being debarred from
further practice, to 'present' any patient under his care
who was in danger of death or permanent disability. The
regulation worked well, for there is no instance of a master
or his wardens having abused their position, though many
family doctors and surgeons were punished for neglecting
to call them in. It made, indeed, for good fellowship, and
it shows incidentally how small a town even London must
have been when patients who were seriously ill could be
visited individually by the busy men at the head of their
profession, who had also to attend to their own work.
With you it would have been impossible, for the distances
and the difficulties of locomotion would have prevented
it, and therefore, as I have said, your conditions made for
entire self-reliance. How splendidly you took it and what
risks you ran! Think of Ephraim McDowell operating
upon Mrs. Crawford in 1809, in a village; or Wright
Post and Valentine Mott tying repeatedly the femoral,
subclavian, and common carotid arteries under the most
primitive conditions; or of William Gibson ligaturing the
common iliac in circumstances which would have appalled
the surgeon of to-day. They had, of course, to deal with
healthy bodies and the absence of those pathogenic organ-
isms which are so much more numerous in crowded tene-
ments than in small towns and villages. In this respect,
and at this time, they were more favourably placed than
our surgeons, when it was openly advertised in London
that, 'Here you can get drunk for a penny, dead drunk
for twopence, and straw to lie upon for nothing'.

The bulk of your profession at this time was poor, for

money, as with us in country places, was scarce, and patients paid rather in kind than in cash. The examinations, even if they were taken, were not very searching, and your surgeons were more learned in experience than book-lore, for books were so extraordinarily scarce that we read of only one or two copies of a text-book existing in a whole state. Distances were great, and a man must either ride or walk where the roads or tracks were not available for wheeled traffic, as was mostly the case. Climatic conditions were severe, and it often happened that a man was so tired at the end of his day's work—which, indeed, more often than not extended into the next day—that he was unable to make any contribution to the literature of his craft. But in spite of this a profession gradually grew up and a tradition was imported. A father who had been somewhat more successful in practice than his fellows determined that if his son was so enamoured of surgery that he *would* follow it, he should at least have a better chance than himself. He would send him to London or Edinburgh or Paris sometimes for the whole of his training, sometimes for a post-graduate course after attendance at one of the American universities. There also came to you from Europe a few anatomists and surgeons who, for a variety of reasons, chose to settle among you, and brought with them surgical knowledge from France, Switzerland, Great Britain, and Ireland.

Among the earliest of these English teachers was Abraham Chovet, whose history has been so excellently elucidated by Dr. William Snow Miller. Chovet was born in 1704, and must have been a good teacher of anatomy, for he published a syllabus of his lectures in 1732 and was a demonstrator of anatomy at the Barber Surgeons' Hall in London from 1734 to 1736, a post which was of first-rate importance in the teaching world of the time. He was thus contemporary with William Cheselden, and was antecedent to Percivall Pott, and, of course, to John Hunter. For some reason he left London rather suddenly and went first to Barbadoes and afterwards to Jamaica, whence he is said to have been driven out by a threatened insurrection of slaves. He fled to Philadelphia and began to lecture there in 1774. The lectures were delivered, he says, 'on his elegant anatomical wax figures and real preparations of the parts beautifully embalmed and prepared'. We may be sure that as an old man of seventy he was *laudator temporis acti*, and that what the barber surgeons had done in London in the early part of the century was good enough for him; he must have been the incarnation of the English tradition. He lived on in Philadelphia until 1790 and was the only one of the twelve senior founders of the College of Physicians who was not born in or near Philadelphia. His anatomical models appear to have been preserved until they were accidentally destroyed by fire in 1888. Stories are told of his sarcastic wit, as, for instance: 'The doctor happening to be overtaken at the house of a member of the Society of Friends by a heavy shower of rain, his patient offered to lend him an overcoat, adding that he must not swear while he wore it—a habit to which he was notoriously addicted. On returning the coat the Quaker asked him, "Friend, didst thou swear while thou hadst on my coat?" "No," replied the doctor, "but there was a damnable disposition to lie."'

In like manner came Granville Sharp Pattison many years later. He had a brother in Pennsylvania, and after lecturing on anatomy and physiology at Glasgow, he arrived at Philadelphia in 1819. He taught anatomy for a few years and then returned to London, to take up a similar appointment at University College. Of a wandering disposition, he came back to the United States and was appointed professor of anatomy at the Jefferson Medical College in 1832. Nine years afterwards he had migrated to New York, and there he died in 1852.

There were doubtless other Englishmen who came over as teachers and brought the English methods of teaching with them, but these are two outstanding examples.

Much more numerous were the sons of successful doctors and business men who were sent to Europe to receive or complete their medical education, and of these there is a long and very distinguished list. Here are some of their names: Wright Post, Philip Syng Physick, John Syng Dorsey, John Collins Warren, Valentine Mott, William Gibson, Benjamin Winston Dudley, John Kearney Rogers, to speak only of the surgeons, who brought with them the English tradition obtained from various sources.

Wright Post was fortunate enough to live with John Sheldon in Great Queen Street, London, from 1784 to 1786. Sheldon at this time had just been elected professor of anatomy at the Royal Society of Arts. He was one of the great teachers in the Hunterian school of medicine, and while Wright Post was living with him he was elected surgeon to the Westminster Hospital. Post had, therefore, ample opportunities to learn clinical surgery as well as anatomy. Whether he profited morally as well as mentally we cannot now tell. John Sheldon was thirty years old and Wright Post was eighteen. Sheldon was engaged in the experimental embalming of dead bodies under the personal supervision of John Hunter, and when his mistress, whom he had picked up in Oxford Street, died of phthisis, he embalmed her and kept her in his bedroom until the lady he afterwards married turned her out. She is now stowed away in a back room of the Royal College of Surgeons, where I often visit her. Wright Post, at any rate, does not seem to have alluded much in his after life to those days, for he is described as a grave and dignified man who never smiled.

Philip Syng Physick was even more fortunate than Wright Post. He came to London in 1789, three years after Wright Post had returned home, became a pupil of John Hunter, and served as his house surgeon at St. George's Hospital. He was so thoroughly imbued with Hunter's teachings that he is rightly called the 'father of American surgery', and for this reason I selected him from all other surgeons to be commemorated on that mace which was presented to the American College of Surgeons as a token of goodwill. Physick afterwards went to Edinburgh, where he graduated doctor of medicine, but possibly our food or the Scotch climate did not agree with him, for we are told that he was 'a cold, dyspeptic, pessimistic and unsociable man'. It is a pleasure to discover that the large family of American surgeons who look upon him as their father have not inherited these traits.

Ephraim McDowell followed Philip Syng Physick at Edinburgh, where he was a pupil of John Bell in 1793. There is, I think, no doubt that John Hunter was the source of inspiration which led him to perform the ovariotomy in 1809, which was destined to become so celebrated in history. Twenty-three years previously John Hunter had stated publicly in the lectures which he delivered in the winter session 1786–7 that 'Tapping is only a palliative cure (for ovarian hydatids) and a large trocar is required as the fluid is generally gelatinous and then only one cell is opened. If taken in the incipient stage they might be taken out as they generally render life disagreeable for a year or two and kill in the end. There is no reason why women should not bear spaying as well as other animals. It would be simply opening the cavity of the abdomen which we often do in healthy constitutions.'

The gods loved the young Quaker, John Syng Dorsey. A man of singular promise, surgeon, artist, and a pioneer in your surgical literature. A nephew of Physick, he spent a year in London and Paris, working at the Windmill Street School of Medicine under Everard Home, the brother-in-law of John Hunter. Returning to Philadelphia, in 1804, he tied successfully the external iliac artery, wrote a textbook of surgery in 1813, which passed through three editions, and died of typhus before he was thirty-five years old.

> For Lycidas is dead, dead ere his prime,
> Young Lycidas, and hath not left his peer.
> Who would not sing for Lycidas?

While McDowell was in Edinburgh, John Collins Warren was sent to London by his father, the professor of anatomy and surgery in the newly founded medical school of Harvard. He arrived in 1799 as a pupil of William Cooper, surgeon to Guy's Hospital, but he was soon transferred to his nephew, Astley Cooper. Warren acted as a dresser at the Borough Hospitals under Astley Cooper for a year and afterwards went to Edinburgh and thence to Paris, returning home in 1802. While he was in London, Sir Astley Cooper and Hey, of Leeds, were busy dissecting and describing the anatomy of the parts concerned in hernia, and it is worthy of note that Warren was one of the earliest surgeons in America to operate for the relief of strangulated hernia.

Valentine Mott, like J. C. Warren, had also the good fortune to be a pupil of Sir Astley Cooper when he visited London in 1806, and, like his master, he became a fearless surgeon and a good anatomist. You will remember how, when there was as yet no chloroform, he spent four hours in excising the clavicle for a huge growth, mentioning the arterial source of each vessel as he tied it. The patient lived afterwards for very many years.

I think it probable that Astley Cooper's republican principles may have influenced the fathers of Warren and Mott to send their sons to him. Cooper had imbibed from his master, Henry Cline, those principles of 'liberty, equality, and fraternity' which nearly wrecked his career in London, for they almost prevented him from being elected to the staff of Guy's Hospital, and sometimes he used to say they gave him a queer feeling in his throat, 'just as though a rope were round it'.

William Gibson, of Baltimore, must have been as much at home in Europe as in this city, where we are meeting. He was a pupil of Wright Post and was sent to Edinburgh when quite a boy. Here he showed such artistic power that he soon attracted the attention of John and Charles Bell, who were equally skilful as artists and surgeons. He followed Charles Bell to London and there came under the influence of Astley Cooper. He had succeeded Dr. Physick at the University of Pennsylvania, and in 1812 he tied the common iliac artery. In 1824 he published

a text-book on surgery, which I have recently read with
pleasure and some profit. It is charmingly written, and is
much more modern in tone than any of the contemporary
treatises.

Benjamin Winston Dudley was another carrier of Euro-
pean tradition to America, but, unlike the surgeons I have
already mentioned, he had to rely on his own resources,
for he had no wealthy father to help him. He was the son
of a captain in the Revolutionary War, and, having a thirst
for knowledge and a desire to see the world, he bought
a cargo of flour at New Orleans, accompanied it across the
Atlantic, sold it at Lisbon and Gibraltar, and then made
his way through Spain to Paris. He spent four years in
Europe, partly with Baron Larrey and partly with Astley
Cooper and Abernethy. It is recorded that after his return
home he cut 225 persons for stone successfully, using
Cline's gorget.

John Kearney Rogers acted in like manner as an inter-
mediary between England and America, devoting himself
more especially to ophthalmic surgery, though he tied the
left subclavian artery medial to the scalenus anticus. He
was in London about the year 1817 and followed the surgical
practice of Sir Astley Cooper and Sir Benjamin Brodie.

I cannot resist telling you of John Peter Mettauer
(1787–1875), although he never visited Europe. He
must have been a very fine surgeon, for he operated 800
times for cataract, and 400 patients he cut for stone. He
did the first operation for the repair of a vesicovaginal
fistula, and he was the first in America to cure a cleft
palate, the operation being performed in 1827. Two years
later he is said to have recognized that typhoid fever was
a separate disease. He practised in Virginia, and excused
himself from writing on the ground that he was never
idle, yet in spite of this he married four times. It is told
of him that he was never seen without his top hat; it was
believed that he slept in it, and it appears certain that he
was buried in it.

I think, gentlemen, you will see from the little sketch

I have just given you how the tradition of British surgery travelled to you and how it influenced your early work. It came chiefly through London and Edinburgh, and in both places a sound knowledge of anatomy obtained by actual dissection was looked upon as the outstanding mark of a surgeon. Your professors of anatomy for many years held a highly distinguished position, and the professorship of surgery was often combined with that of anatomy. The work of John Hunter led your early surgeons to interest themselves in the ligature of the larger arteries. They had many opportunities of practice when syphilis was badly treated and wounds with cutting instruments were not uncommon, so that they left the world a remarkable record of results both in their successful and unsuccessful cases. Sir Astley Cooper was working hard at the subject of fractures, dislocations, and hernia when your younger surgeons came under his influence, and they transported his enthusiasm to your country. These surgical emergencies were constantly arising. You soon made their treatment your own and you greatly advanced our knowledge. Your field of surgery then lay fallow for a time, civil discord prevented any advance, and you fell a little behind. You have more than made up for lost time in recent years, and we are again your debtors, especially in connexion with the surgery of the abdomen, both in men and in women, until at the present time there are a number of American surgeons who in originality, resourcefulness, skill, and wide experience have no superiors and few equals; but you seem to me to be passing from one extreme to the other. Not long ago you were family doctors first and surgeons afterwards; now you appear to be becoming specialists first and general surgeons afterwards. It should surely be the other way round—you ought to be general surgeons first. It is no doubt easier to make money as a specialist and in larger amounts, but it is not good for surgery as a profession to take this view. It is making a trade of one's work. The real surgeon, like the artist, works for the joy of working.

THE PALLIATIVE TREATMENT OF ANEURYSM BY 'WIRING' WITH COLT'S APPARATUS

PATHOLOGICAL aneurysms, the result of chronic inflammation of the large arteries in the chest and abdomen, are of so deadly a nature and run such a distressing course, that any means of relieving the symptoms, even temporarily, must be welcomed by every one who is brought in contact with the unfortunate sufferers, and the means is doubly welcome if it offers even a remote chance of a cure. I make no excuse, therefore, in directing attention to a method of relieving the pain which is so constant a feature of the disease.

The apparatus employed was invented by my former house-surgeon, Mr. G. H. Colt. Its object is to enable a known quantity of wire to be introduced into the sac of an aneurysm with the least disturbance of parts, the maximum of speed, and the certainty of asepsis. Entrance of wire into the aorta, which is known to have occurred in at least seven cases, is also prevented. The instrument (Fig. 10) consists of a trocar and cannula, a ramrod, a tube, and a wisp. The wisp consists of a number of fine steel wires soldered together at one end, each wire being curled over in a separate plane so that it readily expands as soon as it is set free from any controlling force, though under ordinary conditions the wires are packed together and the individual strands lie parallel to each other. The wisp, in fact, is like a miniature umbrella which has a constant tendency to remain open; the end where the wires are soldered together is the handle of the umbrella, and the individual wires are the ribs. Originally a double wisp or 'cage' with the wires soldered together in the middle was intended to be used for a large sac; but it was found that the second half of the cage did not expand with certainty after its insertion, so that its use has been discontinued. Each wisp fits into a hollow metal tube—open at both ends—so fashioned that it can be fitted easily and accurately to the distal end of the cannula after the trocar has been withdrawn. It then forms an extension of the cannula. This tube holds the wisp in its compressed condition as a bundle of wires lying side by side. The wisps are made of different sizes for use with different-sized aneurysms. The amount of wire in each is known, and is always the same for the same size. Thus, No. 1 wisp has a total surface area of $1\frac{3}{4}$ square inches and is composed of 75 inches of wire; wisp No. 2—the one generally used—has a surface of $2\frac{1}{2}$ square inches and the total amount of wire is 105 inches; and wisp No. 3 has $3\frac{1}{2}$ square inches and consists of 150 inches of wire. The wires composing the wisps are dull gilt, and if they be examined under the microscope or passed through the fingers the gilding will be found to have made them slightly granular. This irregularity of surface is intentional, and enables the blood-clot to form more quickly and to adhere more firmly than if the wires were smooth.

Every part of the apparatus can be sterilized by being boiled, and the method of using it is very simple. Care must first be taken to ascertain that the wisp expands freely as soon as it leaves the tube. The skin over the most pulsatile portion of the aneurysm is divided, and the trocar and cannula are thrust into the sac. The trocar is then withdrawn, and a jet of blood issues with considerable force if the cavity of the aneurysm has been reached. The tube containing the wisp is then fitted to the projecting end of the cannula, and the wisp is pushed into the aneurysm by means of the ramrod. If this be done steadily and gently the wisp is entirely released and falls into the cavity of the aneurysm, the expanding wires first and the soldered end last. The cannula is then withdrawn, and the skin incision is closed with a single point suture if necessary. Hitherto, each operation has been performed under a general anaesthetic, but I believe local anaesthesia would be quite sufficient in most cases. I began by making a considerable incision in order to expose the sac, but now I merely puncture the skin to prevent the point of the trocar carrying epithelial cells in front of it into the aneurysm.

Experience has taught me one or two points of importance in performing the operation. In the first place it is necessary to have a free jet of blood issuing from the cannula when the trocar is withdrawn; it is then certain that the whole thickness of the wall of the aneurysm has been pierced, and the wisp will be delivered into the fluid blood, for it will be useless if it merely lies in the active or pre-existing laminated clot.

The introduction of the wisp by means of the ramrod should be done deliberately, and the cannula withdrawn afterwards steadily and without jerking, or the wisp may jump out of the puncture, as happened in one of my cases (*vide* p. 283) when I attempted to operate too quickly. Even in a large thoracic aneurysm the wall of the sac is sufficiently elastic to prevent any escape of blood when the cannula has been withdrawn. This fact had to be learnt by experience. I feared at first that the puncture would continue to bleed, and I used to suture the wall at the seat of puncture and reinforce it in the neighbourhood with a few additional sutures, until I saw this precaution was unnecessary, for there was no bleeding when the cannula was drawn out. I have, therefore, abandoned suturing in my later cases. The operation is attended with so little pain or after-disturbance that narcotics are often not needed; indeed it is better not to give them, because the patient has usually suffered so much that he craves for them, and the operation is a good opportunity to break him of the habit. Where the pain is severe, full doses of aspirin are usually sufficient, especially if the patient can be assured that within a few hours, or at most a day or two, the pain will disappear.

The following are details of my last three cases; the result of the third is still incomplete, for the patient is alive and doing her ordinary housework.

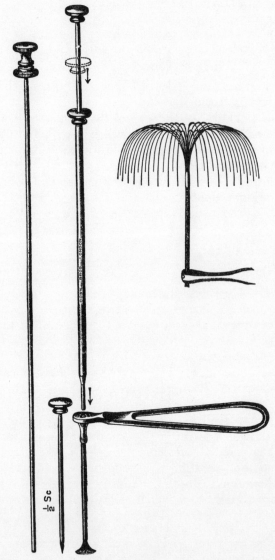

Fɪɢ. 9. Mr. G. H. Colt's apparatus for 'wiring' aneurysms.

CASE 1.—A shopkeeper, age 38, was admitted into St. Bartholomew's Hospital under the care of my colleague, Dr. James Calvert, on 16 July 1915. He stated that he had suffered from a pain in his chest for the last eighteen months, the pain having begun after he had made a sudden muscular effort. It gradually got worse, and during the last seven months it had been severe. He had kept his bed for the past seven weeks. He had served in the army, but on the whole had not led a strenuous life, and he had always been temperate. The patient was a tall, thin, and pale man, who lay curled up in bed on his right side. Movement caused pain in his chest which he said was shooting in character and ran from the scapula down his back. It was made worse by coughing. The cough was dry, and in the later stages was accompanied by stridor; the breathing was oppressed, and deep inspiration caused pain. The pupils were equal and reacted sluggishly to light and accommodation. The Wassermann test was strongly positive.

A well-defined swelling could be seen pulsating on the right side of the chest. It extended from the margin of the sternum to the anterior axillary fold, and from the third to the sixth rib. The pulsation was expansile. Air entry over the right lung was diminished, and the percussion note was impaired all over the back, with occasional patches of bronchial breathing. The apex beat was in the sixth space, and was palpable from the sternum outwards for two inches. The heart sounds were muffled, and a systolic murmur was audible at the apex, in the epigastrium, and over the tumour. The liver reached an inch below the costal margin in the nipple line. The urine contained much albumin. X-ray examination showed a large saccular aneurysm of the ascending part of the arch of the aorta. On 23 July 1915 the patient being under a general anaesthetic, I made an incision $\frac{3}{4}$ in. long over the most prominent part of the swelling and punctured the aneurysm by means of Colt's apparatus. A No. 3 wisp was introduced, but on withdrawing the cannula the wisp shot out of the sac with considerable violence and fell on the floor. Fortunately I had another wisp ready sterilized, so I made a second puncture into the sac and introduced a wisp of the same size. Blood issued freely from each puncture when the trocar was withdrawn, but there was no haemorrhage when the cannula was pulled out, so it was not necessary to suture the sac. The skin was closed with two point sutures of silkworm-gut.

The operation was followed by cough and dyspnoea. The temperature rose to 100·4° F. and the pulse to 120 for a few hours; but the temperature soon fell to normal and the pulse-rate diminished. The pain, however, was not relieved; the dyspnoea increased, and the swelling in the chest got steadily larger. The patient died eleven days after the operation. The post-mortem examination showed the body of a well-developed man with a marked swelling in the right pectoral region, over which was a small and recently healed wound where the aneurysm had been wired. The right lung was collapsed and was lying at the back of the pleural cavity. There were many adhesions of the right pleura, and the cavity contained blood-stained fluid. The chest contents, together with a portion of the thoracic wall involved in the swelling, were removed entire and sent to the museum to be hardened before a more detailed examination was made. The pericardium and heart were evidently not normal, and there appeared to be a large aneurysm of the ascending aorta which projected in part into the pericardium, but for the greater part was external to it and had 'bulged' the chest wall. The aneurysm had not ruptured. Subsequent inquiry showed that the specimen had neither been examined nor preserved. I think that I should have done better not to have operated in this case, but to have let the disease take its natural course. The patient was very ill, he was worn out by pain, and he had albuminuria. I hoped, however, that I might relieve his pain.

CASE 2.—A dock labourer, age 51, was admitted into St. Bartholomew's Hospital under the care of my colleague, Sir Percival Horton-Smith Hartley, on 14 January 1916, complaining of a lump in the front of his chest. He said that in 1914 he had fallen down suddenly in the street whilst on his way home from work and had been taken to the London Hospital, where he was found to be suffering from left hemiplegia. He was kept in the hospital for sixteen days, and his left arm had remained weak ever since the attack. Eight months ago he began to feel a dull pain over the front of the chest, and six months later he noticed a lump in the front of the chest on the right side. The swelling had gradually increased in size. His voice was husky, but he had not experienced any trouble in swallowing. Examination of the chest showed many dilated veins with slight oedema. There was a visible tumour—showing expansile pulsation—situated to the right of the sternum. The note over the tumour was dull, the dullness extending from the second to the fourth rib, and for four inches to the right of the sternum. There was a systolic thrill and a murmur over the swelling, which x-ray examination showed to be an aneurysm of the ascending part of the arch of the aorta measuring 4½ inches vertically and 3 inches horizontally.

The patient was kept in bed under the care of Sir Percival Hartley from 14 January until 21 February on a light diet and with restricted fluids. He was given full doses of potassium iodide, as his Wassermann test was positive. The tumour increased in size steadily in spite of this treatment, and the patient complained bitterly of pain.

I wired the aneurysm on 21 February 1916, using Colt's apparatus and introducing a No. 2 wisp, which presented a clotting surface of 2½ square inches and consisted of 105 inches of wire.

The patient being under a general anaesthetic, a semicircular incision was made over the tumour, beginning at the second right costal cartilage and extending downwards over the third costal cartilage. This was deepened until the pectoralis major was exposed; the fibres of the muscle were separated, and the sac of the aneurysm was seen as a bluish membrane of the consistency of thin parchment. The sac pulsated freely and it was obvious that it did not contain much clot. A trocar and cannula were introduced, and a full stream of dark-coloured blood spurted out for some distance as soon as the trocar was withdrawn. The No. 2 wisp was introduced without difficulty and the cannula was withdrawn. Blood still continued to issue from the puncture, which was closed with a single point suture of No. 2 silk on a round curved intestinal needle. The patient did not sleep much during the night, but he was fairly comfortable by eleven o'clock the next morning. He had a slight bronchitic cough which increased his pain. The temperature was 99·4° and the pulse 84. On 24 February he stated that he was free from pain, and on 6 March he left the hospital. The patient was seen eleven weeks afterwards, when the pulsation was found to be diminished, and on x-ray examination (Plate XVI a) the shadow of the sac was darker than before and very little pulsation was observed in it. The relative density of sac and wire was slight, and the active clot must therefore have been only small in amount.

He was readmitted on 9 February 1917, just a year later, saying that he went home sufficiently well to go back to work. In August 1916, he was employed at Woolwich Arsenal sorting bullets—not an ideal occupation for a man with a large thoracic aneurysm. He worked there for two months, and was summarily dismissed when the Arsenal doctor discovered his condition. The diminution in the size of the aneurysm continued for some months, but in November 1916 the swelling again began to get larger. The pain returned and his cough became more troublesome. He bore this for some months, but the pain and cough had become so much worse early in February that he came back to the hospital and asked to be readmitted for a further operation.

Examination of the chest showed that the respiratory movements were good, and equal on the two sides. There was a swelling over the second, third, and fourth ribs and costal cartilages. The swelling measured 2¼ in. in breadth and 3 in. in length. There was visible and expansile pulsation, and the percussion note over the tumour was dull. The tactile vibrations were diminished over the upper part of the right lung, and the breath sounds in that region were weak. The percussion note was impaired below; the bronchial sounds were harsh, and there were some bronchitic sounds. There was also a slight tracheal tugging, and the voice was hoarse. The pulse was regular and of full volume; the tension was increased, and the left pulse was slightly weaker than the right. Shortly after admission the blood-pressure in the right radial artery was 128 mm. Hg. and in the left 120 mm.; after a rest in bed for twelve days the blood-pressure was 105 on the right side and 115 on the left.

An x-ray picture (Plate XVI b), taken on 13 February showed a large aneurysm of the ascending arch of the aorta and a small bulge on the transverse portion of the arch. The wisp is clearly seen with the wires expanded, and the sac and its contents are much clearer than in the previous radiograph. The note states that the patient began to cough violently on 19 February and brought up a small quantity of bright blood. The aneurysm increased in size during his stay in the hospital until it reached the sixth rib, but there were no physical signs of pressure within the chest, except that the bronchial sounds were greater at the right than at the left apex of the lung.

I again wired the aneurysm on 2 May using Colt's apparatus and introducing a No. 2 wisp. The patient made an uneventful recovery, and was discharged on 30 May with the note, 'The pain is much less than before the operation, and the pulsation in the swelling is less marked'. An x-ray plate, taken on 2 June just showed the wires *in situ*, but it was not easy to determine the degree of expansion of the second wisp. The relative density of the sac and wire was much greater in this plate than in either of the two previous ones, and a considerable amount of clotting must therefore have taken place. The man only lived about a mile from the hospital and often came to report himself. He was able to do a little work as a night watchman, until on 27 August 1919—forty-two months

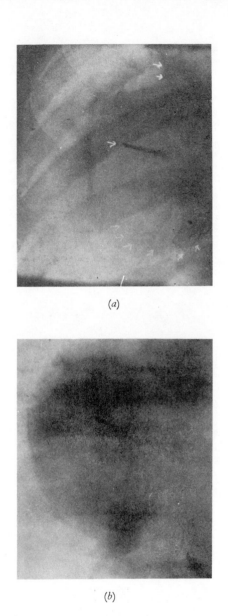

(a)

(b)

XVI. Radiograms of Colt's apparatus in an aneurysm (Case 2)

after the first and twenty-seven months after the second wiring—he fell down in the street on his way home from work and died the same night. There was no post-mortem examination, as we did not hear of his death until some weeks afterwards. A fourth skiagram, however, had been taken on 30 January 1918, in which it was seen that the relative density of the sac and the wisps was not so great as it had been in June 1917, which shows, perhaps, that the sac of an aneurysm fluctuates in size independently of any tendency to rupture.

CASE 3.—The third case was that of a married woman, age 52, who was admitted into St. Bartholomew's Hospital on 25 March 1919, complaining of a constant aching pain in her chest. She said that she struck her breast accidentally about the beginning of December 1918. The pain had been constant ever since, and was now getting unbearable. It was throbbing in character. Examination showed visible pulsation on the right side of the chest over the second interspace close to the sternum. The swelling was pulsatile. The chest-wall was so well covered that it was almost impossible to percuss out the heart. A diastolic and systolic murmur were heard at the apex, and there was a double aortic murmur. The Wassermann test was strongly positive.

The patient was kept under observation in a medical ward from 25 March to 24 April 1919, and during the whole of this time she suffered much pain in her chest in spite of all that could be done to relieve her.

On 24 April I wired the aneurysm under a general anaesthetic, using Colt's apparatus and introducing a No. 2 wisp at the point of maximum pulsation. The patient made an uninterrupted recovery, and a note written on 30 June 1919, records that there was much less pulsation over the swelling and the pain was greatly diminished.

The patient was readmitted to the hospital on 8 June 1920, saying that the pain had returned in November—five months after her discharge—and had again got gradually worse until she decided to apply for another operation. The blood-pressure in her right radial artery at the time of her second admission was 165–160 mm. Hg., and in the left radial 180–170 mm. There was no obvious tracheal tugging. Examination of the chest showed visible pulsation in the second right interspace, and the pulsation could be felt. There was also dullness over an area in the second right interspace close to the sternum. A double aortic murmur was heard at the base of the heart, and a diastolic murmur at the apex—"systolic conducted (?)"

the note says. Both legs were oedematous, and the urine contained a trace of albumin.

The patient was kept in bed from 30 June until 5 July, when I again introduced a No. 2 wisp by means of Colt's apparatus. The patient made a good recovery, and left the hospital on 19 August the last note recording that the pain was much less than it had been before her admission. At the present time (March 1921) the patient is living and doing her housework.

My friend, Mr. G. E. Gask, D.S.O., C.M.G., allows me to publish the following case which was under his care at St. Bartholomew's Hospital:

CASE 4.—C. W., age 35, a cattle-rancher, was admitted on 19 September 1919, complaining of continual pain in the small of his back, and periodic attacks of acute pain in the left hypochondrium. When the pain comes on in the left side he also feels a numb but burning sensation, and the skin becomes so sensitive that he cannot bear the weight of the bedclothes.

One day in May 1917 he was twice thrown from a mule and much shaken, but it was not until two months later that he began to feel pain in the small of the back. The pain was at first slight and intermittent, but it gradually increased and was constant. The patient states that he lost weight at this time and that he often had cramp in his stomach.

He was admitted to a hospital in San Paulo in March 1918, and was treated for rheumatism. He was discharged some weeks later feeling quite well. He remained well for three months, when the pain returned in the back and left side of the abdomen. The cramp in his stomach became bad, and he lost 10 kilos in weight. He was treated by a Spanish doctor for 'nodular peritonitis', and was subcutaneously injected, probably with tuberculin. The patient again improved and gained 8 kilos in weight. The pain, however, returned, and he determined to come to England. He arrived in September, having suffered severe pain during the last eight days of the voyage. He was passing blood and mucus by the bowel and had lost 4 kilos in weight.

Examination showed that the apex of the heart was in the fifth space internal to the nipple, and that the sounds were normal. The abdomen moved well; there was no distention, but the upper third of the abdominal wall was rather resistant. There was a slight swelling in the epigastric region $2\frac{1}{2}$ in. above the umbilicus and just to the left of the middle line. In this region there was a circular area about 2 in. in diameter where pulsation and a slight thrill could be felt. Expansibility could not be definitely made out, but there was dullness on percussion, and a systolic and diastolic bruit could be heard.

At the back, about 1 in. to the left side of the spine of the tenth dorsal vertebra, there was a small circular area of fullness, about the size of a half-crown, which was expansile and pulsated. A faint bruit could be heard over it. There was very great tenderness over the lower part of the abdomen, particularly on the left side, where the patient could not bear the pressure of the bedclothes.

X-ray photographs showed more shadow than normal in the right upper abdomen, and the shadows of the intestines appeared to be pushed away from this part. There was no evidence of erosion of bone. The Wassermann test was strongly positive.

A diagnosis was made of abdominal aneurysm, and on 6 October Mr. Gask passed a No. 4 cage into it by means of Colt's apparatus. The skin was cleaned with ether and picric acid, and a longitudinal incision was made through the skin at the level of the tenth dorsal vertebra and to the left of the middle line. The patient died suddenly from rupture of the aneurysm at 12.30 p.m. on 15 October, nine days after the operation. He rallied well from the operation, and said that he had experienced much relief from the pain, which had previously been unbearable. The pulsation, however, remained unchanged and the femoral pulses were good.

Subsequent examination of the body showed a large aneurysm of the abdominal aorta arising just below the pleural reflection. The primary opening of the sac was at the level of the first lumbar vertebra in the posterior wall of the aorta. The sac had expanded upwards into both sides of the thorax, pushing aside the diaphragm and the parietal pleura, downwards on each side of the spine, and posteriorly amongst the deep muscles of the back on the left side. The greater part of the aneurysm lay in the left pleura, and it had burst through a ragged and bruised-looking opening just above the diaphragm. The sac had made its way amongst the deep muscles of the back and had eroded the last rib, which was fractured. Much of the sac contained laminated clot of old standing, but some more recent clot had formed round the strands of wire which had been introduced nine days before death. The cage of wire had expanded freely at both ends, but the recent clot did not extend to the ends of the wires which, during life, must have been bathed in fluid blood. There was no wire in the right half of the aneurysm where there was no clot. None of the wires were near the seat of rupture. The specimen is preserved in the museum of St. Bartholomew's Hospital (No. F. 272 [o.s. 1551 f]).

More or less pain is a constant feature of all pathological aneurysms. When it occurs quite early in the disease and in deeply-seated arteries the cause is often overlooked or misinterpreted. Here is an example which came under my notice a few years ago:

CASE 5.—A lady, age 46, complained of pain in the chest, loss of appetite, flatulence, discomfort after meals, and constipation. The pain was referred to the lower half of the sternum, going through to the left scapula. It was worse after food, and sometimes prevented her taking a deep breath. These symptoms were prominent throughout her illness, though they varied in intensity. She said that she had always suffered from a weak digestion, and to cure her 'dyspepsia' she was in the habit of taking long walks—preferably uphill—and of bicycling. Her condition remained without material change from February 1907 until August 1910, during which time she took aspirin and bromides to relieve the pain. A physical examination of the chest in August 1910 revealed a soft systolic murmur over the aortic valves, and at this time she was complaining of pain extending to the left shoulder and down the left arm. In January 1911 pulsation was visible in the second left intercostal space near the sternum, and she had a cough with expectoration of mucus, which was occasionally blood-stained. The pain still continued, and was increased by the act of swallowing. A skiagram taken eighteen months later showed a sacculated aneurysm which contained a considerable quantity of clot and sprang from the descending portion of the arch of the aorta. The patient was then kept in bed; but in spite of rest, a low diet, and large doses of potassium iodide, the aneurysm increased in size, while the pain became more severe and was felt in the left axilla. Four months later the second, third, and fourth ribs on the left side, with the corresponding costochondral articulations, had become eroded. The aneurysm was wired on 25 March 1913, and she left the nursing home on 19 April, twenty-five days after the operation, with pulsation in the aneurysm almost imperceptible and the pain greatly diminished. She lived until the aneurysm ruptured on 26 July the pulsation remaining imperceptible from April to July, and with only occasional attacks of pain which she said were quite bearable.

I was fortunate enough to obtain a post-mortem examination of the body, and the specimen is preserved in the museum of St. Bartholomew's Hospital (No. F. 270 [o.s. 1551 e]), with the following description:

'A section through a large aneurysm of the third part of the arch of the aorta which had been treated four months previously by gilt wires inserted by means of a Colt's apparatus. The aneurysm springs from the left side of the descending aorta at its junction with the aortic arch; it has eroded the second, third, and fourth left ribs and costochondral joints, and passes through an aperture in the chest-wall fully 3 in. in diameter. The aneurysmal sac measures 5 in. in diameter, and is more than two-thirds filled with firm laminated clot, embedded in which is a network of gilt wires. The laminated clot is from $2\frac{1}{2}$ in. to 5 in. in thickness, and the double wisp, which has expanded freely, is embedded along its inner aspect.'

It is clear, therefore, that the bulk of the laminated clot has been formed since the introduction of the wisp, or the wires could not have expanded. Some of the free ends of the wires lie in recent clot. This recent clot is $\frac{3}{4}$ in. in thickness and is situated in that part of the sac lying outside the chest-wall. The rupture has taken place as a small slit which allowed the blood to pass into the left pleura. The aneurysm lying inside the chest is cured; that lying external to the chest-wall, and which is of the size of a man's fist, still remains.

This case well illustrates the character of the pain in aneurysm. It is slight and badly localized in the early stages, but it is constant and tends to get worse; in the later stages it often becomes so severe as to render the patient's life intolerable. The less the clotting in the sac, the greater appears to be the pain in the earlier stages of the disease. It may be caused, therefore, by the distention of the inflamed wall of the artery. If this be the case the good results following the wiring of an aneurysm are easily explained. A clot is formed round the wires, the pulsation is diminished, and the pain is lessened because the arterial wall is at rest.

The severe pain of the later stages is felt when the aneurysm is brought into relation with resisting structures which are either absorbed or inflamed by the intermittent pressure. It is usual, therefore, to have severe pain in thoracic aneurysms where the ribs and costal cartilages are being eroded, and in the descending aorta when the vertebral column is involved. I have seen it in subclavian, and less frequently in popliteal, aneurysms; but carotid aneurysms and aneurysms of the coeliac axis may attain a large size without much pain. Even in these, however, no rule can be laid down, as is shown by the following cases.

In February 1912, Sir W. I. de C. Wheeler showed two cases of aneurysm in the coeliac-axis region.[1] Colt's instruments were used in both cases. A cage of 150 in. of gilded wire was introduced in the first case, and a wisp of 105 in. in the second. The prominent symptoms before operation were intense pain in the back, marked epigastric pulsation, and digestive disturbances. A systolic murmur could easily be heard over the tumour. Sir William Wheeler considered that the pain in the back, which was severe enough to require morphia before operation, was more likely due to stretching and heaving of the peritoneum of the posterior abdominal wall than to erosion of the vertebrae. He also wired a third case of abdominal aneurysm, introducing 150 in. of wire and performing a gastro-enterostomy at the same time. The patient shortly afterwards developed symptoms of intestinal obstruction, and on reopening the abdomen a loop of jejunum was found compressed between the tumour formed by the aneurysm and the stomach and abdominal wall. The obstruction was relieved, but the vomiting continued to a less extent, and the patient died in a week from rupture of the aneurysm at a point remote from where the wire was introduced. At the post-mortem examination the wisp of wire was found situated between the layers of laminated clot— formed before operation—and had not expanded to any extent. The aneurysm extended from just below the coeliac axis to the level of the inferior mesenteric artery. An opening about the size of a shilling was found between

[1] *Trans. Roy. Acad. Med. Ireland*, 1912, xxx. 224; and *Dublin Jour. Med. Sci.*, 1912, i. 297.

the anterior wall of the aorta and the sac of the aneurysm. This opening was almost occluded by a valvular arrangement of laminated clot within the sac.

Sir William Wheeler commented upon the intense pain in the back suffered by this and two other patients upon whom he had operated. There was no erosion of the vertebrae in this case, and Sir William Wheeler suggested that the pain in the back, which is so constant a feature of this form of aneurysm, might be due to the stretching plus the heaving of the posterior parietal peritoneum. Stretching alone would not necessarily account for the pain. In each of the three cases the pulsation and pain in the back were more violent for a few days after the operation than they had been previously, but they then improved rapidly and the pain completely disappeared.

Of the two cases which survived, one was shown five years later.[1] The man had worked hard and continuously at his original employment in Guinness's brewery. He was free from symptoms, but a pulsating swelling could still be felt in his abdomen. There was no bruit to be heard over it, and the pulsation was no longer expansile. It may be assumed, therefore, that the aneurysm is cured. Sir William Wheeler tells me (February 1921) that the man is still alive and at work in his usual situation, and that it is now eleven years and a half since the aneurysm was wired.

In the second case[2] the patient was passed as sound for service in the Naval Reserve, and during the war acted as stoker on a patrol trawler. He died of leakage from a secondary dilatation of the aorta below the aneurysm four years and eight months after the operation. The aneurysm itself was about the size of a full-term foetal head, and was apparently completely consolidated. The wires had expanded evenly.

Lieut.-Colonel C. B. Lawson, R.A.M.C., wired an aneurysm as large as a Tangerine orange springing from

[1] *Trans. Roy. Acad. Med. Ireland*, 1916, xxxiv. 266.
[2] *Brit. M. J.*, 1911, ii. 1090; and *Lancet*, 1917, i. 535.

the aorta between the coeliac axis and the superior mesenteric artery. The operation was performed on 6 May 1906, the man's age being 33. He died on 26 November 1916, and was able to perform his duties in the interval. The earlier details of the case are recorded in the Proceedings of the Royal Society of Medicine.[1]

Mr. R. C. B. Maunsell, of Dublin, wired an abdominal aneurysm in a woman, age 30, who lived a year after the operation. She was then readmitted to hospital suffering from acute abdominal pain. Next day she died very rapidly with symptoms of internal haemorrhage. No postmortem examination could be obtained. Mr. Maunsell writes: 'This woman never gave herself a chance of permanent cure, as she drank heavily. The abdominal tumour never disappeared, but after the operation it remained firm, and I could not satisfy myself that there was expansile pulsation.'

The severe pain in the later stages of some forms of aneurysm, therefore, is due to the effect of the pulsatile swelling on rigid structures, and if the pulsation be stopped the pain is relieved.

The effect of wiring in relieving pain in cases of thoracic aneurysm is greater in thin-walled aneurysms than in those which already contain much clot, and the relief follows quickly upon the operation. The introduction of the wire results in extensive coagulation of the blood in the sac, the clot being of the 'passive' variety; that is to say, it is like ordinary blood-clot and is not laminated. A soft and elastic buffer is introduced, therefore, between the pulsating blood-stream and the inflamed and painful structures which have been previously pressed upon intermittently. Presently some of the clot becomes organized and the sac-wall becomes thickened, so that if the patient lives long enough, and the aneurysm is well sacculated, with only a small communication between it and the vessel from which it rises, an actual cure may take place. Unfortunately, however, it is only too often a cure of the

[1] *Proc. Roy. Soc. Med.* (Surg. Sect.), 1913, v. Pt. iii, 175.

aneurysm and not a cure of the patient. The inflammatory processes in the artery which led originally to the formation of the aneurysm continue in other or neighbouring parts. Another aneurysm is formed, or rupture takes place and the patient dies. Still, a few cures have resulted and many patients have been relieved of pain, so that the method is well worthy of more extended application, the more so as the operation is simple and is not attended with excessive danger. I do not see any advantage in combining electrolysis with wiring. It prolongs the operation, it introduces additional factors of danger, and it does not alter the physiological effect of the treatment, which is to obtain clotting within the sac. Admittedly the chief effect of it is to *initiate* the process of clotting, and this we now know is done quickly by the granular surface of the dull-gilt wisp. I have never employed electrolysis, for it has always seemed to me to be reminiscent of a time when little was known of the physiological processes connected with the clotting of blood and too much was expected of electrical treatment.

Duration of Aortic and Abdominal Aneurysms

To enable an idea to be formed of the value of operation in cases of thoracic and abdominal aneurysm, Mr. Colt has investigated the notes of all the fatal cases which occurred in St. Bartholomew's Hospital during the thirty-six years 1871–1907 inclusive, and has included twenty-two cases given by Nunneley[1] and two by Sir William Osler.[2] In the 179 cases collected by J. A. Nixon[3] the duration of the disease is only mentioned in one case, and this is included in the present list. The numbers are those of patients whose records are sufficiently explicit to allow an estimate to be made of the length of time which intervened between

[1] F. P. Nunneley, *Aneurysm of the Abdominal Aorta*. London: Baillière, Tindall & Cox, 1906.
[2] 'Aneurysm of the Abdominal Aorta', *Lancet*, 1905, ii. 1089.
[3] *St. Barth. Hosp. Rep.*, 1911, xlvii. 43.

the first complaint of symptoms and death—no operation having been performed. They are too small to warrant an average, and the median duration of the disease, therefore, has been taken instead. The Registrar-General is unfortunately unable to furnish any data compiled from death certificates. Such data in this and other diseases would be of great value in determining prognosis, and would aid the assessment of the value of operation in any particular case. The table of male cases is as follows:

Site of Aneurysm.	Median Age.	Median Duration of Symptoms.	Number of Cases Analysed.
Ascending arch . .	44	15 months (max. 4 years 4 months) [1]	34
Ascending and transverse arch.	46	9 months (max. 1 year 9 months)	16
Transverse arch . .	39	7½ months (max. 3 years 1 month)	24
Transverse and descending arch.	Number of cases insufficient to generalize		
Descending arch . .	49	15 months (max. 3 years 3 months)	11
Descending aorta . .	39	10½ months (max. 6 years)	6
Abdominal aorta . .	36	10 months (max. 3½ years)	42

[1] An exceptional case in which the disease lasted at least eight years has been omitted.

Aneurysm is much less common in women than in men. Of five cases in which the *ascending* portion of the arch of the aorta was affected, the mean age was 42½ years; the mean duration was 25 months, the maximum being 54 months. In three cases where the *transverse* portion of the arch was involved, the mean duration was 21 months and the average age 46 years. The longer duration of symptoms in women suffering from aneurysm of the transverse part of the arch may, of course, be due to the small number of the cases, but as the pressure symptoms are greatly aggravated when consolidation occurs in this portion of the arch, operation is clearly out of the question.

I have purposely headed this paper, 'The Palliative Treatment of Aneurysm by Wiring', because I do not wish to raise vain hopes about the treatment of a deadly disease. I know quite well that relief from pain is often secured by rest in bed for a prolonged period of time on a low diet with restriction of fluids and the administration of large doses of iodide of potassium. In the cases which have been given in this article, these methods had been tried by competent persons under the best possible conditions of nursing, and had failed. In nearly all the cases the pain was relieved by wiring, and two of the patients returned voluntarily and asked for a second operation. In some of the recorded cases an actual cure of the aneurysm seems to have followed the introduction of the wire, but in spite of the figures which Mr. Colt has been good enough to supply, we do not yet know enough about the natural history of the disease to say whether this great prolongation of life was in consequence of the operation or whether it would have occurred spontaneously. This will form the subject of a future investigation.

The following is a summary of all cases up to March 1921, treated by Colt's apparatus, without electrolysis:

1. Male.—Ascending arch; right carotid and subclavian tied two years previously; sac bulging externally. Died seven days after operation from external haemorrhage.—*Unpublished*.

2. Female.—Descending arch. Died four months after operation from rupture of sac.—*Power*.

3. Male.—Ascending and transverse arch. Died eleven days after operation from dyspnoea.—*Power*.

4. Male.—Ascending arch. Died three and a half years after first and two and a quarter years after second operation, probably from rupture of sac.—*Power*.

5. Female.—Ascending arch. Alive and well two years after first and eight months after second operation.—*Power*.

6. Male.—Abdominal. Died two days after operation from ether pneumonia.—*Holt*.

7. Male.—Abdominal. Died four days after operation from rupture of sac.—*Power*.

8. Male.—Abdominal. Died two months after operation from leakage of sac.—*Unpublished*.

9. Male.—Abdominal. Died of pneumonia some months after operation. No further particulars could be obtained.—*Prof. Conway Dwyer*.

10. Male.—Abdominal (partly dissecting). Died six days after operation. The cage had not expanded.—*Braine Hartnell and Collins*.

11. Male.—Abdominal, causing pyloric obstruction; gastro-enterostomy. Died of rupture of sac seven days after wiring.—*Wheeler*.

12. Male.—Abdominal. Alive and well eleven and a half years after operation.—*Wheeler*.

13. Male.—Abdominal. Died four years eight months after operation from leakage of secondary dilatation. Aneurysm apparently cured.—*Wheeler*.

14. Male.—Abdominal. Died nine days after operation from rupture of sac.—*Gask*.

15. Male.—Abdominal. Died ten and a half years after operation. No details ascertained.—*Lawson*.

16. Female.—Abdominal. Died one year after operation, probably from rupture of sac.—*Maunsell*.

XVI

ON CANCER OF THE TONGUE [1]

Mr. President and Gentlemen,

It was, I think, a wise latitude on the part of Mrs. Bradshaw when she founded this lecture in the year 1882 in memory of her husband—Dr. William Wood Bradshaw, M.A. Oxon., D.C.L.—to lay down no limitations as to its scope. It was to be a lecture on Surgery, and it is thus left to each lecturer to choose his own subject.

When the President invited me to undertake this honourable duty, I hesitated to accept, because in the hurry of these latter days it is difficult to find time for the original research which can alone render it of permanent value. I reflected, however, that you had recently nominated me to serve as one of your representatives on the Executive Committee of the Imperial Cancer Research Fund, and this gave me an opportunity of dealing with a topic which embraces the clinical and scientific sides of that dreadful disease. I have therefore chosen for your consideration this afternoon the subject of 'Cancer of the Tongue', one of the most distressing forms of cancer which afflict the human race. I have done so the more willingly because it brings into close relationship the historical, clinical, and scientific sides of inquiry, and it seems to me that these three lines must be closely followed if any satisfactory conclusion is to be arrived at.

Peculiarities of Cancer of the Tongue

Cancer of the tongue, as is well known, presents several peculiarities which make it worthy of careful consideration. In the first place, it is almost entirely a human disease, and this is remarkable, because the tongues of many animals are more liable to injury than is the human tongue. Secondly, cancer of the tongue is always primary, and is always of one type—a squamous-celled carcinoma.

[1] The Bradshaw Lecture delivered at the Royal College of Surgeons of England, 14 November 1918.

This is noteworthy, because the tongue of all animals contains many varieties of epithelium, any one of which might be expected to undergo malignant change as easily as the squamous epithelium. Cancer of the tongue is unknown in children; it is rare in young people; becomes frequent between the ages of forty and sixty; and, until lately, it has diminished in frequency in extreme old age. It is common in men; rare in women. Moreover, it does not run the same course in men as in women: in men, it generally ends in death within eighteen months of the onset; in women, it appears more often to follow an erratic course. I shall presently mention the cases of women in whom recurrence took place with such rapidity, after a complete operation by a competent surgeon, that nothing more could be done three weeks later, and of others whose sufferings were mercifully ended by death after eighty-four months and one hundred and eight months respectively of constant pain. Lastly, the inherited predisposition to cancer which is thought to be a feature in some forms of carcinoma seems to be nearly absent in cancer of the tongue. Each of these peculiarities is deserving of more careful consideration than it has hitherto received, for each must be due to some discoverable cause. I propose therefore to offer a few suggestions which may be interesting to you and serviceable to those who choose to work further upon the subject.

Historical

I will deal first with the historical side, and in doing so I find a virgin page in the history of medicine. No one, so far, has made any attempt to write about the literary history of surgical disease, though such a study would be of great interest and value. Such a history would be easier to write than that of medical complaints, because visible pathological conditions are more readily observed than those which are hidden.

The classical writers were well acquainted with cancer of the breast, of the uterus, of the penis, and of other parts of the body. From Hippocrates downwards, they give directions for the treatment of these diseases either by medical or surgical means, and state when they may and when they may not be removed. Cancer of the tongue, at any rate in its later stages, is no more difficult to recognize than epithelioma of the penis; yet Dr. E. T. Withington, who is making a special study of the old Greek writers for the new edition of Liddell and Scott's *Lexicon*, tells me that he has noticed a curious absence of any direct mention of cancer of the tongue in the Greek medical writers. The twelfth section of the second book of the *Prorrheticon*[1] contains an injunction to examine the teeth in cases of chronic ulcer on the side of the tongue. The passage immediately preceding it treats of the deep and superficial καρκίνοι occurring in elderly persons, and it looks, therefore, as if the writer thought that chronic ulcers of the tongue might sometimes be of this nature, but did not like to say so definitely.

Galen (b. A.D. 131) describes functional disorders of the tongue, but says that he purposely omits organic diseases because he is considering them elsewhere. This treatise, unfortunately, has not come down to us.[2]

Oribasius (A.D. 326–403) in his *Synopsis* has a chapter on 'Malignant Ulcers', where he mentions cancer and malignant ulcers of the pudenda, testes, and breasts. He also has a chapter on cancer of the vulva, which he says is incurable, and gives some methods of relieving the pain, but gives no hint of any similar affection of the tongue. It is probable, therefore, that he was unfamiliar with cancer of the tongue, and had never seen a case.[3]

[1] Hippocrates, *Opera*, Genevae, 1657, p. 96 E.

[2] The tongue, he says, is liable to 'inflammationes, tumores duri, tumores molles, erysipelata, suppurationes, de his vero, utpote quae tum visu tum tactu discerni possunt, nihil aliud in hisce commentariis dicemus, quippe eas duntaxat affectas partes hoc in libro prosequi proposuimus'. (*Galeni Opera*, Basil., 1549, vol. iv; *De Locis Affectis*, Liber iv, cap. ii, p. 88 C.

[3] The passages occur in the *Synopseos*. Under 'De Ulceribus Malignis', he mentions 'medicamenta ad carcinode, malignaque ulcera, ad pudendorum, testium et mammarum inflammationes'. (Liber vii, cap. xi.) A

In like manner Rufus, commenting on Oribasius (45, ii), gives a detailed account of the different forms of carcinomata and their usual localities, but omits all mention of the tongue.

Rhazes (A.D. 850–923?) says nothing about 'apostema durum' when enumerating the different forms of 'apostema' which occur in the tongue.

Avicenna (A.D. 980–1037), in his *Canon of Medicine*, devotes a long chapter to the tongue. He may have obtained his account of the 'apostema durum' and cancer of the tongue from the lost treatise of Galen. At any rate he mentions cancer as distinct from 'apostema durum'. It is possible, therefore, that he had seen or heard of a case, but he gives no detailed description of one.[1]

Arnold of Villanova (A.D. 1238–1314), who was an epitome of the medical knowledge of the school of Salerno, wrote a chapter on 'Ulcers and Pustules of the Tongue', but without mentioning any condition which can at all be described as cancer.

Bernard Gordon (fl. 1285), his contemporary, devoted a long chapter to 'Diseases of the Tongue' in his *Lily of Medicine*. He there speaks of 'ulcera maligna', but states that they are seen chiefly in children, and are easily cured by simple remedies. In all probability, therefore, they were aphthous ulcers.

William de Salicet (fl. 1245), Lanfranc (d. 1306), Henri de Mondeville (1260–1320), Jan Yperman (1275–1330), Gui de Chauliac (d. 1368), and John Arderne (1307–1390), all writers of the great surgical text-books of the thirteenth and fourteenth centuries, neither mention cancer of the tongue, nor do they describe any condition which in the least resembles it.

little farther on is the chapter 'De Cancro Vulvae', of which he says, 'Hic morbus curationem non recipit'.

[1] Avicenna, *Canon*, Liber iii, fen vi, cap. 14, 'De Apostematibus Linguae'. 'Quandoque accidunt linguae apostemata calida, et apostemata phlegmatica, et apostemata ventosa, et apostemata dura, et cancer. Et signa omnium illorum manifesta erunt cum redierint ad illud quod dictum est in signis apostematum.'

John of Vigo (1460–1517), with his keen surgical instinct, and Fernelius (1497–1558), who wrote on *Universal Medicine and Pathology*, would certainly have alluded to the condition had it been of frequent occurrence in their practice. Both are silent.

Riverius (1589–1655) devoted the fifth book of his *Praxis Medica* entirely to diseases of the tongue. The first edition was published in 1640, and he there says expressly, 'Tumours of the tongue do not for the most part endanger life unless they grow so large as to cause suffocation, or come from a certain malignant or melancholic humour, when a cancerous swelling may be produced which is known by its hardness, blueness, and pricking pain.' It would seem from this passage that Riverius had actually seen cancer of the tongue, but it is noteworthy that he gives no details of any case in the volume which he published containing accounts of the many patients who had been under his care during his long and busy life.

The first definite notice of cancer of the tongue which I have been able to find is in English. It occurs in *The Chirurgicall Lectures of Tumours and Ulcers*, which were given by Dr. Alexander Read to our predecessors, the United Company of Barber Surgeons, in their Hall in Monkwell Street, on Tuesdays in 1635. Dr. Read says:[1]

'It falleth out sometimes that sores in this member (the tongue) prove maligne and very fretting, as it happened to the late Lord Mayor of London, Ralph Freeman. Hee lacked neither Physitians nor Physicke, yet old age, weaknesse and the malignitie of the sore hindered the procuring of his health, which his Physitians and Chirurgeans aimed at and wished for. The ulcer was so corrosive that it fretted asunder the veines and arteries of the tongue on that side which it possessed and caused a great flux of blood which exceedingly weakned him, for that present causing a strong syncope, so that afterward nature could not re-collect her selfe. When such griefes befall great personages their case is worse than that of the

[1] '*The Chirurgicall Lectures of Tumors and Ulcers*, delivered on Tusedayes appointed for these exercises, and keeping of their Courts in the Chirurgeans Hall these three yeeres last past, viz. 1632, 1633, and 1634. Lond. 1635.' Treat. 2, lect. 26, p. 313.

poorest in the like infirmities, because Physitians and Chirurgians are not permitted to use the like libertie in the application of medicaments to the one as to the other. If the like case fall out hereafter at any time, I advise you to use medicaments borrowed of the vegetables so that you contemne not the minerals. What hurt I pray you can come from the use of Merc. Dulcis and Merc. praecipitat. with gold? None I assure you; for these medicaments are familiar to nature and are true balsams for maligne sores.

'But you may aske what was the reason these medicaments were not used? I answer, because there was no mention made of these medicaments at the first, and it was too late to minister them at the last, nature being surprised: for this only would have made the medicaments odious, and the Physitian (who should have advised this course) obnoxious to calumnie and reproach.'

Ralph Freeman died on 16 March 1633–4, during his year of office as Lord Mayor of London, evidently from secondary haemorrhage due to cancer of the tongue. Dr. Read wished to administer mercury, but was overruled. It is possible, therefore, that he thought an antisyphilitic course might have been useful; on the other hand, mercurius dulcis, which was the precursor of calomel, was just coming into vogue, and was being employed in every form of inflammation by those advanced physicians who had adopted the new chemical pharmacy then replacing the treatment by herbs which had been in use from time immemorial.

It is interesting that this first record of a case of cancer of the tongue which I have been able to discover should have been presented just two hundred and eighty-four years ago to an audience similar to that which I am now addressing—the Master, Wardens, and Members of the United Company of Barbers and Surgeons: the only difference being that attendance on Dr. Read's lecture was compulsory, whereas attendance here to-day is voluntary. At that time it was enacted that 'every man of the Company useing the mystery and facultye of surgery—be he freman, fforeyn or alian straunger—shall come unto the lecture, being by the Beadle warned thereto. And for not keepinge their houre both in the forenoone and also in the afternoone and being a ffreman shall forfayt and paye at every tyme iiiid.'

From the middle of the seventeenth century onwards, cancer of the tongue was a well-recognized surgical disease in England, for Wiseman and other writers on surgery make frequent mention of it, and were devising methods for its cure.

It was, however, still rare in Germany, for Paul de Sorbait published a case in 1672. 'We saw', he says, 'an ulcer [of the tongue] degenerating into cancer in the case of the noble Baron Vertemali, which caused such a haemorrhage from destruction of the sublingual arteries and veins that the patient was suffocated. He recognized with great penitence that the cause of this cancer was a divine punishment because he had often abused the clergy.'

Bonetus (1620–89), writing on the tongue and its diseases thirteen years later, seems to have been unable to find another case—unless, indeed, he wished to point a moral—for he quotes the same case with some elaboration of details.

'There was lately', he says, 'a certain Baron who had a very poisonous tongue. He not only directed his jibes against all and sundry, but kept his most venomous shafts for the clergy and those who devoted themselves to God's service. He was caught at last in the very act when he was pealing this cursed bell, by a holy brother of good repute, who said to him, "Your foul tongue has overlong deserved that punishment from an offended God which it will shortly receive." The Baron went off undismayed, but a few days afterwards a small swelling began to grow on the side of his tongue. Little by little it increased in size until it became an inoperable cancer, and at length, the tongue having become incurved, twisted, and drawn back to the fauces, miserably afflicted, but penitent and confessed, he was summoned before the Great Judge who calls his servants to a most strict account.'[1]

I think from the historical side it is fair to assume that cancer of the tongue has always existed; that during the

[1] *Medicina Septentrionalis Collatitia*, Genevae, 1685, vol. i, p. 302. The case is headed 'Tumor Linguae Miraculosus'.

classical and medieval periods it was so rare as hardly to merit attention by the ordinary writers on surgery; in the seventeenth century it became common; and, as I shall show presently, its frequency is still increasing.

During the sixteenth century, therefore, something occurred to increase the frequency of cancer of the tongue; and three causes at once suggest themselves, for they were new factors, and greatly influenced the social life of the time—syphilis, tobacco, and the consumption of alcohol in the form of spirits. Of syphilis I shall speak in greater detail presently.

Tobacco, as is well known, was brought from Cuba by the Spaniards in 1497, and under the name of Petum was introduced into Europe on account of its medicinal properties. Inhalation of the smoke was also learnt from the Indians, but it was not until 1586 that Ralph Lane brought the implements and materials for smoking into England, although a few persons had acquired the habit as early as 1573. It quickly took root amongst the Elizabethan courtiers, the pipes being short and made at first of silver and afterwards of clay, as is known from the pipes and pipe-cases belonging to Sir Walter Raleigh, which are still preserved in the Wallace Collection at Hertford House.

The poor at this time were content with a walnut-shell and a straw. One pipe often sufficed them for a smoking party, the pipe being handed round the table at threepence a pipeful. It is hardly surprising that sore tongues increased rapidly in number. Syphilis at the same time was rife, and the older treatment by mercury was beginning to give place to guaiacum and other less reliable remedies. Syphilis of the tongue, both as a primary lesion and as a late glossitis, soon became well known to the medical profession.

The practice of smoking was at first essentially English, but it quickly spread to the north of Europe, being probably introduced by our sailors. King James I tried to stop the habit, and in 1604 issued his *Counterblaste to*

Tobacco, in which he says that smoking is 'A Custome loathsome to the Eye, hatefull to the Nose, harmefull to the braine, dangerous to the lungs, and in the black-stinking fume thereof neerest resembling the horrible Stigian smoke of the pit that is bottomlesse'. The *Counterblaste* was useless; but although the custom was well established in London, it took a long time to spread through the country, and as late as 1665 it was noted as something unusual that 'such an one was a smoker of tobacco'.

Alcohol.—It is often said that alcohol in the form of spirits plays some part in the production of cancer of the tongue, but history does not appear to show any close interrelation between spirit-drinking and lingual carcinoma. During the seventeenth century social habits remained very much as they had always been. In London, breakfast was not usually eaten, but a piece of bread with a draught of wine or a cup of beer was taken at a tavern some time in the morning. Dinner was the chief meal of the day, and taverns were used for that purpose nearly as often as we now go to restaurants. The fare was simple but ample, and although men were often 'scandalously overserved with liquor', it was usually with wine or beer. Spirits, in the form of Scotch whiskey or French aqua vitae, were esteemed as early as the sixteenth century, but they were not much drunk until the reign of Elizabeth, nor was any excise duty imposed until 1684, and in that year it was only levied upon a little more than half a million gallons.

Habits changed quickly after the introduction of coffee. Men became interested in learning the news, and frequented the coffee-houses. Coffee-houses in turn gave place to social clubs, where, in place of coffee, a bottle of wine or a bowl of punch became the popular beverage, and the use of spirits thus increased so enormously that during the years 1721–91 the consumption of British spirits alone reached an average of 0·62 gallon per head of the population, an amount which did not include foreign and colonial spirits. The eighteenth century was a jovial, sociable, hard-living age, when men drank spirits freely, kept extraordinarily late hours, and yet were obliged to take much physical exercise owing to the poor facilities for travelling both in town and country. Cancer of the tongue increased in frequency during this period, but not out of proportion, so far as can be ascertained. It seems probable, therefore, that spirit-drinking is not an important factor in its causation. During the whole of this period syphilis continued unabated, but it was treated so severely by salivation and diet that many died of the cure.

Zoological Distribution

Cancer, as is well known, occurs in many vertebrate animals, from mammals to fish. Its zoological distribution has been the subject of more than one interesting contribution to the reports of the scientific investigations of the Imperial Cancer Research Fund. The types of carcinoma do not differ materially in human beings and in animals, when similar organs are affected.

I have made inquiries of my friend Sir John M'Fadyean, the Principal of the Royal Veterinary College, and of Dr. J. A. Murray, Director of the Imperial Cancer Research Fund, as to the frequency with which cancer of the tongue occurs in animals. Sir John M'Fadyean had especial facilities for gaining knowledge of this nature, because he asked in 1890 that veterinary surgeons, stock owners, and others would send him all tumours excised by them in order that he might collect information regarding the occurrence of cancer in domesticated animals. The appeal brought him a considerable number of specimens, and he wrote to me in 1918, twenty-eight years after this appeal was issued:

'In 1890 I published in the *Journal of Comparative Pathology* an account of a case of cancer of the tongue in a cat. It was the first case I had seen in any animal, and since then I have only seen one other case, and that was in the tongue of a horse. The tumour in the horse had been diagnosed during life as one of actinomycosis, but the appearance of the tongue after death was different from actinomycosis as seen in the tongue of cattle, and microscopical examination showed that the case was one of quite typical epithelioma.'

The details of Sir John M'Fadyean's first case are as follows:

'*Carcinoma of a Cat's Tongue.*—The tumour grew on the tongue of a cat, and was handed to me by Professor Walley. The cat was a male, and aged twelve years. It had been ill for about two months prior to the date at which it was killed, the symptoms observed being discharge of saliva with occasional streaks of blood, difficulty of mastication and deglutition, and progressive emaciation. Microscopical examination showed that the tumour was composed essentially of masses of epithelium burrowing along the lymphatic spaces of the tongue. The epithelium resembled pretty closely that of the deepest layer of the buccal mucous membrane. Each cell had a large nucleus and a deeply staining (carmine) nucleolus. The central cells in the larger masses of epithelium had undergone a colloid degeneration, probably in consequence of defective nutritive supply.'[1]

In like manner, Dr. Murray wrote: 'I can only recollect two cases of squamous-celled carcinoma linguae in animals in our material, both in cats.'

In 1902 Dr. Anton Sticker published a very elaborate paper 'Ueber den Krebs der Thiere',[2] in which he analysed the occurrence of cancer in 215,037 horses, 5,795 cattle, 91,273 dogs, 1,732 cats, and many pigs. In this vast collection, cancer of the tongue only occurred in one old dog.

The net result, therefore, is that one horse, three aged cats, and one old dog are known to have died of cancer of the tongue, and in each case it was a squamous-celled carcinoma. Nothing is known of the previous history of these animals.

These figures show that cancer of the tongue occurs in domesticated animals, but so rarely that it is negligible,

---

[1] *J. of Comp. Path. & Therap.*, 1890, iii. 41; with an illustration of the microscopic appearances.

[2] *Arch. f. klin. Chir. von Langenbeck*, 1902, Bd. 56, pp. 616, 1023, and 1067.

and that when it occurs it is of the squamous-celled variety, just as it is in the human. It seems fair to assume that cancer of the tongue in domesticated animals at the present time has not increased in frequency, but remains the same as it has always been; and, as I have already said, history appears to show that until the seventeenth century cancer of the tongue was as infrequent in men as it now is in animals.

Statistical

Leaving now the historical and scientific sides of the question, and turning to the statistical aspect, Dr. T. H. C. Stevenson, superintendent of statistics at the Central Register Office, Somerset House, told me that cancer of the tongue had already attracted the attention of the Registrar-General as early as 1909, when he wrote, 'The increase amongst males from cancer of the jaw and especially of the tongue is remarkable, and can scarcely be explained by improved diagnosis. Although cancer of the tongue in its later stages presents little difficulty in diagnosis, the recorded mortality has increased amongst males by no less than 228 per cent. in 41 years. The increase, moreover, is entirely confined to the male sex.'[1] This remarkable statement is based upon the following figures, which show the annual death-rate per million living, 35 years of age and upwards:

			1868	1888	1909
Males	.	.	46·49	77·49	152·54
Females	.	.	17·45	12·46	14·97

The increase in the death-rate from cancer of the tongue continued to increase, until in 1915 it had more than trebled since 1868. There was still no material increase for women, and amongst men the increase was chiefly at the higher ages, that is to say, from 65 years upwards. Thus, the mortality between the ages of 65 and 75 was 283 in 1901, and 432 in 1916; between 75 and 85 it

[1] Seventy-second Annual Report, p. xciii.

was 284 in 1901, and 420 in 1916; whilst in persons over
85 it was 166 in 1901, and no less than 516 in 1916.

It is a pity that statistics of death from cancer of the
tongue are not available before 1868, but Dr. Charles
Singer has done something to remedy the omission. He
states[1] that 'the death registers referring to the Chelsea
Hospital for old soldiers have been examined from the
years 1837 to 1910, and among 4,719 deaths of pensioners of the age of 55 and upwards, at least 62 were
certified as due to oral cancer. Of these 62, at least 28
were carcinomata of the tongue and floor of the mouth,
giving the proportion of deaths due to the last two causes
as 6 per 1,000.'

An examination of the blue-books issued by the General
Registrar shows that of the deaths of males over 55 years
of age registered in England and Wales during the years
1901–9, only 3.5 per 1,000 deaths were due to cancer of
the tongue. Thus, even with the imperfect certification
and greater statistical rarity of carcinoma in earlier years,
cancer of the tongue appears to have been twice as common among this group of old soldiers as among the general
population of comparable age in Britain to-day.

It should be remembered that the pensioners in this
series were long-service men, and that, in the earlier years
at least, many of them must have been serving in 1817, at
a time when Thomas Rose,[2] surgeon to the Coldstream
Guards, had nearly persuaded the army that syphilis could
be cured without mercury, a heresy which was supported
by Guthrie,[3] but was not shared by the soldiers themselves,
many of whom bought Liq. Hyd. Perchlor. privately, and
thereby made the fortune of a druggist living near their
barracks.

Some additional facts can be gleaned from the reports
of the Registrar-General.[4] Here is a table showing the

[1] *Quart. J. Med.*, 1911, v. 20.
[2] *Med.-Chir. Tr.*, 1817, viii. 349.
[3] Ibid., p. 550.
[4] Seventy-second Annual Report, pp. lxxxii–lxxxv.

ages at which death occurred from cancer of the tongue
during the years 1901–9 in 6,257 men and 782 women:

Age at Death.	Males.	Females.
Under 5 years . .	0	1
„ 10 „ . .	1	0
„ 15 „ . .	1	0
„ 20 „ . .	2	3
„ 25 „ . .	33	53
„ 35 „ . .	427	85
„ 45 „ . .	1,626	128
„ 55 „ . .	2,143	167
„ 65 „ . .	1,485	209
„ 75 „ . .	498	121
85 and upwards . .	41	15
Totals . .	6,257	782

This table shows that the true proportion of males to
females affected with cancer of the tongue is 8 to 1. Our
hospital statistics give a proportion of 18 to 1; Sir Henry
Butlin thought it was 6 to 1. The table also shows that at
that time the optimum, or shall I not rather say the pessi-
mum, age for cancer of the tongue is 45–55 in males, and
55–65 in females. The table, to be strictly accurate,
should be headed 'Cases of Malignant Disease of the
Tongue', because the two or three cases occurring in very
young persons are almost certainly sarcomata and not
carcinomata.

The difference in the death-rates of males and females
has already been noticed by Dr. Charles Singer, who
plotted it out in curves on the accompanying chart
(Chart 1) which he has kindly allowed me to reproduce
from his article, 'A Study of some Factors in the Aetiology
of Oral Carcinoma'.[1] He says:

'The death-rate presented by cancer of the tongue has certain
peculiarities which are not shared by that of cancer of other parts
of the body. It differs, in the first place, from the death-rate from
malignant disease of those other parts of the body in which a liability
is shared by both sexes, in the marked differences in character of the

[1] *Quart. J. Med.*, 1911, v. 22.

age incidence of males and of females (Chart 1). The death-rate
from cancer of the tongue in males rises steadily until about the
sixty-fifth year, when the rate remains almost uniform for two
decades, to fall again in extreme old age. In the female cases the
death-rate rises slowly at first, and by no means parallel to the male;

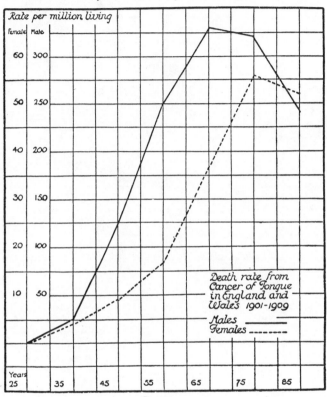

CHART I.

then, becoming accelerated about the sixtieth year, it rises rapidly
to a maximum at or about the eightieth year, and again falls slightly
(though less than the male curve) at the extreme limit of life.

'The chart illustrating the death-rate from lingual cancer thus
presents the following characteristic features: (a) The dissimilarity
of the male and female curves; (b) The approximately equal rates
for males in the decades 65–75 and 75–85; (c) The drop in extreme
old age in both sexes. As regards the general form of the curves

presented by this group of cases, it may be said that, while the male curve is a type of its own, the female curve accords fairly well with

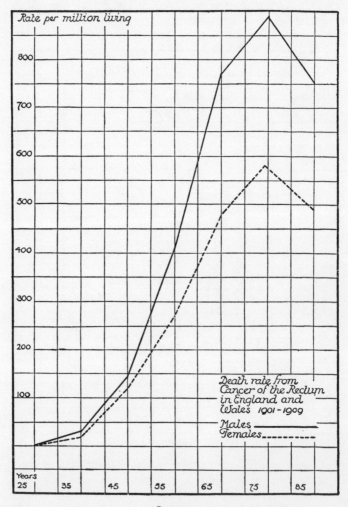

CHART 2.

those for cancer of several other parts of the body, and is, for example, closely similar to the curve for cancer of the rectum in either sex (Chart 2).'

Possible Factors Causing the Increase in
Cancer of the Tongue

It is clear from the historical and statistical evidence that cancer of the tongue is increasing in frequency, and at the present time it is increasing more rapidly in men than in women. It is of interest, therefore, to try to discover some of the factors which have caused this increase. Irritation is thought to be an important factor in the causation of cancer, and I have been at some pains to ascertain whether the state of the teeth has altered materially since cancer of the tongue became rife, because many patients state that injury to the tongue by a tooth was the origin of the cancer.

Pyorrhoea Alveolaris vel Periodontitis

Pyorrhoea is widely distributed throughout the human race, and is often met with in animals under domestication, as well as in wild animals kept in captivity. The animals which have been most carefully observed in regard to pyorrhoea are the horse, the cat, and the dog—the three animals in which cancer of the tongue has occasionally occurred.

Amongst 600 horses working in London, it was found that approximately one-third presented some degree of periodontal disease, mainly of local origin and the result of injury to the mucoperiosteum by foreign bodies in the diet.

Periodontal disease is also extremely prevalent in domestic cats and dogs. It is most frequent in highly-bred cats, because they are fed on soft food, whilst the ordinary domestic cat, which has to get its own living and feeds upon a meat diet, is comparatively free. The same holds true for dogs. Pyorrhoea is seen most commonly in lap-dogs and dogs with short muzzles, and especially in the functionless incisor teeth of bulldogs. Dogs living on a good flesh diet which gives plenty of exercise to the jaws are invariably free from the disease. It is clear, therefore,

that whilst pyorrhoea may act as a source of irritation to
the tongue, it is only of minor importance in producing
cancer, as otherwise cats and dogs should be affected much
more often than is actually the case.

Caries

Caries of the teeth, in like manner, seems to be only of
slight importance as a factor in causing cancer of the
tongue, although it is often put forward prominently as
an exciting cause.

Dental surgeons have done much good work in determining the existence of caries in the teeth of different races
from prehistoric times to our day. The late Mr. Mummery examined over 3,000 skulls to determine the pre-
valence of dental caries, and tabulated the results of 1,658
cases. Caries occurs from the earliest times, varying in
frequency in different districts. Among 68 skulls obtained
from Wiltshire barrows, there was only a single case of
decay; whilst in 44 skulls from similar long barrows in the
more northern parts of England, there were 9 cases of
caries.

During the Bronze Age caries was more frequent, for
there were 7 instances in 32 skulls, whilst in the York-
shiremen of this period there were no less than 26 cases
of caries in the 60 skulls examined.

During the Roman period the teeth were often diseased,
and in 143 Roman skulls 41 were thus affected, the
amount of caries in some individuals being very great;
thus, in one woman, aged about thirty, every molar and
every bicuspid was diseased. If such a large proportion of
Romans in Britain suffered from caries, there is no reason
to suppose that the Romans at home were exempt; and if
dental caries and stumps were an important cause of cancer
of the tongue, it must certainly have attracted the attention
of the classical writers on surgery. Yet Celsus, in speaking
of ulcers of the tongue, contents himself with following
the statement in the *Prorrheticon* of Hippocrates, saying,
'Those on the side of the tongue last a very long time, and

it should be noticed whether there is a sharp tooth, for this often prevents healing and must be filed.' [1]

In Anglo-Saxon times the proportion of teeth affected with caries was certainly less than in Roman times, and Mr. Mummery states that he only met with it in 12 out of 76 Anglo-Saxon skulls. We have no knowledge of the incidence of dental caries in England from the time of the Conquest until the beginning of the seventeenth century. Mr. J. F. Colyer has now taken up the investigation, and has been examining skulls obtained from the Clare Market district in the immediate neighbourhood of this college. Large numbers of Londoners were buried in the graveyard which occupied this site between the years 1600 and 1800. He tells me that 3,443 teeth were present in the skulls which he examined, and 319 of these were carious, the percentage of carious teeth being therefore 9·2 per cent., as against 28 per cent. in the Romano-British period. In the skulls and mandibles examined by Mr. Colyer, 669 teeth had been lost from disease. If these specimens are examined more in detail, 'we find in the complete dentures 1,683 teeth were present, of which 68 were carious, or just over 4 per cent., while in the incomplete dentures there were 1,760 teeth present, of which 251 were carious, that is, 14·2 per cent. In the latter group 669 teeth were missing, and of these it would be a generous estimate to assume that half were lost from caries, and the other half from periodontal disease. If the estimated carious teeth be added to the known carious teeth, the figures would indicate about one-third carious.'

It seems, therefore, as though the proportion of carious teeth amongst modern Londoners is about the same as in Romano-British times. A fallacy lies in the smallness of the numbers under consideration; but if it be assumed for the sake of argument that they are substantially correct, the conclusion must be drawn that, whilst the number of cases of caries has not increased, there has been a very rapid increase in cases of cancer of the tongue. Caries, therefore,

[1] Celsus, *De Medicina*, Lib. vi, cap. xii.

is not an important factor in causing lingual carcinoma.

Syphilis and Tobacco

None of the factors so far enumerated exercises a preponderating influence upon the increase of cancer of the tongue. It remains, therefore, to consider in somewhat greater detail the two factors pointed out by the history of the disease—syphilis and tobacco.

I have recently examined the records of patients admitted into St. Bartholomew's Hospital suffering from cancer of the tongue during the years 1909–16. During that period 169 persons entered the Hospital with this disease. Most of them submitted to operation, a few were inoperable, and some discharged themselves after a preliminary examination. The diagnosis of 'squamous-celled carcinoma' was verified in every case operated upon, by an independent microscopical examination carried out in the Pathological Institute attached to the Hospital.

Women.—Of the patients, 9 were women, and 160 men. The proportion of women to men, therefore, was nearly one to eighteen, which, as I have already said, is much smaller than the true proportion as shown—by the returns of the Registrar-General—viz. one woman to eight men.

Seven of the nine women were married, one was unmarried, and the social state of the other is not given. Of the seven married women, one gave a history of syphilis; two had healed syphilitic scars on the body; one was a widow who had only one child alive out of a family of five —the note adds 'she looks as if she drank'; one had suffered from leucoplakia of the tongue from the age of 17, and stated that her father had suffered from 'an abscess of the brain', of which he was cured by medicine—this was probably a gummatous meningitis, the patient herself being the subject of inherited syphilis; there was no history of syphilis, either acquired or inherited, in the other two married women. The unmarried woman, a nurse aged 42, said that her father died of aneurysm, and that one sister had cancer of the breast. The patient herself, during the same month in which she first noticed the ulcer on her tongue, found that her right eye was fixed in such a manner that she could not turn it outwards—abducent paralysis. This affection of the eye was cured by medicine, and was probably syphilitic in origin.

All the women had bad teeth, and attributed the cancer of the tongue to irritation caused either by the teeth or by a badly-fitting or broken denture. None of them smoked. In none of these cases was a Wassermann test done.

The duration of the disease had varied greatly in these women. In one, a woman of 52, the cancer grew so rapidly that the tongue was removed three weeks after the first occurrence of symptoms; whilst in another patient the tongue had been painful for eleven years before an operation was considered necessary.

There was also an interesting case which may be mentioned here, though it does not belong to the series, as it was under the care of Sir Henry Butlin. The patient was a married woman, age 24, with pyorrhoea. She was admitted to the hospital with a cancer of the tongue dating, as she said, from the irritation of a carious tooth in May 1898. Sir Henry Butlin removed her tongue on 9 December 1898. She was discharged from the hospital on 7 January 1899, and returned on 23 January of the same year—i.e. only sixteen days later—with such extensive recurrence that no farther operation could be undertaken. This woman had suffered repeatedly from small ulcers of the tongue before the cancerous ulcer was observed. These ulcers had appeared in crops three or four at a time, but were curable. The case is remarkable, both on account of the youth of the patient and the rapidity of recurrence after removal of the tongue by a surgeon who was especially careful not to do things by halves.

Men.—The men admitted with cancer of the tongue presented some additional and noteworthy points. Their teeth were nearly always bad, but not worse than is usual in the class to which they belong. Many were edentulous, some from age, some because they had their teeth removed after the appearance of the ulcer for which they sought advice. Of the 160 patients, 93, that is to say 58·5 per cent., were syphilitic. Of the 93, 62 gave a history of syphilis, and the remaining 31 showed signs of syphilis in the form of chronic glossitis, aortic disease, scars of healed ulcers, tabes, &c. The syphilis was invariably of long standing and, taking a few cases in the series without selection, the primary infection was said to have been 26 years, 30 years, 29 years, 40 years, 28 years, 23 years, and 43 years previously. Twenty-six of the patients stated definitely that they had never contracted syphilis, but of these one had suffered from gonorrhoea, and two had a positive Wassermann test. Many of the patients had drunk beer to excess, but did not as a rule acknowledge that they had taken spirits freely. There is no doubt, however, that many were, or had been, alcoholic. For instance, one was a farmer who stated that he took thirty glasses of strong beer daily and smoked continuously; he had cancer of the tongue which was removed at the age of 74. Another man, who said that he smoked eighty cigarettes a day, was usually drunk six days a week, and had contracted syphilis twenty years previously, suffered from a richly deserved cancer of the tongue at the age of 42. On the other hand, a teetotaller and non-smoker, who denied that he had ever suffered from syphilis, had his tongue removed for carcinoma at the age of 51.

A Wassermann test was performed 26 times, with the result that in 12 cases it was negative, in 6 positive, in 5 it was doubtfully negative, and in 3 doubtfully positive. These results may be compared with those obtained by Captain Arnold Renshaw, in the Department of Pathology at the Manchester University Medical School (who wrote to me at the kind request of Dr. C. H. Browning, Director of the Bland-Sutton Institute of Pathology, Middlesex Hospital), and by Captain Archibald Leitch, at the Cancer Hospital, Brompton. Captain Renshaw wrote: 'Seventeen cases of squamous-celled carcinoma of the tongue were examined, and only two cases showed a positive Wassermann reaction. Two of the negative cases gave negative reactions before and after (twenty-four hours before and forty-eight hours after) an intravenous injection of neosalvarsan, this being repeated in each case after a second injection had been given. In one of these cases there was a definite history of syphilis twenty-five years previously.' Captain Leitch wrote: 'I regret that I cannot give you any definite figures. All I can say is that the majority of cases I tested gave a positive reaction. The numbers tested were comparatively few, merely sufficient to establish in my own mind the fact that the result of a Wassermann reaction was of no service whatever in assisting a diagnosis between syphilis of the tongue and carcinoma of the tongue. Of that I am certain. Strangely enough, I did a few reactions in advanced lingual syphilis, and some of these were quite negative.' Carl Bruck[1] says that he obtained ten positive Wassermann tests in twelve cases of leucoplakia of the tongue.

The Wassermann results are interesting, but too much importance must not be attached to them as signs of active syphilis, because, as Lieutenant-Colonel L. W. Harrison wisely says,[2] 'Although the Wassermann test looks deeper into the patient's condition than the naked eye, it is not an absolute guide to a decision regarding the absence of syphilis.'

As regards the influence of syphilis upon cancer of the tongue, the number of cases under review is too small to generalize upon, and is only useful to point out the direction in which future work is advisable. There is, moreover, a possible fallacy. It is a matter of common belief that syphilis is in some way associated with cancer of the tongue. Every patient, therefore, is asked as a matter of routine whether or not he has previously suffered from syphilis. This is not done in other surgical diseases, and there is consequently no means of determining what pro-

[1] *Die Serodiagnose der Syphilis*, Berlin, 1909, p. 70.
[2] *The Diagnosis and Treatment of Venereal Diseases in General Practice.* Oxford Medical Publications, 1918, p. 280.

portion of patients admitted into hospital would acknowledge previous syphilitic infection.

It is not uncommon in a family for two or more members
of the same generation to suffer from lingual carcinoma,
but it is very rare for a father and son to die of the disease.
There is one case in the records at St. Bartholomew's
Hospital, but I can find no other. This may mean that
the son, born whilst the father has active syphilis, is thereby protected if he does not happen to have leucoplakia; or
it may imply that the tissue changes in the tongue which
are sufficient predisposing causes in the first generation
are compensated in the second generation. The first
assumption is the less likely, because inherited syphilis, as
has been shown, is actually a factor in cancer of the tongue.
The point is in need of further investigation, first as to
whether it is a fact, and secondly as to the explanation.
Another point for investigation is to determine whether
cancer of the tongue occurs more frequently in syphilized
members of families predisposed to cancer than in those with
no such history. Personally I do not believe that it does.

The evidence seems to point at present to a close association between syphilis and cancer of the tongue. The
syphilis may be active; it is more often quiescent or even
extinct. It may be inherited; it is more often acquired.
In every case the syphilitic infection has preceded the
appearance of cancer by very many years, and the preliminary syphilitic changes therefore are slow and prolonged. Of these preliminary changes I know nothing.
I have examined many sections of cancerous tongues, but
there are no constant histological changes in the deeper
tissues which are attributable to the effects of spirochaetal
infection. Tongues which were leucoplakic at the time of
removal show a thickening and fibrosis of the walls of the
arterioles, but in others there was no manifest change
either in the blood-vessels, the lymphatics, or the con-
nective tissue. An examination for such changes needs
more care, a larger amount of material, and much more
prolonged study than I have been able to give in the

limited time at my disposal. All that can be said at present is that syphilis in some way alters the resisting power of the epithelium of the tongue, and allows the squamous cells to run riot; in other words, that lingual carcinoma is born on the bed prepared by syphilis. A similar relationship has long been known to exist between syphilis and tubercle, but in tuberculosis there is a definite infective agent; as yet there is no proof of any such exciting cause in cancer.

When mercury fell into temporary disrepute in the treatment of syphilis at the end of the sixteenth century, and again in the army at the beginning of the nineteenth century, it seems that cancer of the tongue increased in frequency. It would be interesting to determine whether the present increase can be associated with the very imperfect treatment of syphilis which was in vogue during the mid-Victorian period. The sound teaching of John Pearson (1758–1826), surgeon to the Lock Hospital, that mercury in sufficient doses was the proper treatment for syphilis,[1] regulated the practice of most surgeons during the earlier decades of the last century. The introduction of potassium iodide, and its obvious utility in the later stages of syphilis, led to the very imperfect mercurial treatment which continued until our own day. Several of the patients who were treated for syphilis at St. Bartholomew's Hospital, and were admitted for cancer of the tongue forty and fifty years afterwards, stated that they had been given mercury for a fortnight or three weeks only. As late as 1880 the old dread of salivation still lingered, and it was quite usual in the out-patient room to hear a patient protest that he would not take mercury on any account. The treatment at that time was merely a treatment of symptoms, and minute doses of the red and green iodides of mercury were frequently prescribed. Is the present great increase in cancer of the tongue amongst old syphilitic patients the aftermath of this treatment?

[1] *Observations on the Effects of Various Articles of the Materia Medica in the Cure of Lues Venerea*, London, 1800.

But if syphilis is a predisposing cause of cancer of the tongue, the exciting cause must be looked for elsewhere, and it ought to be some form of long-continued local irritation. The provocative irritation is sometimes, but not so often as might be expected, syphilitic—the fissures and abrasions of chronic glossitis or the soreness of leucoplakia. Pyorrhoea and carious teeth, as I have shown, are very frequently associated with cancer of the tongue; but had there been no previous syphilis, lingual. carcinoma should not have occurred in men and women more often than in the domesticated animals, whose teeth are equally affected by disease. Pyorrhoea and caries are at least as frequent in women as in men, and it is probable that syphilis is just as common, yet cancer of the tongue in women has not yet increased in the same ratio as in men.

It remains, therefore, to inquire whether any change has taken place in the habits of men within the last fifty years which has not affected women to the same extent.

Before 1868, any one who looks at the pictures in *Punch* will see that snuff-taking was on the wane, and that whilst cigars might be smoked openly in the streets, pipes were taboo in public, and cigarettes were unknown except to foreigners, and travellers who had learnt to smoke them on the Continent or in America. Smoking after dinner was not usual amongst gentlemen who still drank a glass or two of port wine, and in the various Senior Common Rooms to which I was hospitably invited at Oxford during the years 1874–80, the Fellows of the older school only smoked after going to their own rooms. On the other hand, long clay or churchwarden pipes, with a mug of home-brewed beer, solaced the leisure of many country parsons and doctors at the bowling greens and quoit grounds in summer, and round the hearth in winter. The labourer smoked a short clay or cutty as a matter of course. On the whole the upper classes smoked a great deal less than they do at present, whilst the lower classes smoked about the same, but in a more irritating manner so far as the tongue was concerned. From 1877 onwards the smoking of cigarettes has become an ever-increasing habit, until now it is wellnigh universal amongst men, women, and boys.

Amongst the patients suffering from cancer of the tongue admitted into St. Bartholomew's Hospital whose cases I analysed, 37 men stated they had been great smokers, whilst only 2 were non-smokers. It seems possible, therefore, that smoking acts as the exciting cause of cancer in a tongue which has been sufficiently prepared by previous syphilitic infection of the tissues. Smoking acts as an irritant in two ways. My friends have kindly experimented for me, as I do not myself smoke, and they tell me that it causes a definite rise of temperature in the mouth, registerable by the thermometer; and there is also the irritant action of the nicotine itself. Smoking may thus bear the same relation to the production of lingual carcinoma as the brazier does to Kangri cancer.

To sum up, then, I think the following conclusions can be safely arrived at from the evidence I have obtained. Cancer of the tongue has always existed both in men and in animals, the actual cause being as yet unknown. Its rapid increase in men within historical times is the result of two causes: the first predisposing, the second the exciting.

The predisposing cause is the degenerative change taking place as a result of spirochaetal infection, the change being accentuated by lapse of years and by indulgence in alcohol. The form in which the alcohol is taken does not seem to be important; beer, spirits, and wine are equally harmful. It is the amount consumed, not the quality, which matters.

The exciting cause is local irritation. The most effective local irritant is tobacco, although pyorrhoea and carious teeth often act as minor exciting causes. The exciting causes may act for long periods of time, but will not produce cancer, except in the rarest instances, without the long-continued action of the predisposing cause—syphilis.

The occasional·occurrence of cancer of the tongue in animals and in non-syphilized people shows that, as in cancer
generally, there is a *tertium quid* as yet undiscovered, which
is called for convenience the predisposition to cancer. This
predisposition manifests itself in the varying resistance to
cancer shown by different persons. Sometimes the course
of the disease is rapid, and an accidental injury to the
tongue is quickly followed by a carcinomatous ulcer; at
other times, when every factor seems to be present and the
individual ought to have cancer of the tongue, he lives to
a good old age, and dies of some wholly different disease.

It is this *tertium quid* which we should seek, by corre-
lating, as I have tried to do this afternoon, historical,
clinical, and pathological results; for it is only by a wide
survey on all sides that it is possible to discover where
experimental research is likely to be most useful. Years
ago[1] I carried out a series of experiments to ascertain
whether irritation by itself had any influence in producing
cancer in animals; but the results were uniformly negative,
and some other factor was clearly necessary to make the
epithelial cells change their natural method of growth.

Conclusion and Forecast

In conclusion, some points of great practical importance
are obtainable from what has been stated.

In the first place, it ought to be possible to reduce
cancer of the tongue to the subordinate position which it
occupied before the seventeenth century in men, and
which it still holds amongst the domesticated animals.

At the present time syphilis is more prevalent than it
has been for many years, and the consumption of tobacco
has risen from seven and a half million pounds in 1914 to
eight and a half million pounds in 1915. Much of this
tobacco is smoked in the form of cigarettes, and women
now smoke on a much larger scale than they used to do.
It follows, therefore, that if matters are allowed to continue
as they are doing, there will be a huge increase in the

[1] *J. Path. & Bacteriol.*, 1897, iv. 69.

number of patients suffering from cancer of the tongue. The increase should begin about 1950, and it should affect women as well as men.

Such an increase can be prevented by a thorough and systematic treatment of syphilis in its initial stages; for, as has been shown, cancer of the tongue has always increased in frequency some years after syphilis has been treated inadequately. Persons who are being treated for syphilis, therefore, should be told never to smoke, not to drink to excess, and to pay regular visits to a dentist in order that their teeth may be kept in the best possible state, and that any dentures they may have to wear should be maintained well-fitting and free from rough edges.

Such advice should be given whilst the patient is actually under treatment for syphilis. It is useless to defer it until the tongue has become sore, because it is then too late in a large number of instances. Many patients, of course, will say that they would rather run the risk of having cancer of the tongue than put up with such a restriction as is involved in renouncing tobacco. It may be so; but at any rate it is our duty to put the matter plainly before them, and to point out the risk they run, in the hope that a few will take advice and be saved from a painful disease and a miserable death.

THE WRITINGS OF SIR D'ARCY POWER

In 1877 appeared Sir D'Arcy Power's first published writing. Entitled *On the albuminous substances which occur in the urine in albuminuria*, it was written with Dr. Lauder Brunton for *Saint Bartholomew's Hospital Reports*. Physiology and biology busied his pen for the next five years, to which period belongs his first book, a manual for the physiological laboratory, written with Dr. Vincent Harris. His first clinical paper, also in the *Reports*, the notes of a case of congenital locomotor ataxy from Dr. Gee's Wards, bears the date 1882, the year of his qualification.

The editing of South's *Memorials of the Craft of Surgery* was his first venture into the History of Medicine, and was followed by a long series of unsigned historical articles in the *British Medical Journal*. Of this time he writes: 'Both of us [Sir Dawson Williams and himself] were keeping our heads above water by devilling for Ernest Hart, a past-master in the art of extracting "copy" from those he was accustomed to call his young men—"copy" in the form of articles or abstracts often demanded at a moment's notice and criticized by a somewhat caustic tongue.' This hard apprenticeship served him in good stead, and on many of these short articles he founded his longer works.

From these sources flow the three streams of his writings, in science, in practice, and in letters. Certain subjects, notably cancer and the surgery of the abdomen, like the traditions of St. Bartholomew's and of the College of Surgeons, have held his imagination captive. In 1893 the first of his one hundred and eighty-four biographies appeared in the *D.N.B.* Scarcely a number of *The British Journal of Surgery*, since the first in 1913, has lacked an 'Eponym', an 'Epoch-making Book', or the biography of a bygone surgeon.

This bibliography is based on that in the *Life History and Abstract of Work of Sir D'Arcy Power*, typed copies of which are to be found in a few reference libraries. For our lapses from accuracy and from completeness we apologize.

A. H. T. Robb-Smith.
Alfred Franklin.

A SHORT-TITLE BIBLIOGRAPHY OF THE WRITINGS OF SIR D'ARCY POWER

HISTORICAL, BIOGRAPHICAL, AND BIBLIOGRAPHICAL

MEDICINE AND SURGERY

General

1. How Surgery became a Profession in London. *Med. Mag.*, 1899, viii. 413, 483, 582, 645, 814.
2. The Serjeant Surgeons of England and their Office. *Janus*, 1900, v. 174.
   (Reprinted, *Brit. M. J.*, 1900, i. 583; and *St. Barth. Hosp. J.*, 1901, viii. 81.)
3. Early Surgical Consultations. *St. Barth. Hosp. J.*, 1908, xv. 138.
4. An Early English Surgeon and what he knew. *Med. Mag.*, 1910, xix. 406.
5. The Evolution of the Surgeon in London. *St. Barth. Hosp. J.*, 1912, xix. 83.
6. Early Books on Naval and Military Surgery. *Tr. M. Soc. Lond.*, 1915, xxxviii. 157.
7. The History of Surgery in London. (Reported.) *St. Barth. Hosp. J.*, 1921, xxviii. 146.
8. CHRONOLOGIA MEDICA A Handlist of Persons, Periods and Events in the History of Medicine. By Sir D'Arcy Power . . . and C. J. S. Thompson . . . London: John Bale, Sons & Danielsson, Ltd., 1923. Pages iv, 278. Illustrated. 18 × 11·5 cm.
*9. How the British Tradition of Surgery came to America. *Tr. Am. S.A.;* 1924, xlii. 14.
10. Humour and the Surgeon. *St. Barth. Hosp. J.*, 1925, xxxii. 166.
11. MEDICINE IN THE BRITISH ISLES [Clio Medica II]. Paul Hoeber, New York, 1930. Pages ix, 84. Plate i. 16·5 × 10·5 cm.

Medieval

*12. English Medicine and Surgery in the Fourteenth Century. *Lancet*, 1914, ii. 176.

Sixteenth Century

13. Stricture and its Treatment in the Reign of Elizabeth. *Brit. M. J.*, 1896, ii. 1836.
    (Reprinted, *M. J. & Rec.*, 1926, cxxiii. 21.)
14. The Elizabethan Revival of Surgery. *St. Barth. Hosp. J.*, 1902, x. 1, 18.

---

* Reprinted in *Sir D'Arcy Power Selected Writings* (1877–1930). Oxford, at the Clarendon Press, 1930.

*15. The Education of a Surgeon under Thomas Vicary (The Vicary Lecture.) *Brit. J. Surg.*, 1920–1, viii. 240.

16. The Place of the Tudor Surgeons in English Literature. *Proc. Roy. Soc. Med.* (Hist. Sect.), 1927, xx. 1075.

17. The Beginnings of the Literary Renaissance of Surgery in England. *Proc. Roy. Soc. Med.* (Hist. Sect.), 1928, xxii. 77.

Seventeenth Century

18. The Brave Soldier: an operation for the removal of a fatty tumour in the year 1665. *M. J. & Rec.*, 1926, cxxiii. 258.

Eighteenth Century

19. Articles on the History of Medicine and Surgery in Trail's *Social England*, vols. 5 and 6. Cassell, London, 1896–7.

Nineteenth Century

20. The Royal College of Physicians during the Victorian Era. *Brit. M.J.*, 1897, i. 1587.

21. Medicine at Oxford during the Victorian Era. *Brit. M. J.*, 1897, i. 1594.

22. The Medical Profession in 1837. *Brit. M. J.*, 1897, i. 1671.

23. Pathology in 1800. *Brit. M. J.*, 1900, ii. 1846.

The Barber-Surgeons, the Royal College of Surgeons, and the Apothecaries

24. MEMORIALS OF THE CRAFT OF SURGERY IN ENGLAND. From materials compiled by J. F. South. Edited by D'Arcy Power. Cassell, London, 1886. Pages xxx, 412. Plates vi. 22 × 14 cm.

25. The Ordinances of the Barber-Surgeons of Oxford. *Brit. M. J.*, 1896, ii. 1392.

26. The Barber-Surgeons of Newcastle-on-Tyne and the Durham School of Medicine. *Brit. M. J.*, 1897, i. 213.

27. The College Medal and Early Anatomical Teaching in England. *Brit. M.J.*, 1897, i. 1185.

28. Lecturers and Lectures at the Royal College of Surgeons of England. *Brit. M.J.*, 1900, i. 518.

*29. The Centenary of the Royal College of Surgeons of England. *Phys. & Surg.*, London, 1900, i. 1043.

An article with the same title was printed in the *Practitioner*, 1900, lxv. 11.

30. Speech at the Sex-centenary Dinner of the Worshipful Company of Barbers of London. *Lancet*, 1908, ii. 1836.

31. A Precept of the Archbishop of Canterbury forbidding barbers to carry on their trade on Sundays. *Lancet*, 1909, i. 262.

32. The Debt of the Medical Profession to the Barbers of London. *Med. Mag.*, 1910, xix. 538.

33. Early Portraits of John Banister, William Harvey, and the Barber-Surgeons' Visceral Lecture in 1581. *Proc. Roy. Soc. Med.* (Hist. Sect.), 1913, vi. 18.

34. PLARR'S LIVES OF THE FELLOWS OF THE ROYAL COLLEGE OF SURGEONS OF ENGLAND. Revised by Sir D'Arcy Power, with the assistance of W. G. Spencer and Professor G. E. Gask. Printed and published for the Royal College of Surgeons by John Wright, Bristol, 1930. 2 vols. Pages xxvi, 752, 596. 25·5 × 16 cm.

35. The Society of Apothecaries of London. *Brit. M.J.*, 1895, i. 1349.

HOSPITALS AND PRIVATE MEDICAL SCHOOLS

36. The Rise and Fall of the Private Medical Schools in London. *Brit. M.J.*, 1895, i. 1388, 1451.

37. The Hospitals with Medical Schools. *Brit. M.J.*, 1895, ii. 140.

38. The Future of the City Hospitals in London. In *Contributions to Medical and Biological Research dedicated to Sir William Osler in honour of his seventieth birthday.* 2 vols. Paul Hoeber, New York, 1919. Vol. i. 146.

*39. Notes on the Bibliography of three sixteenth-century English Books connected with London Hospitals. *The Library*, 1921, 4th ser., ii. 73.

40. Some Early Hospital Statistics. *Proc. Roy. Soc. Med.* (Hist. Sect.), 1921, xiv. 21, and (Epid. Sect.), 1924, xvii. 76.

41. Pawnbroking and Hospitals. *Sixth Annual Report of the Voluntary Hospitals in Great Britain*, 1925, pp. 132–4.

St. Bartholomew's Hospital

42. History of the Surgical Teaching at St. Bartholomew's Hospital during the Nineteenth Century. *St. Barth. Hosp. J.*, 1897, iv. 163, 183; 1898, v. 10, 17.

43. St. Bartholomew's and Christ's Hospitals. *Brit. M.J.*, 1901, ii. 1607.

44. St. Bartholomew's Hospital and School. *Practitioner*, 1905, lxxiv. 111, 243.

45. London in the Early Days of the Hospital. (Reported.) *St. Barth. Hosp. J.*, 1905, xii. 71.

46. The Lecturers on Surgery at St. Bartholomew's Hospital, 1731–1906. *Brit. M.J.*, 1907, i. 211.

47. Some Past Worthies of the Surgical Staff. (Reported.) *St. Barth. Hosp. J.*, 1908, xv. 22.

48. The School Prize Medals. *St. Barth. Hosp. J.*, 1911, xviii. 166, 181.

*49. Some Episodes in the History of the Hospital. *St. Barth. Hosp. J.*, 1918, xxv. 28, 37.
    An amplified form of this entitled 'Smithfield', read before the Friday Club on 16 March 1928, has remained in manuscript.

50. St. Bartholomew's and the War, 1914–1919. *St. Barth. Hosp. Rep.*, 1920, liii. 5.
51. The Debt of Fleet Street to the Hospital. *St. Barth. Hosp. J.*, 1922, xxix. 61.
52. The Octocentenary of the Foundation. *St. Barth. Hosp. J.*, 1922, xxix. 139, 156, 170, 184; 1923, xxx. 6, 19, 34, 54, 68, 85, 100, 116.
53. A SHORT HISTORY OF ST. BARTHOLOMEW'S HOSPITAL 1123–1923. Past and Present by Sir D'Arcy Power. The Future by H. J. Waring. London Printed for the Hospital 1923. Pages xv, 201. Plates xxxiv. Text-figures. 22·5 × 18 cm.
54. Our Tradition: The Past. *St. Barth. Hosp. J.*, 1924, xxxi. 20.
55. The Passing of the Little Britain Gate. *St. Barth. Hosp. J.*, 1925, xxxii. 3.
56. The Rebuilding of the Hospital in the Eighteenth Century. *St. Barth. Hosp. Rep.*, 1926, lix. 9; 1927, lx. 7.
57. St. Bartholomew's Hospital. *Camb. Univ. Med. Soc. Mag.*, 1928, v. 109.
58. Some Books by Bartholomew's Men. *St. Barth. Hosp. J.*, 1928, xxxv. 148, 164.
59. The Philosopher's Stone. *Observer*, 29 June 1930.

Various

60. The Human Foot in Art. *Brit. M.J.*, 1898, i. 29.
61. Lithontriptics. *Brit. M.J.*, 1901, ii. 1476.
*62. The Fees of Our Ancestors. *Janus*, 1909, xiv. 287.
   Modified as 'The Fees of Our Predecessors' in *Proc. Roy. Soc. Med.* (Hist. Sect.), 1920, xiii. 76.
63. Medical Baronets, 1645–1911. *Brit. M.J.*, 1912, i. 1188.
64. The Scamnum Hippocratis. *Proc. Roy. Soc. Med.* (Hist. Sect.), 1925, xviii. 15.
65. Five greatest contributors to Medical Progress. (A letter.) *M. Press*, 1926, o.s., clxxii. 52.
66. The Food of Mankind treated Historically and Geographically. In *The Importance of Diet in Relation to Health.* London, Routledge, 1926, pp. 12–64.
   First given in shortened form under the title of 'The Meals of Our Ancestors' to the London Institute in 1896, and then to the Sheffield Literary and Scientific Institute in 1897, it remained in manuscript until 1926.

BIOGRAPHIES

67. Abernethy, John (1764–1831). *Brit. J. Surg.*, 1913–14, i. 549.
68. — 'My Book'. *Brit. J. Surg.*, 1929–30, xvii. 369.
69. Acland, Sir Henry Wentworth (1815–1900). *D.N.B.*, Suppl. 1901.

70. [Alexis Pedemontanus.] The Secrets of Alexis. *Brit. M.J.*, 1897, ii. 90.
71. Althaus, Julius (1833–1900). *D.N.B.*, Suppl., 1901.
72. Annandale, Thomas (1838–1907). *D.N.B.*, 2 Suppl., 1913.
73. [Archer, John (fl. 1768).] John Archer, M.B., The First American Graduate in Medicine. *Brit. M.J.*, 1900, ii. 452.
74. [Arderne, John (fl. 1370).] TREATISES OF FISTULA IN ANO HAEMORRHOIDS, AND CLYSTERS BY JOHN ARDERNE, FROM AN EARLY FIFTEENTH-CENTURY MANUSCRIPT TRANSLATION. Edited, with introduction, notes, etc., by D'Arcy Power,... London:... *Early English Text Society* [o.s., 139] ... Kegan Paul, ... 1910. Pages xxxvii, 156. Plates iv. 21·5 × 13·5 cm.
75. — The Lesser Writings of John Arderne. *XVII Internat. Congr. of Med.*, London., 1914, sect. xxiii, Hist. Med., p. 107.
76. — John Arderne. *Brit. J. Surg.*, 1917–18, v. 519.
77. — DE ARTE PHISICALI ET DE CIRURGIA OF MASTER JOHN ARDERNE, ... DATED 1412. Translated by Sir D'Arcy Power [*Wellcome Research Studies*, No. 1]. London John Bale, Sons & Danielsson, Ltd. 1922. Pages xii, 60. Plates xiv. 24·5 × 18·5 cm.
78. — 'A System of Surgery', by Master John Arderne. *Brit. J. Surg.*, 1927–8, xv. 1.
79. Arnald of Villanova (1235–1313). The Mystic Physician. *Brit. M.J.*, 1897, i. 1001.
80. [Baker, William Morrant (1839–96).] 'Baker's Cysts', and Baker's Tracheotomy Tubes. *Brit. J. Surg.*, 1921–2, ix. 200.
81. Banester, John (1533–1610). *Brit. J. Surg.*, 1917–18, v. 8.
82. Banks, Sir William Mitchell (1842–1904). *D.N.B.*, 2 Suppl., 1913.
83. [Baulot, Frère Jacques (1651–1719).] Frère Jacques, Rupture Curer and Lateral Lithotomist. *Brit. M.J.*, 1897, ii. 1349.
84. [Bayley, Dr. Walter (1529–92).] Dr. Walter Baily. (A letter.) *Lancet*, 1906, ii. 1764.
85. — Dr. Walter Bayley and his Works. *Med.-Chir. Tr.*, 1907, xc. 414; and *The Library*, 1907, 2nd ser., viii. 370.
86. Bell, Sir Charles (1774–1842). *Brit. J. Surg.*, 1920–1, viii. 389.
87. — Bell's Palsy. *Brit. J. Surg.*, 1923–4, xi. 405.
88. Bellew, Henry Walter (1834–92). *D.N.B.*, Suppl., 1901.
89. [Bernard, Charles (1656?–1710).] Two Unpublished Letters of Charles Bernard. *St. Barth. Hosp. J.*, 1906, xiii. 147.
90. Blandford, George Fielding (1829–1911). *D.N.B.*, 2 Suppl., 1913.
91. Blizard, Sir William (1743–1835). *Brit. J. Surg.*, 1920–1, viii. 3.
92. [Boerhaave, Hermann (1668–1738).] The Letters of Boerhaave to Cox Macro. *Proc. Roy. Soc. Med.* (Hist. Sect.), 1918, xi. 21.
93. Bowman, Sir William (1816–92). *D.N.B.*, Suppl., 1901.
94. Bristowe, John Syer (1827–95). *D.N.B.*, Suppl., 1901.
95. Brodie, Sir Benjamin (1783–1862). *Brit. J. Surg.*, 1918–19, vi. 157.

96. — Brodie's Tumour, and Brodie's Abscess. *Brit. J. Surg.*, 1921–2, ix. 334.

97. [Browne, John (1642–1700).] John Browne and the Royal Gift of Healing. *Brit. M. J.*, 1895, ii. 555.

98. Brown-Séquard, Charles Edward (1817–94). *D.N.B.*, Suppl., 1901.

99. Brunton, Sir Thomas Lauder (1844–1916). Obituary notice. *St. Barth. Hosp. Rep.*, 1916, lii. 1.

100. [Bryant, Thomas (1828–1914).] Bryant's Ilio-Femoral Triangle. *Brit. J. Surg.*, 1925–6, xiii. 201.

101. Buchanan, Sir George (1831–95). *D.N.B.*, Suppl., 1901.

102. Buchanan, George (1827–1905). *D.N.B.*, 2 Suppl., 1913.

103. Bucknill, Sir John Charles (1817–97). *D.N.B.*, Suppl., 1901.

104. Bullar, John Follett (1855–1929). Obituary notice. *St. Barth. Hosp. J.*, 1929, xxxvi. 51.

105. Carlisle, Sir Anthony (1768–1840). *Brit. J. Surg.*, 1919–20, vii. 147.

106. Carpenter, Alfred John (1825–92). *D.N.B.*, Suppl., 1901.

107. [Cellini, Benvenuto (1500–71).] The Medical Experiences of Benvenuto Cellini. *Quart. Med. J.*, 1898, vi. 199.

108. [Charcot, Jean-Martin (1825–93).] Charcot's Joints. *Brit. J. Surg.*, 1925–6, xiii. 1.

109. [Charles I (1600–49).] The Cure of the King's Evil. (Reported.) *St. Barth. Hosp. Rep.*, 1891, xxvii. 282; and *St. Barth. Hosp. J.*, 1894, ii. 130.

110. — The Royal Cure for the King's Evil. *Brit. M. J.*, 1899, i. 1182.

111. — The Head of Charles I. *Brit. M. J.*, 1906, i. 209.

112. Cheselden, William (1688–1752). *Brit. J. Surg.*, 1915–16, iii. 157.

113. — Cheselden's Anatomy. *Brit. J. Surg.*, 1928–9, xvi. 533.

114. Clay, Charles (1801–93). *D.N.B.*, Suppl., 1901.

115. Cline, Henry (1750–1827). *Brit. J. Surg.*, 1918–19, vi. 12.

116. [Clowes, William (1540–1604).] 'A Proved Practise for all Young Chirurgians by William Clowes Maister in Chirurgery.' *Brit. J. Surg.*, 1927–8, xv. 353.

117. Clutton, Henry Hugh (1850–1909). *D.N.B.*, 2 Suppl., 1913.

118. [Cock, Edward (1805–92).] 'Cock's Operation.' *Brit. J. Surg.*, 1926–7, xiv. 201.

119. Colles, Abraham (1773–1843). *Brit. J. Surg.*, 1914–15, ii. 351.

120. — Colles's Fracture. *Brit. J. Surg.*, 1921–2, ix. 4.

121. Cooper, Sir Alfred (1838–1908). *D.N.B.*, 2 Suppl., 1913.

122. Cooper, Sir Astley Paston (1768–1841). *Brit. J. Surg.*, 1913–14, i. 341.

123. — Sir Astley Cooper's 'Treatise on Dislocations and Fractures'. *Brit. J. Surg.*, 1929–30, xvii. 573.

124. Corfield, William Henry (1843–1903). *D.N.B.*, 2 Suppl., 1913.

125. [Cowper, William (1666–1709).] William Cowper, the Anatomist. *Brit. M. J.*, 1898, i. 160.

126. Crampton, Sir Philip (1777–1858). *Brit. J. Surg.*, 1919–20, vii. 299.
127. Croft, John (1833–1905). *D.N.B.*, 2 Suppl., 1913.
128. Cumston, Charles Greene (1868–1928). Appreciation. *Brit. M.J.*, 1928, i. 734.
129. Cunningham, James McNabb (1829–1905). *D.N.B.*, 2 Suppl., 1913.
130. [Currie, James (1756–1805).] James Currie, Physician. *Brit. M.J.*, 1903, i. 880.
131. Depage, Antoine (1863–1925). *Brit. M.J.*, 1925, i. 1198.
132. [Dover, Thomas (1660–1742).] Dover's 'Ancient Physicians' Legacy'. *Brit. M.J.*, 1897, i. 671.
133. [Doyley, Thomas (1548–1603).] Dr. Thomas Doyley: An Elizabethan Medical Opinion. *St. Barth. Hosp. J.*, 1921, xxviii. 179.
134. Dudgeon, Robert Ellis (1820–1904). *D.N.B.*, 2 Suppl., 1913.
135. Dutton, Joseph Everett (1874–1905). *D.N.B.*, 2 Suppl., 1913.
136. Erichsen, Sir John Eric (1818–96). *D.N.B.*, Suppl., 1901.
137. Fergusson, Sir William (1808–77). *Brit. J. Surg.*, 1918–19, vi. 479.
138. FitzGerald, Sir Thomas Naghten (1838–1908). *D.N.B.*, 2 Suppl., 1913.
139. [Floyer, Sir John (1649–1734).] Sir John Floyer, the Teller of the Pulse. *Brit. M.J.*, 1898, i. 1601.
140. [Fludd, Robert (1574–1637).] Robert Fludd, The Mystical Physician. *Brit. M.J.*, 1897, ii. 408.
141. Gale, Thomas (1507–87). *Brit. J. Surg.*, 1920–1, viii. 145.
142. — 'Certain Works of Chirurgerie by Thomas Gale, Maister in Chirurgerie.' *Brit. J. Surg.*, 1927–8, xv. 177.
143. Gamgee, Arthur (1841–1909). *D.N.B.*, 2 Suppl., 1913.
144. [Gamgee, Sampson (1828–86).] Gamgee's Tissue. *Brit. J. Surg.*, 1926–7, xiv. 557.
145. [Goldsmith, Oliver (1728–74).] On the Cause of Oliver Goldsmith's Death. *Proc. Roy. Soc. Med.* (Hist. Sect.), 1914, vii. 97.
146. Gore, Albert Augustus (1840–1901). *D.N.B.*, 2 Suppl., 1913.
147. Green, Joseph Henry (1791–1863). *Brit. J. Surg.*, 1919–20, vii. 7.
148. Guthrie, George James (1785–1856). *Brit. J. Surg.*, 1915–16, iii. 5.
149. [Hales, Stephen (1677–1761).] Stephen Hales, A pioneer in Modern Physiology. *Brit. M.J.*, 1897, ii. 1191.
150. [Hall, Marshall (1790–1857).] Dr. Marshall Hall and the Decay of Bloodletting. *Practitioner*, 1909, lxxxii. 320.
151. Halle, John (1529–68). *Brit. J. Surg.*, 1917–18, v. 181.
152. — John Halle and Sixteenth-Century Consultations. *Proc. Roy. Soc. Med.* (Hist. Sect.), 1918, xi. 55.
    The reprint contains some additional matter.
153. [Haller, Albert von (1708–1777).] Haller and Some Bygone Observations in Pathology. *M.J. & Rec.*, 1925, cxxii. 45.

154. — Albert von Haller and the Disputationes Chirurgicae Selectae. *V Congr. Internat. d'Hist. de la Méd.*, Genève, 1926, p. 9.
155. Hanbury, Sir James Arthur (1832–1908). *D.N.B.*, 2 Suppl., 1913.
156. [Harman, Edmund (1509 ?–76).] Notes on Edmund Harman, King's Barber. *Proc. Roy. Soc. Med.* (Hist. Sect.), 1916, ix. 67.
157. Harrison, Reginald (1837–1908). *D.N.B.*, 2 Suppl., 1913.
158. Hart, Ernest Abraham (1835–98). *D.N.B.*, Suppl., 1901.
159. [Harvey, William (1578–1657).] WILLIAM HARVEY. [Masters of Medicine.] London T. Fisher Unwin 1897. Pages xi, 283. Plates i. 19 × 12.5 cm.
160. — William Harvey's Diploma. *Brit. M.J.*, 1908, ii. 1700.
161. — PORTRAITS OF DR. WILLIAM HARVEY. Published for the Historical Section of the Royal Society of Medicine by Humphrey Milford, Oxford University Press, 1913. Pages v, 50. Plates xx. 32 × 22·5 cm.
*162. — A revised Chapter in the Life of Dr. William Harvey, 1636. *Proc. Roy. Soc. Med.* (Hist. Sect.), 1917, x. 33.
163. — Dr. William Harvey as a Man and an Art Connoisseur. *C.r. II Congr. Internat. d'Hist. de la Méd.*, Évreux, 1922, p. 452.
*164. — Dr. William Harvey and St. Bartholomew's Hospital. *St. Barth. Hosp. Rep.*, 1924, lvii. pt. ii, 96.
Reprinted in a modified form. *St. Barth. Hosp. Rep.*, 1928, lxi. 1.
165. — A Memorial Group of the Harvey Family. *Ann. M. History*, 1929, n.s., i. 241.
166. [Havers, Clopton (d. 1702).] Clopton Havers, M.D., An Early English Histologist. *Brit. M.J.*, 1898, i. 224.
167. Heath, Christopher (1835–1905). *D.N.B.*, 2 Suppl., 1913.
168. Hewett, Sir Prescott Gardner (1812–91). *D.N.B.*, Suppl., 1901.
169. Hey, William (1736–1819). *Brit. J. Surg.*, 1914–15, ii. 517.
170. — William Hey, of Leeds. *Brit. J. Surg.*, 1921–2, ix. 473.
171. Hilton, John (1805–78). *Brit. J. Surg.*, 1919–20, vii. 435.
172. Hogg, Jabez (1817–99). *D.N.B.*, Suppl., 1901.
173. Holden, Luther (1815–1905). *D.N.B.*, 2 Suppl., 1913.
174. Holmes, Timothy (1825–1907). *D.N.B.*, 2 Suppl., 1913.
175. Humphry, Sir George Murray (1820–96). *D.N.B.*, Suppl., 1901.
176. [Hunter, John (1728–93).] John Hunter's Family. (A letter.) *Brit. M.J.*, 1895, ii. 1463.
177. — John Hunter. *Brit. J. Surg.*, 1913–14, i. 153.
*178. — JOHN HUNTER: A MARTYR TO SCIENCE. The Hunterian Oration Delivered at The Royal College of Surgeons of England, on Saturday, February 14th, 1925. Bristol: John Wright & Sons Ltd. ... 1925. Pages 26. Figs. 10.
Reported *Lancet*, 1925, i. 369.
179. — Hunter's Operation for the Cure of Aneurysm. *Brit. J. Surg.*, 1929–30, xvii. 193.

180. Hunter, Sir William Guyer (1827–1902). *D.N.B.*, 2 Suppl., 1913.
181. [Hutchinson, Sir Jonathan (1828–1913).] Hutchinson's Triad. *Brit. J. Surg.*, 1926–7, xiv. i.
182. Ireland, William Wotherspoon (1832–1909). *D.N.B.*, 2 Suppl., 1913.
183. Jago, James (1815–93). *D.N.B.*, Suppl., 1901.
184. Jenner, Sir William (1815–98). *D.N.B.*, Suppl., 1901.
185. Keetley, Charles Robert Bell (1848–1909). *D.N.B.*, 2 Suppl., 1913.
186. Kerr, Norman (1834–99). *D.N.B.*, Suppl., 1901.
187. [Kymer, Gilbert (d. 1463).] Dr. Kymer and the University of Oxford. *Brit. M.J.*, 1899, i. 821.
188. Langton, John (1839–1910). Obituary. *St. Barth. Hosp. Rep.*, 1912, xlvii. 1.
189. Lister, Joseph, Lord (1827–1912). *Brit. J. Surg.*, 1913–14, i. 3.
190. Liston, Robert (1794–1847). *D.N.B.*, xxxiii, 1893.
191. — Robert Liston. *Brit. J. Surg.*, 1918–19, vi. 333.
192. [Lowe, Peter (1550–1610).] 'Peter Lowe, John Smith and King Solomon's Portraiture of Old Age.' *Brit. M.J.*, 1895, i. 106.
193. — Maister Peter Lowe. *Brit. J. Surg.*, 1915–16, iv. 557.
194. — 'The Whole Course of Chirurgerie compiled by Peter Lowe, Scotchman.' *Brit. J. Surg.*, 1927–8, xv. 533.
195. Macartney, James (1770–1843). *D.N.B.*, Suppl., 1901.
196. MacCormac, Sir William (1836–1901). *D.N.B.*, 2 Suppl., 1913.
197. McDonnell, Robert (1828–89). *D.N.B.*, xxxv, 1893.
198. [Macewen, Sir William (1848–1924).] Macewen's Osteotomy. *Brit. J. Surg.*, 1924–5, xii. 413.
199. Mackenzie, Sir Morell (1837–92). *D.N.B.*, xxxv, 1893.
200. Mackenzie, William (1791–1868). *D.N.B.*, xxxv, 1893.
    [Macro, Cox (1683–1767).] *vide* No. 92.
201. Manley, William George Nicholas (1831–1901). *D.N.B.*, 2 Suppl., 1913.
202. Mapother, Edward Dillon (1835–1908). *D.N.B.*, 2 Suppl., 1913.
203. Marsden, Alexander Edwin (1832–1902). *D.N.B.*, 2 Suppl., 1913.
204. Marsden, William (1796–1867). *D.N.B.*, xxxvi, 1893.
205. Marsh, Frederick Howard (1838–1915). In Memoriam. *St. Barth. Hosp. Rep.*, 1916, li. 1.
206. Marshall, John (1818–91). *D.N.B.*, xxxvi, 1893.
207. Mason, Francis (1837–86). *D.N.B.*, xxxvi, 1893.
208. Meadows, Alfred (1833–87). *D.N.B.*, xxxvii, 1894.
209. Miller, James (1812–64). *D.N.B.*, xxxvii, 1894.
210. Moore, Langford (d. 1929). Obituary. *St. Barth. Hosp. J.*, 1929, xxxvi. 51.
211. Moore, Sir Norman (1847–1922). *St. Barth. Hosp. J.*, 1923, xxx. 51.
212. Morton, Thomas (1813–49). *D.N.B.*, xxxix, 1894.

213. Moyle, John (d. 1714). *Brit. J. Surg.*, 1915–16, iii. 585.
214. Needham, Walter (1631–91). *D.N.B.*, xl, 1894.
215. Northcote, William (d. 1783). *D.N.B.*, xli, 1895.
216. Nunn, Joshua Arthur (1853–1908). *D.N.B.*, 2 Suppl., 1913.
217. Nunneley, Thomas (1809–70). *D.N.B.*, xli, 1895.
218. Orton, Reginald (1810–62). *D.N.B.*, xlii, 1895.
219. Outram, Sir Benjamin Fonseca (1774–1856). *D.N.B.*, xlii, 1895.
220. Paget, Sir James (1814–99). *D.N.B.*, Suppl., 1901.
221. — Sir James Paget, Bart. *Brit. J. Surg.*, 1914–15, ii. 4.
222. — (On Disease of the Mammary Areola.) *Brit. J. Surg.*, 1922–3, x. 1.
223. — (On Osteitis Deformans). *Brit. J. Surg.*, 1922–3, x. 161.
224. [Paré Ambroise (1510–90).] Johnson's Ambrose Parey. *Brit. J. Surg.*, 1928–9, xvi. 181.
225. — The Iconography of Ambroise Paré. *Brit. M.J.*, 1929, ii. 965.
226. Parker, Samuel William Langston (1803–71). *D.N.B.*, xliii, 1895.
227. Partridge, Richard (1805–73). *D.N.B.*, xliii, 1895.
228. Pavy, Frederick William (1829–1911). *D.N.B.*, 2 Suppl., 1913.
229. Pearson, John (1758–1826). *D.N.B.*, xliv, 1895.
230. Pearson, John Norman (1787–1865). *D.N.B.*, xliv, 1895.
231. Penrose, Francis (1718–98). *D.N.B.*, xliv, 1895.
232. [Pepys, Samuel (1633–1703).] The Medical History of Mr. and Mrs. Samuel Pepys. *Lancet*, 1895, i. 1357. Expurgated. The complete version appears in the *Occasional Papers* (*v. inf.*).
233. — Who performed Lithotomy on Mr. Samuel Pepys ? *Lancet*, 1904, i. 1011.
*234. — Why Samuel Pepys discontinued his diary. *Lancet*, 1911, i. 1687. Nos. 232, 233, and 234 were reprinted in *Occasional Papers of the Samuel Pepys Club.* Edited by the President. Vol. i. 1903–1914, London, 1917, pp. 78, 58, 64.
235. — Samuel Pepys and the Royal Society. *Brit. M.J.*, 1912, ii. 184.
236. — Mr. Samuel Pepys. An address. *Trans. Lond. and Middlesex Arch. Soc.*, 1927, n.s., v. part iv.
237. Pettigrew, James Bell (1834–1908). *D.N.B.*, 2 Suppl., 1913.
238. Pettigrew, Thomas Joseph (1791–1865). *D.N.B.*, xlv, 1895.
239. [Phayer, Thomas (1510–60).] Thomas Phayer, Lawyer, Physician, and Poet. *Brit. M.J.*, 1897, i. 925.
240. Pilcher, George (1801–55). *D.N.B.*, xlv, 1895.
241. Pott, Percivall (1714–88). *D.N.B.*, xlvi, 1896.
242. — Percivall Pott: his own fracture. *Brit. J. Surg.*, 1922–3, x. 313.
243. — Pott's Fracture. *Brit. J. Surg.*, 1922–3, x. 433.
244. — Pott's Disease of the Spine. *Brit. J. Surg.*, 1923–4, xi. 1.
245. — Pott's Puffy Tumour. *Brit. J. Surg.*, 1923–4, xi. 197.
246. — The Works of Percivall Pott. *Brit. J. Surg.*, 1929–30, xvii. 1.
247. Potter, John Phillips (1818–47). *D.N.B.*, xlvi, 1896.

248. Priestley, Sir William Overend (1829–1900). *D.N.B.*, Suppl., 1901.
249. Propert, John Lumsden (1834–1902). *D.N.B.*, 2 Suppl., 1913.
250. Pym, Sir William (1772–1861). *D.N.B.*, xlvii, 1896.
251. Quain, Jones (1796–1865). *D.N.B.*, xlvii, 1896.
252. Quain, Richard (1800–87). *D.N.B.*, xlvii, 1896.
253. Quain, Sir Richard (1816–98). *D.N.B.*, Suppl., 1901.
254. Radcliffe, Charles Bland (1822–89). *D.N.B.*, xlvii, 1896.
255. Rae, James (1716–91). *D.N.B.*, xlvii, 1896.
256. Ranby, John (1703–73). *D.N.B.*, xlvii, 1896.
257. [Raynalde, Thomas (fl. 1540–51).] 'The Byrth of Mankynd, other-
     wyse named the Womans Boke.' *Brit. M.J.*, 1894, ii. 1436.
258. — The Birth of Mankind or the Woman's Book. A bibliographical
     study. *The Library*, 1927, 4th ser., viii. 1–37.
     The reprint contains, in addition, tables of 'comparison of the
     ornamental initial letters as a means of distinguishing the various
     issues'.
259. Read, John (fl. 1588). *D.N.B.*, xlvii, 1896.
260. Reece, Richard (1775–1831). *D.N.B.*, xlvii, 1896.
261. Reid, Alexander (1586–1641). *D.N.B.*, xlvii, 1896.
262. — A Seventeenth century Teacher of Anatomy and Surgery, Dr.
     Alexander Reid. *Brit. M.J.*, 1895, ii. 678.
263. Reid, Thomas (1791–1825). *D.N.B.*, xlvii, 1896.
264. Richardson, Sir Benjamin Ward (1828–96). *D.N.B.*, Suppl., 1901.
265. Ring, John (1752–1821). *D.N.B.*, xlviii, 1896.
266. Roberts, Sir William (1830–99). *D.N.B.*, Suppl., 1901.
267. Robertson, Douglas Moray Cooper Lamb Argyll (1837–1909).
     D.N.B., 2 Suppl., 1913.
268. Robertson, Sir William Tindal (1825–89). *D.N.B.*, xlviii, 1896.
269. Roe, George Hamilton (1795–1873). *D.N.B.*, xlix, 1897.
270. Rolleston, George (1829–81). *D.N.B.*, xlix, 1897.
271. Roose, Edward Charles Robson (1848–1905). *D.N.B.*, 2 Suppl.,
     1913.
     [Rosslin, Eucharius.] *vide* Nos. 257, 258.
272. Rowe, George Robert (1792–1861). *D.N.B.*, xlix, 1897.
273. Rushworth, John (1669–1736). *D.N.B.*, xlix, 1897.
274. Rutherford, John (1695–1779). *D.N.B.*, l, 1897.
275. Rutherford, William (1839–99). *D.N.B.*, l, 1897.
276. Sainbel, Charles Vial de (1753–93). *D.N.B.*, l, 1897.
277. St. André, Nathanael (1680–1776). *D.N.B.*, l, 1897.
278. Saints Cosmas and Damian. (A letter.) *Lancet*, 1895, i. 725.
279. [Saint Cuthbert (636–87).] The Bones of St. Cuthbert. *Brit. M.J.*,
     1901, ii. 42.
280. Saumerez, Richard (1764–1835). *D.N.B.*, l, 1897.
281. Saunders, Sir Edwin (1814–1901). *D.N.B.*, 2 Suppl., 1913.
282. Saunders, John Cunningham (1773–1810). *D.N.B.*, l, 1897.

283. Sawrey, Solomon (1765–1825). *D.N.B.*, l, 1897.
284. Scott, John (1798–1846). *D.N.B.*, li, 1897.
285. Sharp, Samuel (1700–78). *D.N.B.*, li, 1897.
286. Sharp, William (1805–96). *D.N.B.*, li, 1897.
287. Sharpey, William (1802–80). *D.N.B.*, li, 1897.
288. Shaw, Alexander (1804–90). *D.N.B.*, li, 1897.
289. Shaw, John (1792–1827). *D.N.B.*, li, 1897.
290. Sheldon, John (1752–1808). *D.N.B.*, lii, 1897.
291. — John Sheldon, Anatomist and Surgeon. *Brit. M.J.*, 1899, i. 1342.
292. Shipton, John (1680–1748). *D.N.B.*, lii, 1897.
293. Sims, James (1741–1820). *D.N.B.*, lii, 1897.
294. Skey, Frederic Carpenter (1798–1872). *D.N.B.*, lii, 1897.
295. Smee, Alfred (1818–77). *D.N.B.*, lii, 1897.
296. Smith, Henry Spencer (1812–1901). *D.N.B.*, 2 Suppl., 1913.
297. Smith, John Gordon (1792–1833). *D.N.B.*, liii, 1898.
298. Smith, Sir Thomas (1833–1909). *D.N.B.*, 2 Suppl., 1913.
299. Snow, John (1818–58). *D.N.B.*, liii, 1898.
300. Solly, Samuel (1805–71). *D.N.B.*, liii, 1898.
301. South, John Flint (1797–1882). *D.N.B.*, liii, 1898.
302. Spence, James (1812–82). *D.N.B.*, liii, 1898.
303. Stafford, Richard Anthony (1801–54). *D.N.B.*, liii, 1898.
304. Stanley, Edward (1793–1862). *D.N.B.*, liv, 1898.
305. Stevenson, John (1778–1846). *D.N.B.*, liv, 1898.
306. Stevenson, William (1719–83). *D.N.B.*, liv, 1898.
307. Stewart, Charles (1840–1907). *D.N.B.*, 2 Suppl., 1913.
308. Stewart, Isla (1855–1910). *D.N.B.*, 2 Suppl., 1913.
309. — Miss Isla Stewart. In Memoriam. *St. Barth. Hosp. J.*, 1910, xvii. 106.
310. Stokes, Sir William (1839–1900). *D.N.B.*, Suppl., 1901.
311. Stratton, John Proudfoot (1830–95). *D.N.B.*, lv, 1898.
312. Struthers, Sir John (1823–99). *D.N.B.*, Suppl., 1901.
313. Swan, Joseph (1791–1874). *D.N.B.*, lv, 1898.
314. Syme, James (1799–1870). *Brit. J. Surg.*, 1914–15, ii. 189.
315. — Syme's Amputation. *Brit. J. Surg.*, 1924–5, xii. 1.
316. Tait, Robert Lawson (1845–99). *D.N.B.*, Suppl., 1901.
317. Tanner, Thomas Hawkes (1824–71). *D.N.B.*, lv, 1898.
318. Taunton, John (1769–1821). *D.N.B.*, lv, 1898.
319. Taylor, Charles Bell (1829–1909). *D.N.B.*, 2 Suppl., 1913.
320. [Teale, Thomas Pridgin (1801–67).] Teale's Amputation. *Brit. J. Surg.*, 1923–4, xi. 605.
321. [Thomas, Hugh Owen (1834–91).] Thomas's Hip Splint. *Brit. J. Surg.*, 1925–6, xiii. 405, 601.
322. Thompson, Sir Henry (1820–1904). *D.N.B.*, 2 Suppl., 1913.
323. Thomson, Allen (1809–84). *D.N.B.*, lvi, 1898.
324. Thomson, Anthony Todd (1778–1849). *D.N.B.*, lvi, 1898.

325. Thomson, John (1765–1846). *D.N.B.*, lvi, 1898.
326. Thomson, William (1802–52). *D.N.B.*, lvi, 1898.
327. Thorne, Sir Richard Thorne- (1841–99). *D.N.B.*, Suppl., 1901.
328. Thornhill, William (fl. 1737–55). *D.N.B.*, lvi, 1898.
329. Tilt, John Edward (1815–93). *D.N.B.*, lvi, 1898.
330. [Tofts, Mary (1701–63).] Mary Tofts, the Rabbit Breeder. *Brit. M.J.*, 1896, ii. 209.
331. Towne, Joseph (1808–79). *D.N.B.*, lvii, 1899.
332. Toynbee, Joseph (1815–66). *D.N.B.*, lvii, 1899.
333. Travers, Benjamin (1783–1858). *D.N.B.*, lvii, 1899.
334. Trye, Charles Brandon (1757–1811). *D.N.B.*, lvii, 1899.
335. Tufnell, Thomas Joliffe (1819–85). *D.N.B.*, lvii, 1899.
336. Turner, James Smith (1832–1904). *D.N.B.*, 2 Suppl., 1913.
337. Turner, Thomas (1793–1873). *D.N.B.*, lvii, 1899.
338. Tyrrell, Frederick (1793–1843). *D.N.B.*, lvii, 1899.
339. Vicary, Thomas (1490–1562). *Brit. J. Surg.*, 1917–18, v. 359.
340. [Vigo, John of (1460–1520).] John of Vigo: His English Translator and Bookseller. *Brit. M.J.*, 1894, i. 1141.
341. Vincent, John Painter (1776–1852). *D.N.B.*, lviii, 1899.
342. Wadd, William (1776–1829). *D.N.B.*, lviii, 1899.
343. Wade, Sir Willoughby Francis (1827–1906). *D.N.B.*, 2 Suppl., 1913.
344. Waller, Augustus Volney (1816–70). *D.N.B.*, lix, 1899.
345. Walsham, William Johnson (1847–1903). *D.N.B.*, 2 Suppl., 1913.
*346. [Ward, John (1629–81).] John Ward and His Diary. *Tr. M. Soc. Lond.*, 1917, xl. 1. Presidential address.
347. — The Oxford Physic Garden. *Ann. M. History*, 1919, ii. 109.
348. — The Rev. John Ward and Medicine. *Tr. M. Soc. Lond.*, 1920, xliii. 253. The Annual Oration
349. — An Eighteenth [Seventeenth] Century Operation for Torticollis. *St. Barth. Hosp. J.*, 1922, xxix. 30.
350. — The Rev. John Ward, M.A. and Stratford-upon-Avon. *Stratford-upon-Avon Herald*, 23 Feb. 1923.
       This is a synopsis of a paper read before the Shakespeare Club at Stratford-upon-Avon in February 1923; the complete text remains in manuscript.
351. Wardrop, James (1782–1869). *D.N.B.*, lix, 1899.
352. Ware, James (1756–1815). *D.N.B.*, lix, 1899.
353. Warner, Joseph (1717–1801). *D.N.B.*, lix, 1899.
354. Warren, John Taylor (1771–1849). *D.N.B.*, lix, 1899.
355. Warren, Richard (1731–97). *D.N.B.*, lix, 1899.
356. Watson, Sir Patrick Heron (1832–1907). *D.N.B.*, 2 Suppl., 1913.
357. Wells, Sir Thomas Spencer (1818–97). *D.N.B.*, lx, 1899.
*358. — Spencer Wells' Forceps. *Brit. J. Surg.*, 1926–7, xiv. 385.
359. Wheeler, Thomas (1754–1847). *D.N.B.*, lx, 1899.

360. Wheelhouse, Claudius Galen (1826–1909). *D.N.B.*, 2 Suppl., 1913.
361. — Wheelhouse's Operation. *Brit. J. Surg.*, 1924–5, xii. 209.
362. White, Anthony (1782–1849). *D.N.B.*, lxi, 1900.
363. Whitehead, John (1740–1804). *D.N.B.*, lxi, 1900.
364. — Whitehead's Operation. *Brit. J. Surg.*, 1924–5, xii. 625.
365. Williams, Sir Dawson (1854–1928). Appreciation. *Brit. M.J.*, 1928, i. 420.
366. Williams, Robert (1787–1845). *D.N.B.*, lxi, 1900.
367. Willis, Browne (1682–1760). The Willis Patronal Lecture at Fenny Stratford, 1929. *In manuscript.* Reported in *The North Bucks. Times*, 12 November 1929.
368. Wilson, Sir William James Erasmus (1809–84). *D.N.B.*, lxii, 1900.
369. Wiseman, Richard (1622–76). *D.N.B.*, lxii, 1900.
370. — Richard Wiseman. *Brit. J. Surg.*, 1915–16, iii. 349.
371. — 'Severall Chirurgicall Treatises by Richard Wiseman, 1676.' *Brit. J. Surg.*, 1928–9, xvi. 357.
372. Wood, Alexander (1817–84). *D.N.B.*, lxii, 1900.
373. Wood, John (1825–91). *D.N.B.*, lxii, 1900.
374. [Woodall, John (1556–1643).] John Woodall: The Status and pay of Land and Sea Surgeons under the Early Stuarts. *Brit. M.J.*, 1894, i. 600.
375. — John Woodall. *Brit. J. Surg.*, 1916–17, iv. 369.
376. — 'The Surgeons Mate by John Woodall.' *Brit. J. Surg.*, 1928–9, xvi. 1.
377. Woolhouse, John Thomas (1650–1734). *D.N.B.*, lxii, 1900.
378. Wormald, Thomas (1802–73). *D.N.B.*, lxiii, 1900.
379. Wright, William (1735–1819). *D.N.B.*, lxiii, 1900.
380. Wyatt, John (1825–74). *D.N.B.*, lxiii, 1900.
381. Yearsley, James (1805–69). *D.N.B.*, lxiii, 1900.
382. Yeo, Gerald Francis (1845–1909). *D.N.B.*, 2 Suppl., 1913.

SURGICAL WORKS

A. ABDOMINAL SURGERY

General

383. Vanishing Tumours. *Lancet*, 1899, i. 583.
384. A Year's Abdominal Operations. *St. Barth. Hosp. Rep.*, 1902, xxxvii. 27.
385. The Abdominal Emergency Cases met with in Six Months' Hospital Practice. *Med. Chron.*, 1901, 4th ser., i. 81.
386. On Surgical Danger Signals in Acute Abdominal Disease. *Clin. J.*, 1907, xxix. 246.
387. On some Misleading Abdominal Cases. *Brit. M.J.*, 1908, i. 185.
388. The After-treatment of Some Surgical Cases. *Practitioner*, 1920, cv. 1.

389. Some Surgical Emergencies, with special reference to the Abdominal Region. *Practitioner*, 1923, cx. 26.

Peritonitis

390. A Case of Peritonitis with Effusion treated by Laparotomy. *Lancet*, 1893, ii. 1563.

Stomach and Duodenum

391. Two Cases of Perforated Gastric Ulcer. (Notes by Mr. G. V. Bull.) *Brit. M.J.*, 1901, i. 705.

392. Some Cases of Gastric and Intestinal Perforation and the Lessons they teach. *St. Barth. Hosp. Rep.*, 1903, xxxviii. 5.

393. Four Cases of Duodenal Ulcer perforating acutely. *Brit. M.J.*, 1903, i. 67.

394. On Some Cases of Gastric Surgery and their Results. *Clin. J.*, 1904, xxiii. 97.

395. Some Cases of Gastric Surgery. *St. Barth. Hosp. Rep.*, 1904, xxxix. 19.

396. Discussion on the Operative Treatment of Gastric and Duodenal Ulcers. *Med.-Chir. Trans.*, 1903, xxxvi. 555.

397. Four Cases of Gastro-jejunostomy. *St. Barth. Hosp. Rep.*, 1905, xl. 67.

398. On the After-history of Patients who have undergone the Operation of Gastro-jejunostomy. *Clin. J.*, 1905, xxvi. 257, 283.

399. The Causes, Symptoms, and Treatment of Pyloric Obstruction. *Practitioner*, 1905, lxxv. 642.

400. Duodenal Ulcer and its Treatment. *Tr. M. Soc. Lond.*, 1905, xxviii. 37.

401. A Year's Gastro-jejunostomies. *St. Barth. Hosp. Rep.*, 1906, xli. 169.

402. On Acute Duodenal Perforation. *Lancet*, 1906, ii. 1195.

403. The Symptoms, Treatment and Sequelae of Non-malignant Duodenal Ulcer. *XV Congr. Internat. de Méd.*, Lisbonne, 1907, sect. ix, fasc. 2, p. 310.

404. Discussion of the Operative Treatment of Gastric Ulcers. *Med.-Chir. Trans.*, 1907, xc. 289.

405. On a Case of Duodenal Ulcer. *Clin. J.*, 1910, xxxv. 209.

406. Case of Acute Duodenal Perforation. Operation. Death. *M. Press*, 1912, o.s., cxlv. 112.

407. On Five Cases of Acute Duodenal Perforation. *Lancet*, 1912, ii. 67.

408. Discussion on the Remote Results of the Surgical Treatment of Gastric and Duodenal Ulcers. *Proc. Roy. Soc. Med.* (Surg. Sect.), 1920, xiii. 165.

Intestinal Obstruction

409. An unusual Case of Acute Intestinal Obstruction in an Infant. *Brit. M.J.*, 1895, ii. 1356.

410. A Case of Intestinal Obstruction. *M. Press*, 1911, o.s., cxliii. 502.
411. Three Cases of Intestinal Obstruction. *M. Press*, 1912, o.s., cxliv. 489.
412. Two Cases of Acute Intestinal Strangulation by Bands. *M. Press*, 1914, cxlviii. 546.

Intussusception

413. A Case of Multiple Intussusception. *Trans. Path. Soc.*, 1886, xxxvii. 240.
414. Some Points in the Minute Anatomy of Intussusception. *J. Path. & Bact.*, 1897, iv. 484. (First Hunterian Lecture.) *vide* No. 418.
415. On the Pathology and Surgery of Intussusception. *Brit. M.J.*, 1897, i. 381, 453, 514. (Hunterian Lectures.) *vide* No. 418.
416. Ileo-caecal Intussusception and its Treatment. *Edinburgh M.J.*, 1897, n.s., i. 592.
417. A Case of Recurrent Intussusception with Remarks. *Treatment*, 1897–8, i. 418.
418. SOME POINTS IN THE ANATOMY, PATHOLOGY, AND SURGERY OF INTUSSUS-CEPTION. London: The Rebman Publishing Company, 1898. Pages 88. Illustrated. 21 × 14 cm.
    Based on The Hunterian Lectures, *vide* Nos. 414, 415.
419. Two Unusual Cases of Intussusception. *Trans. Path. Soc.*, 1899, l. 121.
420. Two Cases of Colo-Colic Intussusception; Operation; Recovery. *Brit. M.J.*, 1901, i. 1404.
421. Intussusception and its Treatment. *Clin. J.*, 1901, xviii. 268.
422. A Case of Ileo-Ileac Intussusception spontaneously cured. (Remarks.) *Brit. M.J.*, 1903, i. 964.
423. Editor of section 'On Invagination of the Intestine'. Nöthnagel's *Encyclopaedia of Practical Medicine*. Engl. ed. Eds. i and ii, Philadelphia and London, 1904–7.
424. On Intussusception. *Clin. J.*, 1906, xxvii. 321.
425. On a Case of Sarcoma causing Chronic Intussusception. *Clin. J.*, 1912, xl. 193.
426. Acute Irreducible Intussusception in a Child aged six months; Resection; Recovery. (By G. S. Hughes.) Note. *Lancet*, 1912, ii. 879.

Hernia

427. Three Specimens of Encysted Hernia. *Trans. Path. Soc.*, 1885, xxxvi. 216.
428. A Case of Congenital Umbilical Hernia. *Trans. Path. Soc.*, 1888, xxxix. 108.
429. Strangulated Omphalocele; Operation; Death. (Remarks.) *Lancet*, 1894, ii. 1217.

430. Strangulated Inguinal Hernia in a boy aged two and a half years. (Remarks.) *Brit. M.J.*, 1899, i. 788.
431. Strangulated Inguinal Hernia in a boy aged ten and a half months. (Notes.) *Lancet*, 1899, ii. 889.
432. A Case of Strangulated Hernia in a premature child, aged five weeks. (Remarks.) *Lancet*, 1901, i. 1536.

Appendicitis

433. The Prognosis and Modern Treatment of Appendicitis. *Brit. M.J.*, 1899, ii. 1467.
434. Haemophilia complicating Appendicectomy. *M. Press*, 1912, o.s., cxlv. 633.
435. On Some Pitfalls in Appendicitis. *Practitioner*, 1915, xcv. 729.

Volvulus

436. On Volvulus. *Am. J. Surg.*, 1916, xxx. 178.

Colitis

437. The Causes, Sequelae, and Treatment of Pericolic Inflammation. *Brit. M.J.*, 1906, ii. 1171.
438. The Surgical Treatment of Chronic Colitis. *Brit. M.J.*, 1911, i. 863.
439. Report upon the Treatment of Chronic Colitis. *3me Congr. de la Soc. Internat. de Chir.*, Bruxelles, 1911, pt. ii. 419.
   Ann. Internat. de Chir. Gastro-intestinale, 1911, v. 65.
440. On the Treatment of Ulcerative Colitis. *M. Press*, 1911, o.s., cxliii. 414, 440.
441. A Case of Appendicostomy for Chronic Colitis. *M. Press*, 1913, o.s., cxlvi. 689.
442. Appendicostomy. *M. Press*, 1913, o.s., cxlvii. 532.
443. Ulcerative Colitis and its Surgical Treatment by Appendicostomy. *St. Barth. Hosp. Rep.*, 1914, xlix. 59.

Rectum

444. Imperforate anus; (A) male, (B) female. *Trans. Path. Soc.*, 1887, xxxviii. 149.
445. Some Cases of Chronic Ulceration of the Rectum. *Practitioner*, 1909, lxxxiii. 136.

Liver

446. A Case of Non-alcoholic Cirrhosis of the Liver. *Trans. Path. Soc.*, 1890, xli. 152.
447. Gall-stones: a plea for earlier operation. *Brit. J. Surg.*, 1913–14, i. 21.

Spleen

448. Repair after Rupture of the Spleen and Kidney. *Trans. Path. Soc.*, 1890, xli. 162.
449. Successful Removal of an Enlarged and Displaced Spleen. *Brit. M.J.*, 1900, ii. 1428.
450. On some Cases illustrating the Surgery of the Spleen. *Clin. J.*, 1907, xxix. 97; *St. Barth. Hosp. Rep.*, 1909, xliv. 95.

Urinary System

451. A Case of Partial Laceration of the Urethra successfully treated by continuous dilatation. *Brit. M.J.*, 1885, ii. 912.
452. Congenital Pelvic Cyst, probably of Postanal origin leading to Retention of Urine. *Trans. Path. Soc.*, 1894, xlv. 216.
453. A Case of Suppression of Urine associated with a single Kidney. (Remarks.) *Lancet*, 1900, i. 25.
454. Prostatectomy. (Two cases.) *M. Press*, 1912, o.s., cxliv. 64.
455. Discussion on the Treatment of Subacute Nephritis by Kidney Decapsulation. *Proc. Roy. Soc. Med.* (Urol. Sect.), 1921, xiv. 19.

Generative Organs

456. A Case of Successful Ovariotomy in a child four months old. *Brit. M.J.*, 1898, i. 617.
457. Ovarian Cyst from a child aged four months. *Trans. Path. Soc.*, 1898, xlix. 196.
458. A Dermoid Cyst of the Right Testis. *Trans. Path. Soc.*, 1887, xxxviii. 224.
459. On the Diseases and Displacements of the Testicle. *Brit. M.J.*, 1907, ii. 716.

B. ARTERIAL SURGERY

460. Aneurysm of the Abdominal Aorta treated by the introduction of silver wire, with a description of instruments invented and constructed by Mr. G. H. Colt to facilitate the introduction of wire into aneurysms. (With G. H. Colt, B.A.) *Lancet*, 1903, ii. 808; *Med.-Chir. Trans.*, 1903, lxxxvi. 363; *Brit. M.J.*, 1903, i. 1493.
461. Recent Advances in the Surgery of the Blood Vessels. *XV Congr. Internat. de Méd.*, Lisbonne, 1907, sect. ix, fasc. 1, p. 1; *Lancet*, 1906, i. 1159.
462. On Varicocele. *M. Press*, 1909, o.s., cxxxix. 654.
463. Discussion of the Surgical Treatment of Aneurysms. (Jointly with Mr. Colt.) *Proc. Roy. Soc. Med.* (Surg. Sect.), 1912, v. 169.
464. Intrathoracic Aneurysm wired with Colt's Apparatus. (Jointly with Sir A. Bowlby.) *Clin. J.*, 1914, xliii. 113; *Tr. M. Soc. Lond.*, 1915, xxxvii. 68.
*465. The Palliative Treatment of Aneurysm by 'Wiring' with Colt's Apparatus. *Brit. J. Surg.*, 1921–2, ix. 27.

C. DISEASES OF THE BREAST (NON-MALIGNANT)

466. True Adenoma of the Breast. *Trans. Path. Soc.*, 1885, xxxvi. 411.
467. Cystic Disease of the Breast in a boy aged three years. *Trans. Path. Soc.*, 1899, l. 225.
468. The Diagnosis and Treatment of Cystic Disease of the Breast. *Lancet*, 1910, ii. 1604.

D. DISEASES OF CHILDREN

469. A Case of Symmetrical Gangrene of the Feet. (In a child.) *Lancet*, 1893, ii. 249.
470. THE SURGICAL DISEASES OF CHILDREN AND THEIR TREATMENT BY MODERN METHODS. London H. K. Lewis, 1895. Pages xvi, 548. Illustrated. 18 × 12 cm.
471. Results of a Year's Experience in the Surgical Treatment of Hydrocephalus in Children. *Internat. Clinics*, Philadelphia, 1895–6 (5th) ser., iii. 254.
472. Meningitis in its Surgical Aspects. *Clin. J.*, 1896, viii. 49.
473. On Cystic Lymphangioma in Childhood. *Brit. M.J.*, 1896, i. 1189.
474. A Case of Spontaneous Disappearance of a Congenital Cystic Lymphangioma. *Brit. M.J.*, 1897, ii. 1633.

E. MALIGNANT DISEASE

475. A Case of Fibro-sarcoma of the Dura Mater. *Trans. Path. Soc.*, 1886, xxxvii. 12.
476. Multiple Sarcomata in the Cerebral Hemispheres and Pons Varolii with entire absence of Cerebral Symptoms. *Trans. Path. Soc.*, 1886, xxxvii. 54.
477. A Psammoma involving the Superior Frontal Gyrus of the Right Side. *Trans. Path. Soc.*, 1886, xxxvii. 55.
478. Sarcoma involving the Left Fifth Nerve with Multiple Sarcomata of the Body. *Trans. Path. Soc.*, 1886, xxxvii. 62.
479. Primary Carcinoma of the Cerebellum, Left Lateral Hemisphere. *Trans. Path. Soc.*, 1886, xxxvii. 66.
480. Primary Round-celled Sarcoma of the Inferior Vermiform Process of the Cerebellum. *Trans. Path. Soc.*, 1886, xxxvii. 67.
481. Central Sarcoma of the Shaft of the Femur. *Trans. Path. Soc.*, 1886, xxxvii. 377.
482. Round-celled Sarcoma of the Spinal Cord and Brain. (With Sir W. Herringham.) *Trans. Path. Soc.*, 1887, xxxviii. 43.
483. A Case of Sarcoma of the Urinary Bladder. *Trans. Path. Soc.*, 1888, xxxix. 172.

484. A Complete Case of Ossifying Sarcoma. *Trans. Path. Soc.*, 1889, xl. 293.
485. Some effects of Chronic Irritation upon Living Tissues, being first steps in a rational study of Cancer. *Brit. M.J.*, 1893, ii. 830.
486. A Case of Sarcoma occurring in a Tar-worker. *Trans. Path. Soc.*, 1894, xlv. 211.
487. Cancer Houses and their Victims. *Brit. M.J.*, 1894, i. 1240.
488. An Experimental Investigation into the Causation of Cancer. *Brit. M.J.*, 1894, ii. 636.
489. A Comparison of the Results obtained from Inoculation of Portions of Tissue affected with Paget's Disease and of Coccidia. *J. Path. & Bact.*, 1894, ii. 251.
490. The Infectivity of Cancer: A Retrospect and a Forecast. *Brit. M.J.*, 1895, i. 910.
491. The Heredity of Cancer. *Clin. J.*, 1895, vi. 186.
492. Primary Sarcoma of the Vagina in Children. *St. Barth. Hosp. Rep.*, 1895, xxxi. 121.
493. Epithelial Changes produced by Irritation. *J. Path. & Bact.*, 1896, iii. 124.
494. Sarcoma of the Vagina in a Child. *Trans. Path. Soc.*, 1896, xlviii. 169.
495. Some Morphological Changes occurring in epithelial cells as a result of disease. *J. Path. & Bact.*, 1897, iv. 69.
496. The Local Distribution of Cancer and Cancer Houses. *Practitioner*, 1899, lxii. 418.
497. Notes of three Cases of inoperable cancer of the breast treated by removal of the ovaries. *Lancet*, 1902, ii. 933.
498. The Origin of Cancer. *The Hospital*, 1902, xxxii. 37.
499. A Further Investigation into the Causation of Cancer. *Edinburgh M.J.*, 1902, n.s., xii. 39.
500. Remarks in a Debate on Cancer at the Chelsea Clinical Society. *Clin. J.*, 1902, xx. 123.
501. A Further Contribution to the distribution of Cancer. *Practitioner*, 1903, lxx. 697.
502. Have the Locality and Surroundings an influence upon the Recurrence of Malignant Disease after Operation? *Lancet*, 1903, ii. 221.
503. On Some Cases of Malignant Disease from the Department for Diseases of the Throat and Nose. (Jointly with Dr. Jobson Horne.) *St. Barth. Hosp. Rep.*, 1904, xxxix. 219.
504. The Progress of Cancer Research. *The Hospital*, 1904, xxxv. 5.
505. Notes on an Ineffectual Treatment of Cancer, being a Record of Three Cases injected with Dr. Otto Schmidt's Serum. *Brit. M.J.*, 1904, i. 299.
506. Up-to-date Surgery and the Treatment of Cancer. (A letter.) *Brit. M.J.*, 1905, ii. 1236.

507. The Diagnosis and Treatment of Cancer of the Large Intestine. *Med. Mag.*, 1906, xv. 242, 313.

508. Primary Sarcoma of the Spleen. *2me Congr. de la Soc. Internat. de Chir.*, Bruxelles, 1908, i. 178.

509. On the Early Diagnosis and Surgical Treatment of Cancer of the Stomach. *M. Press*, 1909, o.s., cxxxviii. 295.

510. Multiple Inflammation of the Tongue. Unusual Case of Carcinoma. *M. Press*, 1913, o.s., cxlvi. 201.

511. The Predisposition to Cancer of the Tongue. (A letter.) *Lancet*, 1918, i. 781.

*512. On Cancer of the Tongue. (The Bradshaw Lecture.) *Brit. J. Surg.*, 1918–19, vi. 336.

513. Cancer. *M. Press*, 1922, o.s., clxiv. 281.

F. MILITARY SURGERY

514. The Wounded in the War: Some Surgical Lessons. *Lancet*, 1914, ii. 1084.

515. Discussion on the Treatment of Wounds in War. *Tr. M. Soc. Lond.*, 1915, xxxviii. 66.

516. WOUNDS IN WAR THEIR TREATMENT AND RESULTS [Oxford War Primers] London . . . Oxford University Press, 1915. Pages 108. 16·5 × 10·5 cm.

517. Gold Coins carried into the Back by a Shell Fragment. *Brit. J. Surg.*, 1914–15, ii. 510.

G. ORTHOPAEDIC SURGERY

518. An Account of Four Cases of Intramuscular Synovial Cysts associated with Joint Disease. *Trans. Path. Soc.*, 1885, xxxvi. 337.

519. Knee Joints seventeen months after Ogston's Operation. *Trans. Path. Soc.*, 1885, xxxvi. 345.

520. A Case of Osteitis Deformans. *Trans. Path. Soc.*, 1886. xxxvii. 239.

521. Interosseous or Central Necrosis of the Femur. *Trans. Path. Soc.*, 1886, xxxvii. 372.

522. A Neglected Point in the Pathology of Colles' Fracture. *Trans. Path. Soc.*, 1887, xxxviii. 250.

523. Congenital Dislocation of the Hip. *Trans. Path. Soc.*, 1887, xxxviii. 299.

524. Further Specimens of Intramuscular Synovial Cysts. *Trans. Path. Soc.*, 1887, xxxviii. 381.

525. Simple Comminuted Fracture of the Head of the Tibia. *Trans. Path. Soc.*, 1888, xxxix. 237.

526. A Parosteal Lipoma connected with the Periosteum of the Femur. *Trans. Path. Soc.*, 1888, xxxix. 270.

527. A Case of Talipes. *Trans. Path. Soc.*, 1889, xl. 247.

528. Notes on a Case of Dislocation of the Shoulder with Rupture of the Capsule. *Trans. Path. Soc.*, 1889, xl. 235.

529. Discussion on Strumous Arthritis. (Reported.) *St. Barth. Hosp. Rep.*, 1889, xxv. 271.

530. On Intramuscular Synovial Cysts. *Illust. Med. News*, 1889, ii. 145.

531. The Varying effects of Violence in producing Fractures. *Trans. Path. Soc.*, 1890, xli. 232.

532. An Analysis of Seventy-two Cases of Ununited Fracture occurring in the Long Bones of Children. *Med.-Chir. Trans.*, 1892, lxxv. 119. Abstracted in *Internat. Journ. Med. Science*, 1892, ciii. 531.

533. The Relationship between Wryneck and Congenital Haematoma of the Sterno-mastoid Muscle. *Med.-Chir. Trans.*, 1893, lxxvi. 137.

534. On the Value of Bursal Enlargements as indications of Incipient Tuberculous Arthritis. *Brit. M.J.*, 1894, ii. 412; *Clin. J.*, 1894, iv. 229.

535. [DISEASES OF THE JOINTS AND SPINE BY HOWARD MARSH, F.R.C.S. New and revised [2nd] edition. Cassell, London . . . 1895.] 'In the preparation of the volume I have received very valuable assistance from Mr. D'Arcy Power, who has also prepared a copious index.'

536. A Case of Sciopedy. *Brit. M.J.*, 1895, ii. 712.

537. Remarks in Discussion on Non-suppurative Ankylosis of Joints. *Trans. Path. Soc.*, 1896, xlvii. 211.

538. On·Fractures at the Wrist. *M. Press*, 1907, o.s., cxxxv. 656.

539. On the Results of the Surgical Treatment of Displaced Semilunar Cartilages of the Knee. *Brit. M.J.*, 1911, i. 61.

540. On Chronic Joint Disease. *M. Press*, 1913, o.s., cxlvi. 516.

541. Chronic Ulcers of the Tibia. (Reported.) *Lancet*, 1927,i . 495.

H. PATHOLOGY

542. Elephantiasis Arabum. (Jointly with Sir Joseph Fayrer.) *Trans. Path. Soc.*, 1879, xxx. 488.

543. Descriptive List of Specimens added to the Museum. *St. Barth. Hosp. Rep.*, 1884–9, xx–xxv.

544. Angioma of the Cerebral Membranes. *Trans. Path. Soc.*, 1888, xxxix. 4.

545. A Submaxillary Gland removed with an unusually large Salivary Calculus. *Trans. Path. Soc.*, 1888, xxxix. 103.

546. A HANDBOOK OF SURGICAL PATHOLOGY FOR THE USE OF STUDENTS IN THE MUSEUM OF ST. BARTHOLOMEW'S HOSPITAL. Second Edition. By W. J. Walsham, M.B., F.R.C.S., assisted by D'Arcy Power . . . London: Baillière, Tindall, and Cox, 1890. Pages xx, 634. 18·5 × 12·5 cm.

I. SCIENCE

547. On the Albuminous Substances which occur in the Urine in Albuminuria. (Jointly with Dr. T. Lauder Brunton.) *St. Barth. Hosp.
Rep.*, 1877, xiii. 283.
548. Reports on the Progress of Physiology. *Lond. Med. Rec.*, 1878–80.
549. On the Endothelium of the Body-Cavity and Blood-Vessels of the
Common Earthworm. *Quart. J. Micr. Sc.*, 1878, n.s., xviii. 158.
550. Calberla's New Embedding Mixture. *Quart. J. Micr. Sc.*, 1878,
n.s., xviii. 208.
551. Abridgement of Bütschli's Researches on the Flagellate Infusoria.
Quart. J. Micr. Sc., 1879, n.s., xix. 63.
552. On the Present State of our Knowledge in regard to Ferments. *St.
Barth. Hosp. Rep.*, 1880, xvi. 135.
553. MANUAL FOR THE PHYSIOLOGICAL LABORATORY. By Vincent Harris,
M.D., M.R.C.P., and D'Arcy Power, B.A. London: Baillière,
Tindall, and Cox, 1880. Pages 124. Illustrated. 17·5 × 12 cm.
Five editions were published—1880, 1882, 1884, 1888, 1892.
554. [CARPENTER'S PRINCIPLES OF HUMAN PHYSIOLOGY EDITED BY HENRY
POWER, M.B., F.R.C.S. Ninth edition London: J. & A. Churchill
1881.]
'I have to thank my son, Mr. D'Arcy Power, for working up the
Chapter on Development, for revising many of the sheets, and for
aid in completing the Index . . .'
555. Notes of an Experiment on the Induction of False Albuminuria. *St.
Barth. Hosp. Rep.*, 1887, xxiii. 173.
556. Letterpress of AN ATLAS OF THE ANATOMY AND PHYSIOLOGY OF THE
CHILD. London, Baillière, Tindall, & Cox,1902. Pages 23. Plates v.

J. SURGERY

557. The Operations of Sixteen Months and their Lessons. *St. Barth.
Hosp. Rep.*, 1900, xxxv. 37.
558. The Lessons of a Year's Surgical Experience. *St. Barth. Hosp. Rep.*,
1901, xxxvi. 37.
559. On Some Disappointments in Surgery. *Lancet*, 1900, ii. 1789.
560. Some Interesting Surgical Cases. *Clin. J.*, 1913, xlii. 262.
561. Surgical Aphorisms. *St. Barth. Hosp. J.*, 1919, xxvi. 25, 35.
Reprinted with additions. *Clin. J.*, 1920, xlix. 28.
562. Editor of THE PRACTITIONER'S SURGERY. [Oxford Medical Publica-
tions] Oxford University Press, 1919. 3 vols. Pages xii, 672;
viii, 528; viii, 588. 25 × 16 cm.
563. On Prognosis in Surgery. *Lancet*, 1919, ii. 861.
564. The Making of a Surgeon. *St. Barth. Hosp. J.*, 1922, xxix. 4.
565. On Operations in Surgical Emergencies. *Practitioner*, 1924, cxiii. 137.
566. The Training of a Surgeon. *Practitioner*, 1927, cxix. 205.

K. SYPHILIS

567. A Case illustrating some Manifestations of Congenital Syphilis in a Boy. *Lancet*, 1894, i. 1618.

568. A SYSTEM OF SYPHILIS IN SIX VOLUMES EDITED BY D'ARCY POWER AND J. KEOGH MURPHY ... [Oxford Medical Publications] ... Oxford University Press, 1908–10. 2nd ed., 1914.

569. Recent Advances in the Surgical Knowledge of Syphilis. *Tr. M. Soc. Lond.*, 1908, xxxi. 309.

570. On Heredo-Syphilis. *M. Press*, 1909, o.s., cxxxix. 110.

571. Syphilitic Disease of the Joints. *The Hospital*, 1907–8, xliii. 411.

572. The Influence of Syphilis on Tuberculous Infections of the Human Body. *Tr. M. Soc. Lond.*, 1911, xxxiv. 269; *Clin. J.*, 1911, xxxviii. 333.

573. Syphilis with especial reference to the Treatment of the Disease. *Proc. Roy. Soc. Med.*, 1912, v. 38.

574. On the Treatment of Syphilis. *Brit. M.J.*, 1912, i. 1418; *M. Press*, 1912, o.s., cxliv. 641.

575. On Recent Progress in connexion with Syphilis. *Brit. M.J.*, 1912, ii. 1603.
   Abstract in French. *La Presse Médicale d'Égypte*, 1912, 343.

576. Evidence before the Royal Commission on Venereal Diseases. *Lancet*, 1914, i. 846.

577. Venereal Disease in its Surgical and Social Aspects. *Clin. J.*, 1914, xliii. 183.

578. 'Against His Own Body'. (A Clinical Lecture at St. Bartholomew's Hospital.) *Lancet*, 1915, i. 171.
   Reprinted (i) from the *Lancet*. 8vo. 11 pp.
   (ii) anonymously. 8vo. Purple paper cover. 15 pp.
   (iii) Church Army. Long 8vo. 23 pp.
   (ii) and (iii) were circulated throughout the army.

579. A Section on Venereal Disease in *Gask and Wilson's Surgery*. Churchill, London, 1920. Pages 93–105.

580. Syphilis in General Practice. *Lancet*, 1922, i. 1035.

581. The History of Syphilis. *St. Barth. Hosp. Rep.*, 1923, lvi. 105.

DISEASES OF THE THROAT, NOSE, AND EAR

582. A Rhinolith. *Trans. Path. Soc.*, 1887, xxxviii. 321.

583. Recurrent and Severe Haemorrhage after the Operation for Cleft Palate. *Brit. M.J.*, 1894, ii. 1174.

584. Empyema of the Antrum in a child aged eight weeks. *Brit. M.J.*, 1897, ii. 808; *Trans. Path. Soc.*, 1898, xlix. 200.

585. Otitis Media followed by Mastoid Abscess in an Infant aged five weeks. (A case.) *Brit. M.J.*, 1898, ii. 1551.

586. Abstract of a Lecture on the Tonsils. *St. Barth. Hosp. J.*, 1902, x. 28.
587. On Inflammation of the Accessory Sinuses of the Nose. *Clin. J.*, 1903, xxii. 321.
588. Case of Impacted Tooth-plate in Oesophagus. Oesophagotomy. *M. Press*, 1913, o.s., cxlvi. 501.

VARIOUS

589. Case of Hereditary Locomotor Ataxy. (From Dr. Gee's Wards.) *St. Barth. Hosp. Rep.*, 1882, xviii. 305.
590. On the Dangers of Artificial Teeth. *Brit. J. Dent. Sc.*, 1883, xxvi. 545.
591. A Note on Picric Acid in the Treatment of Superficial Burns and Scalds. *Brit. M.J.*, 1896, ii. 651.
592. Editor in Chief of the Surgical Section of *Treatment*. The Rebman Publishing Company, London, 1897.
593. Suggestions for a Veterinary Sanitary Service. Introductory Address at the Royal Veterinary College, 1897–8. *J. Comp. Path. & Therap.*, 1897, x. 276; *Brit. M.J.*, 1897, ii. 998; *Lancet*, 1897, ii. 847.
594. Editor of *Saint Bartholomew's Hospital Reports*. (Jointly with Dr. Norman Moore.) 1898–1902, xxxiv–xxxviii.
595. Articles in the *Encyclopaedia Medica*, Edinburgh, 1899, and subsequent editions. Viz. Artificial Limbs, Bandages, Fractures, Hip-Joint, Parotid Gland, Military Surgery, Peritoneum, Salivary Glands, Shoulder-Joint, Syphilis, Urethra, Venereal Disease, &c.
596. With Mr. D'Arcy Power in the Out-Patient Room at St. Bartholomew's Hospital. *Clin. J.*, 1903, xxii. 287, 383; xxiii. 13.
597. Articles in *Quain's Dictionary of Medicine*. 3rd ed., 1902. Viz. Lumbar Puncture; Diseases of the Nipples; Sordes.
598. Actinomycosis of the Skin in Children. (A case.) *Lancet*, 1904, ii. 1216.
599. On a Case of Haemophilia. *Clin. J.*, 1908, xxxii. 225.
600. In *Dangerous Trades edited by Thomas Oliver* ... London, John Murray, 1902.
    Chapter XV. Agriculture; Horses; Cattle. Pages 232–49.
601. The Nurse in Private Practice. *St. Barth. Hosp. League News*, 1909, iii. 54.
602. Note sur l'usage de la tuberculine comme traitement curatif en Chirurgerie. (With C. H. S. Taylor.) *La Presse Médicale d'Égypte*, 1909, i. 89.
603. The Value of New Tuberculin (T.R.) in Surgical Tuberculosis. *Brit. M.J.*, 1909, ii. 766.
604. Operating Theatre Methods and their Evolution. *The South African Nursing Record*, 1913, p. 9.

605. Follicular Cystic Odontome. *M. Press,* 1914, o.s., cxlviii. 255.
606. Injection of Iodine in the Treatment of Varicose Veins. *M. Press,* 1914, o.s., cxlviii. 255.
607. Embolism. (A letter.) *M. Press,* 1922, o.s., clxiv. 403.
608. The Classical Ideas of Physical Fitness. *Harmsworth's Home Doctor and Encyclopaedia of Good Health,* London, 1924, i, pp. 27–32.
*609. Presidential Address: Section of Comparative Medicine. *Proc. Roy. Soc. Med.* (Sect. Compar. Med.), 1927, xx. 85.

THE IDEA OF THIS BOOK
WAS CONCEIVED BY THE OSLER CLUB
OF WHICH SIR D'ARCY POWER WAS ELECTED
A FRIEND ON 4 JUNE 1928
IT WAS CARRIED OUT FOR THE SUBSCRIBERS
BY THIS COMMITTEE

✳

W. R. BETT · E. FARQUHAR BUZZARD
ALFRED FRANKLIN · G. E. GASK
GEOFFREY KEYNES · G. H. MAKINS
A. L. P. NORRINGTON · A. W. POLLARD
H. E. POWELL · A. H. T. ROBB-SMITH
HUMPHRY ROLLESTON
WILFRED TROTTER

INDEX

INDEX